MEDICAL AND
DENTAL HYPNOSIS
AND
ITS CLINICAL
APPLICATIONS

MEDICAL AND DENTAL HYPNOSIS

AND ITS CLINICAL APPLICATIONS

JOHN HARTLAND

B.Sc., M.B., Ch.B., M.R.C.S., L.R.C.P.
Consulting Psychiatrist (Private Practice);
Formerly Visiting Psychiatrist, Hallam Hospital, West Bromwich;
President of the British Society of Medical and Dental Hypnosis;
Life President of the Midlands Branch of the British Society for Medical
and Dental Hypnosis; Honorary Fellow of the American Society of
Clinical Hypnosis; Fellow of the International Society for Clinical and
Experimental Hypnosis; Editor of the 'British Journal of Clinical Hypnosis'

with a chapter on

THE USES OF HYPNOSIS
IN DENTAL SURGERY

by

STANLEY TINKLER

L.D.S., R.C.S. (Eng.)
Demonstrator, Department of Prosthetics, Birmingham Dental
Hospital; Chairman of the Midlands Branch of the British Society for
Medical and Dental Hypnosis

Second Edition

Baillière Tindall · London

Published by BAILLIÈRE TINDALL
a division of Cassell Ltd,
1 St. Anne's Road, Eastbourne, East Sussex BN21 3UN
ISBN 0-7020-0646-7

First published 1966
Second edition 1971
Reprinted 1973
Reprinted 1975
Reprinted 1977
Reprinted 1979
Reprinted 1980
Reprinted 1982 (twice)

Published in the United States of America by
the Williams & Wilkins Company, Baltimore

Printed in Great Britain
from negatives supplied by
The Anchor Press Ltd,
Tiptree, Colchester, Essex

Contents

Foreword by Milton H. Erickson

To write a foreword to this book is a most unusual pleasure and privilege. The book is not one primarily based upon other men's ideas with special interpretations elaborately evolved to explain the work of those others. Nor is it simply a survey of current literature on hypnosis. It is, rather, an earnest, sincere, objective account of one medical practitioner's experience over a period of twenty-five years, detailing instructively, in an orderly systematic fashion, the learnings he has derived from his day-by-day encounters with all manner of patients in his busy medical practice.

One realizes while reading this book that the author had a much greater purpose in mind than adding just another book to the literature on hypnosis, or a recounting of varied experiences solely for their interest. Each page makes clear that a long overlooked and seriously neglected need is being fulfilled, one of great importance in the furtherance of the scientific modality of hypnosis as an important adjunct in the healing arts. A methodology of the medical use of hypnosis of great value to the patient himself and to medicine as a whole is developed and adequately elucidated in this book. This is achieved by centring around a clear-cut well-ordered basic orientation which acquaints the medical practitioner with the varieties of hypnotic understandings pertinent to the clinical practice of medicine as the author himself has learned from one patient to another, from one kind of medical problem to another. Every effort is made to present clearly, comprehensively and understandably the multitude of problems and questions encountered in a busy twenty-five years, yet to do this simply, concisely, most informatively.

Wherever necessary the literature is adequately cited for content and meaning in relation to specific medical problems, not for speculative purposes; and the author does not hesitate to give full credit to others.

In brief, this book is one which the medical man, even though he may be a novice in hypnosis, can read with interest and intellectual gain. He will be inspired to improve his art of medicine, and after each trial he will return to the book to learn what more he needs to understand in order to care more adequately for his patients and to develop a better understanding of the personal values in the medical development of human welfare.

The writer of this foreword is medically trained and well experienced in hypnosis, and the manuscript of this book was read with a feeling of intense interest, of personal gain and of profound satisfaction that Dr Hartland had written so well this much-needed volume on the use of hypnosis in medicine.

MILTON H. ERICKSON, M.D.

1201 East Hayward
Phoenix, Arizona 85020
U.S.A.

Editor Emeritus of the
American Journal of
Clinical Hypnosis

Foreword by Eric E. Wookey

There is general agreement over the value of hypnosis as an analgesic agent in dentistry where, however, a deep stage of hypnosis is desirable whenever possible. It is the great merit of this book to the dental surgeon that the techniques of induction and deepening are so well described.

The authors of most works on hypnosis prior to 1940 seem almost to be jealous of disclosing the secrets of induction, and volumes are filled with discussions of theory (all speculative), phenomena and case treatments, the latter uncontrolled and inadequate in quantity. Dr Hartland, even more than most modern writers, keeps no secrets from us, and his language is simple and clear—no small advantage to the dental surgeon whose student memories of the brain and nervous system in general have become somewhat dim with the passage of years and his preoccupation with a limited and highly technical field. As he reads this book he will realize, perhaps for the first time, the real meaning of the word 'psychosomatic': he is treating a human being. Undergraduate dental teaching still tends to ignore the interaction between mind and body, and concentrates on turning out good technicians. Hence the value of a book such as this to the dental graduate.

The section on the use of hypnosis in dentistry has been written by a practitioner with wide experience. Mr Tinkler's language, in keeping with the rest of the book, is clear and concise. The practical applications are described so well that, in conjunction with the earlier parts of the book, the beginner can feel thoroughly confident in making a start with a new weapon in his armamentarium. How much use he will make of it will depend largely on his own enthusiasm and his ability to organize the initial extra time needed. The appreciation of his patients will be well worth the effort, whilst the therapeutic effects in dentistry are still largely unexplored.

It is not too much to say, however, that no dentist entirely ignorant of hypnotic techniques can consider himself properly equipped for his professional work.

ERIC E. WOOKEY
M.C., L.D.S., F.C.S.

51 Lake View, Edgeware,
Middlesex
June 1971

*Honorary Consultant, Royal Free
Hospital, London. Past President, British
Society for Medical and Dental Hypnosis*

Preface to the Second Edition

Since the first edition of this book was published four years ago, interest in the medical and dental uses of hypnosis has greatly increased. The general public seems to be much more aware of the possibilities offered by this form of therapy, and judging from the attendances throughout the country at instructional courses held by the various branches of the British Society of Medical and Dental Hypnosis, professional interest is also steadily growing, since increasing numbers of medical and dental practitioners and psychiatrists are nowadays beginning to realize the potentialities of hypnotherapy in their various fields of activity.

Naturally, during this period, techniques have become expanded and improved so that a certain amount of revision and the inclusion of fresh material has become necessary to bring the text up to date. Consequently, although in this new edition the original format has been retained, numerous changes and additions have been made to comply with the views of various critics, to whom I should like to express my appreciation of their helpful suggestions. It should be borne in mind, however, that the book was written primarily to meet the needs of the general practitioner and physician, and thus I do not feel it necessary or even advisable to give a detailed account of the dynamic aspects of the use of hypnosis in the psychiatric field, an omission which has been commented upon in certain reviews. Nevertheless, to meet this objection to a certain extent, the chapter on hypno-analysis and analytical psychotherapy has been considerably expanded. Also, to correct any impression that the hypnotic state can be equated solely with 'hyper-suggestibility', a final chapter has been added to bring the subject into its true perspective.

Further methods of induction, deepening and investigation have been included, and certain of the techniques formerly described have been revised and brought up to date. Moreover, in view of the frequency with which these conditions are seen in general practice, the sections on the use of hypnosis in the treatment of obesity, smoking, and dermatological complaints have been enlarged and re-written to conform with the modern approach. Attention has been drawn to the fact that many conditions that can also be treated successfully by hypnotherapy have not been included in the text. Amongst these, the psycho-sexual disorders such as frigidity, impotence etc, have been specifically mentioned. In my experience, I have found that these conditions frequently require an analytical approach and are consequently likely to be too time-consuming to be treated frequently in general practice. Moreover, considerations of space rendered it necessary for a selection to be made from those complaints that are regularly encountered in the course of an average surgery. Those that are not mentioned can still be treated successfully by a judicious application of the various principles, fully described throughout the text.

Since the 'ego-strengthening technique' has become so widely accepted in many countries, as a result of numerous requests, the opportunity has been taken to describe it and analyse it in much more detail. Although some criticism has been made of the repetitive nature of certain sections of the book, a sufficient weight of opinion has been received appreciating the usefulness of this to the beginner in facilitating the learning process, to persuade me to leave it unaltered.

I should like to express my thanks for the way in which this book has been received, and to those who have shown such a deep interest in the first edition. I hope that the present one will prove even more acceptable and helpful in promoting a deeper understanding of the usefulness of hypnosis in the fields of medicine and dentistry.

Deganwy, North Wales   JOHN HARTLAND
July 1971

Acknowledgements

I would like to express my gratitude for the assistance and encouragement I have received from many of my friends and colleagues, and the courtesies of the many authors and publishers who have granted me permission to quote from their works.

I am particularly indebted to Dr Milton H. Erickson for generously giving up his valuable time in reading my manuscript, for the very helpful criticisms he made and for his willingness to write the foreword. I should also like to thank Mr Eric Wookey for his help and contribution of a foreword; and Dr A. Spencer Paterson for many useful suggestions.

My thanks are also due to Mr Stanley Tinkler for writing the chapter on
'Hypnosis in Dental Surgery'.

The following authors and publishers have generously given me
permission to use quotations: George Allen & Unwin for the quotation
from *Psychological Healing* by Pierre Janet; Edward Arnold (Publishers)
for quotations and material from *The Common Neuroses* and *Analytical
Psychotherapy* by Dr T. A. Ross; The Dental Items of Interest Publishing
Co. for the description of a basic picture-visualization technique from
Hypnodontics by Aaron Moss, D.D.S.; Dr Milton H. Erickson for material
derived from his numerous writings and lectures, especially from his
article, 'Confusion technique', in the *American Journal of Clinical Hypnosis*,
and also for permission to quote the article 'The effects of hypnosis on a
complicated obstetric case', written by myself and Mr Wilfrid Mills and
originally published in the *American Journal of Clinical Hypnosis*; The
Julian Press Publishers for various quotations from *The Study of Hypnosis*
by Albert Moll; Dr André Weitzenhoffer, Grune & Stratton and John
Wiley & Sons for material from *General Techniques of Hypnotism* and
Hypnotism; Dr Lewis R. Wolberg, Grune & Stratton and William
Heinemann for permission to quote freely from *Medical Hypnosis* and
Hypnoanalysis; Dr Calvert Stein and Charles C. Thomas, Illinois, for
quotations from *Practical Psychotherapy in Non-psychiatric Specialities*;
Dr Michael Scott and Charles C. Thomas, Illinois, for permission to
quote from *Hypnosis in Skin and Allergic Diseases*; Dr Herbert Mann for
material from his A.S.C.H. lecture, 1970, 'Hypnosis in the treatment of
obesity'; Dr T. E. A. von Dedenroth for material on the use of hypnosis
with 'Tobaccomaniacs' in the *American Journal of Clinical Hypnosis*; and
Dr Erika Fromm for material from 'Dissociative and integrative processes
in hypnoanalysis' in the *American Journal of Clinical Hypnosis*. My thanks
are also due to Dr Wm. E. Edmonston, jun., Editor of the *American
Journal of Clinical Hypnosis* for permission to draw upon these two articles;
and also to Dr Jay Haley and Grune & Stratton for quotations from
Strategies of Psychotherapy and *Advanced Techniques of Hypnosis and Therapy:
Selected Papers of Milton Erickson*.

Finally, I should like to thank my son, John, for the invaluable help and
advice he gave me in the preparation of my manuscript.

Introduction: Hypnosis and the General Practitioner

For many years, hypnosis was condemned by the medical profession as being unscientific and bordering upon charlatanism and quackery. With few exceptions, its investigation and exploitation were left in the hands of unqualified operators and showmen, by whom so many extravagant and unsubstantiated claims of successful cures were made that it inevitably fell into further disrepute. Such objections, however, are no longer valid, for during the past 20 years so much valuable work and research has been carried out in this particular field that, even in medical circles, hypnosis has at last begun to assume the mantle of respectability. It is now accepted as a legitimate form of medical treatment and is employed with success in a variety of conditions, many of which fall within the scope of general medical practice. Despite this, its possibilities in this field are still too widely neglected, largely because of certain misconceptions that tend to deter the general practitioner from taking a serious interest in the subject. This lack of interest in a method which could often prove invaluable in dealing with many troublesome conditions that are seen in any average surgery seems to arise from the mistaken idea that the induction of hypnosis is not easy to learn, that too few patients are capable of achieving sufficient depth, and that the whole procedure is too time-consuming to be of use in a busy practice.

The art of hypnotic induction is certainly not difficult to acquire, and it does not take long to learn the essential techniques. Most people can do this, although some will naturally prove more successful than others. Nevertheless, it should be realized that this difference will depend far more upon the personality of the individual doctor and the sympathetic contact he can establish with his patient than it will upon the mastery of the simple principles of hypnotic induction. Almost anyone can learn those.

The second objection is easily met by the fact that great depth is rarely necessary to obtain satisfactory results. Many cases will respond successfully when only light or medium depth hypnosis has been achieved. Since approximately 90 per cent of the population can be induced into the light hypnotic state, and some 50 per cent to 60 per cent can attain medium depth with little difficulty, it is obvious that this form of treatment has much more scope than might have been thought. Even these figures can often be improved upon and greater depth obtained if the patient is trained to enter the trance state gradually. I find that, in the course of two or three half-hourly sessions, most adults can be induced deeply enough to enter the hypnotic state immediately it is suggested that they should do so. Subsequent treatments can easily be administered in 7 or 8 minutes. I induce as deep a hypnotic state as possible, for the greater the depth of hypnosis, the more implicitly the patient will accept what is said to him and the less critical he will be. Consequently, whilst treatment may often be undertaken with success in the lighter stages, there is little doubt that the deeper the trance the more rapidly it will take effect. The treatment of children's complaints occupies much of the general practitioner's time, and it is fortunate that most children are very good subjects. Except for the very timid or nervous, the majority can usually be induced into deep or even somnambulistic trances. In comparison the average adult is less responsive, so that both the induction of hypnosis and subsequent treatment are likely to require rather more time and patience than in the case of a child.

In dealing with the third objection that hypnosis is too time-consuming to be of use in general practice, I can best quote from my own experience. In the early 1940s, I was regularly using hypnosis in an industrial general practice with a personal list of some 3500 patients. It was obviously impossible to teach patients to enter the hypnotic state in the course of an average surgery, so that special sessions had to be arranged whenever possible, either during the day's work or at the end of a routine surgery. But once the patient was trained, he could be given his hypnotic treatment during ordinary surgery hours in just as short a time as it formerly took to listen to his latest complaints and write out prescriptions. Moreover, I found that far from being too time-consuming, hypnosis often resulted in an actual saving of time, whilst also affording a steady improvement in the patient's condition.

It is seldom realized what a wide and varied field can be covered by the use of hypnosis in general practice. Many of the common conditions that are regularly seen in the practitioner's surgery can be successfully treated by this method. These include bad habits in children such as nail-biting, thumb-sucking, bed-wetting and tics; complaints such as asthma, migraine, constipation, insomnia and dysmenorrhoea; and certain disorders of the skin such as warts and neurodermatoses, to name but a few. Most of these are particularly responsive to hypnotic suggestion, since the symptoms are often distressing to the patient whilst having no great protective value in themselves. Hypnosis can also be invaluable in allaying fears, removing anxiety and producing both mental and physical relaxation. It can sometimes be used for the relief of pain in minor surgical procedures, but rarely can it be employed to secure complete anaesthesia for major surgical operations. But in obstetrics, with which the general practitioner is usually much concerned, it can frequently succeed in reducing the pain, apprehension and even the duration of the average confinement. Its scope can also include many of the milder yet obstinate psychosomatic symptoms and illnesses, so that its application in general practice is much more extensive than might have been imagined.

Despite this, there is nothing magical or even remarkable about hypnotic treatment. It is just an additional weapon in the struggle against illness and must take its proper place beside other well-established and better known therapeutic measures. The skilled craftsman first sizes up the job and then selects the most appropriate tool from his rack: so should it be with hypnosis. Less than 70 per cent of the cases referred to me for hypnotic treatment are actually accepted for this particular therapy; the remaining 30 per cent are usually found to require some more orthodox procedure. (Selection is based solely upon the suitability of the complaint for treatment by hypnotherapy, and not upon the probable susceptibility or otherwise of the patient.) It cannot be too strongly emphasized that whenever psychological or neurotic illnesses are involved, the general practitioner should exercise the greatest care in selecting the cases he proposes to treat unless he possesses a sound working knowledge of psychopathology.

Many doubts are still expressed from time to time regarding the possible dangers of hypnosis. These are completely unjustifiable for hypnosis in itself is certainly not dangerous. But hypnotists who are ill-advised enough to stray outside their own particular line of country are undoubtedly asking for trouble. The human mind is an extremely delicate piece of mechanism, the normal working of which can quite unwittingly be thrown out of gear by the inexpert though well-intentioned operator. For this reason alone, I consider that apart from the medical and dental professions, no one should attempt to practise hypnosis unless they have received adequate training in both normal and abnormal psychology. Even then, care should be taken not to employ it for purposes outside the normal field of activity of the operator. General practitioners should normally use it only in the course of their daily work. Dental surgeons would be wise to restrict its use to the production of relaxation, the removal of apprehension and anxiety, and the alleviation of pain in the dental chair. Bad habits in children, such as thumb-sucking, nail-biting or even bed-wetting, often yield so readily to direct hypnotic suggestion that dentists may sometimes be tempted to undertake their treatment. It should be remembered, however, that these apparently harmless conditions are occasionally the outward expressions of un-conscious mental conflicts, in which case their removal may well be followed by exaggerated feelings of anxiety and insecurity. It is similarly inadvisable to try to hypnotize one's relatives or close friends, for once hypnosis is removed from the purely professional field many undesirable emotional involvements and difficulties may result, no matter how good the intentions may be.

The question also arises as to whether the patient who is treated regularly by hypnosis is likely to become too dependent upon it. It is my own view that should this occur, it would be entirely the fault of the hypnotist. No conscientious practitioner would ever allow a patient to become so dependent upon habit-forming drugs that drug-addiction ultimately occurred. Whilst the danger is infinitely less with hypnosis, the same principle must surely apply. Furthermore, the whole aim of effective psychotherapy is to establish the patient's feeling of independence and to enable him to stand upon his own feet as quickly as possible, and this can be greatly facilitated by the regular use of appropriately worded hypnotic suggestion.

At the present time, the general public seems to be becoming in-creasingly aware of the possibilities offered by hypnotic treatment. Whether the present demand is likely to increase in the future is difficult to predict, but even at the present time there are far too few facilities available. It is consequently encouraging to note that an increasing number of doctors and dental surgeons are beginning to show more interest in the subject. In certain areas requests for lectures and in-structional courses are becoming more frequent, and it is a healthy sign that these are now being attended by final-year medical and dental students. It is to be hoped that this present trend will continue.

Many practitioners who might otherwise feel inclined to study medical hypnosis fail to do so because they do not know where to begin. Whilst many excellent books are available on the subject, some are far too technical and involved for the beginner, others do not explain how to apply hypnosis therapeutically or are mainly restricted to the analytical approach and do little to help the beginner. The information that the general practitioner needs most in order to encourage him to make a start, is a full description of the precise techniques employed in hypnosis, and the methods that are most effective in each of the conditions that the practitioner is likely to encounter. It has consequently been my intention in writing this book to try to bridge this gap not only by simplifying the approach to the induction and deepening of hypnosis, but also by describing the exact techniques and suggestions that I have found most effective in dealing with each individual complaint.

I have not attempted to write a complete treatise upon hypnosis, for the book is deliberately restricted to a limited field and is based upon a personal experience of some 25 years, much of it gained in general practice and the rest from conducting psychiatric clinics and from lectures and demonstrations given throughout this period. I have confined myself to the essential principles upon which I have relied for many years, and much historical and theoretical material has been omitted which can be found elsewhere. The basic needs of the general practitioner and the individual approach to the treatment of his patient, in so far as I can assess them, have been the primary considerations. I should point out that many of the facts I have stated and the conclusions I have drawn are based wholly upon clinical reports and evidence, and not upon controlled experimental studies. Since the book is directed to the general practitioner for his own use in clinical practice, my own orientation and statements have been entirely clinical in nature.

The objection may well be raised that, in the preliminary explanation of the nature of hypnosis and the way in which it works, I have been guilty of over-simplification in confining myself solely to the suggestion and dissociation theories. Whilst this may be true, I consider that such a step is fully justified in introducing an admittedly difficult and mis-understood subject for the first time. In my experience, it certainly helps to make hypnosis more understandable even to unprofessional audiences, and thus does a great deal to dispel misconception and prejudice. Moreover, the reader is afforded ample opportunity to formulate his own views and get matters in the right perspective when alternative theories are discussed in a later chapter.

Although in recent years I have used hypnosis mainly in psychiatric work, I have restricted consideration of its therapeutic applications largely to the treatment of those ordinary conditions that the general practitioner will most frequently encounter in his daily work. I have tried to deal with these as fully as possible, and have included no more psychopathology and psychiatry than is likely to help the practitioner to understand and select for himself the cases that he feels competent to treat. I have, however, included a brief description of the various hypno-analytic techniques, without which no survey of the therapeutic possibilities of hypnosis would be complete.

Whilst it is possible to learn and even practise medical hypnosis successfully without having undertaken practical instruction in the subject, there is not the slightest doubt that just as medicine is best learned at the bed-side and dentistry beside the dental chair, proficiency in hypnosis is best acquired by watching the actual induction and treatment of patients. The ideal method would be to attend a clinic regularly where hypnosis was being used, but this unfortunately is seldom possible. The initial mastery of trance-induction and trance-deepening techniques, however, can be gained whenever a suitable instructional course can be attended. Such courses are regularly organized by the British Society of Medical and Dental Hypnosis and its Branches in various parts of the country, and can prove extremely useful in the initial stages. The number of these is steadily increasing, and every year Basic, Intermediate and Advanced Courses in Hypnotherapy are being held by the individual Branches. Whilst it is hoped that the demand for these will continue, it is unfortunate that the opportunity for individual tuition still remains much more limited.

In conclusion, I should like to make a strong personal recommendation. I have always held the opinion that it is not wise for medical and dental practitioners to demonstrate the induction or phenomena of hypnosis to a lay audience. When asked to talk about the subject, it is very tempting to illustrate this by demonstration, and it might even be contended that this would help to dispel prejudice. For years, I have lectured to Rotary Clubs and other public bodies, but I have always firmly declined any request to demonstrate. No matter how scientifically it is done, the demonstration of hypnosis and its phenomena will always have a strong entertainment value. Since as a profession we have always deplored and condemned the use of hypnosis on the stage, it is my view that any doctor or dental surgeon who demonstrates it before the general public is not only placing himself in an invidious position, but is doing the cause of hypnosis a profound disservice.

PART ONE

THE HISTORY, NATURE AND TECHNIQUES OF HYPNOSIS

CHAPTER 1

The Development of Hypnosis

It would be difficult to find a more controversial and generally misunderstood subject than hypnotism which, throughout its many vicissitudes, has always simultaneously aroused more enthusiasm and prejudice than almost any other in the whole field of medicine. Even today, these opposing attitudes are just as strongly maintained, for amongst certain sections of the general public and in uninstructed medical circles the practice of hypnosis is still thought to be rather disreputable and to savour of quackery. The medical profession itself must accept a certain amount of responsibility for this state of affairs since it was its own reluctance to investigate the subject scientifically that caused it to pass mainly into the hands of public entertainers and charlatans.

Healing in a trance state is one of the oldest of the medical arts. It was practised even by primitive man, who firmly believed that the trance was divine and that the miraculous cures were religious in nature. He consequently conceived the mysterious forces that produced them as Gods, who behaved however in an extremely irregular and unpredictable manner. Because of this, the cures were both uncertain and capricious in nature. But as scientific knowledge slowly progressed, men began to learn how to treat certain of the simpler ailments themselves, and handed over such elementary matters as fractures and dislocations to the surgeons. But many diseases remained for the relief of which the aid of the Gods still had to be invoked. This often entailed travelling long distances to one of the healing shrines such as the Temple of Aesculapius at Epidaurus, which contained a statue believed to be endowed with miraculous powers of healing. The sufferers, after their long and arduous journeys, used to lay valuable offerings at the gates of the Temple, after which they were cleansed in the waters of the fountain. They then spent one or two nights in prayer and supplication, following which they were admitted to the Temple itself. Here, advice was given by oracles, or in the form of prophetic dreams. This atmosphere of mysticism and ceremonial was highly important, and its significance will presently become clear.

Even in the Middle Ages, miraculous cures were thought to be effected by sacred statues, healing springs, fragments of the true cross or the bones of a saint. Miracles could also be performed by virtue of the exalted rank of an individual. The kings both of England and of France were believed to have the power of curing by the ' laying-on of hands '. This practice was known as ' touching for the King's Evil '. Indeed, this belief in miraculous healing has persisted into the twentieth century. Even today, the cures reported from the miraculous spring at Lourdes are hardly less remarkable than those which occurred at the Temple of Aesculapius, many centuries before Christ. The power of suggestion was also known in Biblical times, and it seems probable that many of the cures produced by the prophets and saints were based upon this power. But though the phenomena of the trance state, which we recognize today as being hypnotic in character, had all been observed as isolated facts, it never occurred to anyone that they might be due to a common or natural cause. They were consequently thought to be supernatural religious manifestations, the results of magical spells or the work of evil spirits. No further explanation was sought until the year 1530, when Paracelsus formulated his theory concerning the effect of the heavenly bodies upon mankind—especially on their diseases. From this, there developed the further theory that not only did the stars influence men, but that men could mutually influence each other through the agency of magnetic powers.

In 1765, Franz Mesmer passed his medical examination with honours, having submitted a thesis based upon the influence of the planets on human health. He believed this to occur through the medium of a magnetic fluid—a kind of invisible gas in which all bodies were immersed—and he began to investigate the effect of these magnetic forces by treating patients with magnets shaped to fit the various parts of the body. The results were both dramatic and surprising. Patients suffering from retention of urine, toothache, earache, depression, trances, temporary blindness and attacks of paralysis, who had hitherto been considered to be incurable, lost their symptoms completely. Such astounding cures, however, could not be effected without a good deal of notoriety. Indeed, they aroused so much hostility among his medical colleagues that Mesmer was soon forced to leave Vienna. He moved to Paris, where he set up one of the most famous clinics in Europe, in which he treated all kinds of diseases. A brief consideration of what took place at this clinic will help us to understand later developments and the essential principles underlying the cures. Pierre Janet, in his book *Psychological Healing*, gives the following description of Mesmer's procedure:

Mesmer used an elaborate apparatus, and *his practice was attended with a ceremonial similar to that employed at miraculous shrines.* The patients were ushered into a hall of which all the windows were thickly curtained, so that darkness prevailed. The air was filled with plaintive strains from a pianoforte. In the middle of the room was a large oaken tub, Mesmer's famous ' baquet '. This was filled with a mixture of water, iron filings and powdered glass. It had a lid pierced with holes, and coming up through the holes were jointed iron rods. The patients, upon whom absolute silence was enjoined, linked hands and applied the rods to the ailing spot. Mesmer, the great magnetizer, now appeared, wearing a silken robe of a pale lilac colour, and holding in his hand a long iron wand. He passed slowly through the ranks, fixing his eye upon the patients, passing his hand over their bodies or touching them with his iron wand. Many patients were unable to notice much result and declared that they could feel absolutely nothing. But some of the patients coughed, spat and felt as if insects were running over their skin. Finally some, especially young women, would fall down and go into convulsions, so that the hall certainly deserved the name of the ' Hell of Convulsions '. This convulsive state, attended by hiccoughs, outbursts of laughter and sometimes delirium, constituted what was known as the crisis, and was supposed to be most salutary. After two or three sittings of the kind, many persons declared that they had been cured of the most multiform disorders.

Now, theatrical though this procedure may have been, it should be borne in mind that although Mesmer failed to understand the real character of the phenomena he induced, he at least perceived that they were due to a common cause. He supposed the human body to be influenced by the planets through the instrumentality of an invisible magnetic fluid. He also believed that human will was able to set this fluid at work—to withdraw it from one area and to concentrate it at another, thereby producing remarkable effects on living creatures. He called this fluid, which had many properties resembling those of a magnet, the fluid of animal magnetism. He considered disease to be caused by an inharmonious distribution of this fluid in the patient's body. Consequently, in making his ' passes ' a few inches from the body-surface, Mesmer believed that invisible magnetic fluid flowed out of his finger-tips into the patient's body, achieving the necessary redistribution and restoring the balance. Once this had been effected, the patient regained his health.

There is no doubt whatever that Mesmer did actually succeed in curing a great many people who had been given up as incurable, and naturally his fame spread rapidly. Patients attended his clinic from all over Europe, much to the disgust of the medical profession which once again became exceedingly hostile. In 1784 this resulted in Louis XVI appointing a Commission to investigate Mesmerism, or animal magnetism as it was then called. Amongst its members were Lavoisier, the famous chemist, Dr Guillotine, the inventor of the machine that bears his name, and Benjamin Franklin, the American scientist. Naturally enough, the Commission failed to discover any concrete evidence of animal magnetism or of the existence of the supposed invisible fluid. It consequently concluded that the phenomena embraced nothing that could not be explained by imitation and imagination, and that in the long run the effects of the treatment could not fail to be harmful.

Today, it seems unfortunate that the Commission chose to investigate the wrong aspect of Mesmer's work. Had it attempted to discover whether Mesmer's cures were in fact genuine and what part imagination had played in effecting them, much light might have been thrown upon the subject and future developments would not have been retarded, as in fact they were, for the next 60 years or so. The Commission's report damaged Mesmer's reputation severely and fashion turned against him. The final blow fell when the Medical Faculty of the University of Paris issued a decree that any physicians found guilty of practising animal magnetism would be excluded from the profession, and lose their licence to practise. This compelled Mesmer to leave France, and when subsequently he wished to return, his place had been filled. Animal magnetism had undergone changes and had entered into a new phase.

The second period of animal magnetism dates from around the year 1787. Two significant discoveries were made at this time. One of Mesmer's followers, the Marquis de Puységur, described a state which became known as artificial somnambulism. The chief characteristic of this state was a kind of sleep in which the ideas and actions of the magnetized person could be directed by the magnetizer. Then, at the beginning of the nineteenth century, Bertrand described this as being entirely due to the working of the subject's imagination. This was put to good use by the Abbe Faria who was the first to induce somnambulism in his subjects by simply saying to them, ' I wish you to go to sleep '. Despite this, however, the unyielding opposition of the medical profession forced Mesmerism to lie dormant for over 60 years. During this period it was exploited only by showmen at travelling fairs who used to demonstrate the phenomena of the trance.

In 1841 the French magnetizer, Lafontaine, visited Manchester and gave a demonstration of magnetic experiments. James Braid, a well-known local surgeon, happened to be present with a colleague. They saw a girl apparently put into a trance, and Braid was so incensed that he went upon the stage himself to expose it as a complete fake. To his intense astonishment he found that the trance was perfectly genuine. He consequently began a series of experiments upon his relatives and friends, and found that he could soon produce a similar trance state quite easily by inducing them to fix their eyes upon a bright object, such as his lancet case. He also discovered that he obtained excellent results when he used the trance for medical and surgical purposes, and in 1842 he offered to read a paper on the subject for the British Association (for the Advancement of Science) which was meeting in Manchester. Needless to say his offer was rejected and his paper branded as ridiculous, together with his reports of cures of contractures and disorders of sensibility such as deafness.

Several years later the same uncomprising opposition of the medical profession caused the physician, Elliotson, to be dismissed from his professorial post at the University College Hospital, London, because he chose hypnotism as the subject for his Harveian Oration. At about the same time James Esdaile, who was practising surgery in India, sent a report to the Medical Board of 75 operations performed painlessly under hypnotic anaesthesia, but his letter was never even acknowledged.

The importance of Braid's work lies in the fact that he was quick to realize that no mysterious magnetic fluids were involved in the production of the trance. Instead he came to the conclusion that the results were purely subjective in nature: *the phenomena were due to suggestion alone, acting upon a subject whose suggestibility had been artificially increased.*

If we examine the implications of this statement, we shall see quite clearly how Mesmer actually obtained his results. The impressive ritual, the ceremonial, Mesmer's own personality, his striking robe and above all his great reputation strongly suggested to his patients that something marvellous was going to happen, and of course it did. Bernard C. Gindes summed up the situation admirably when he suggested the following formula:

Misdirected Attention + *Belief* + *Expectation* = *The Hypnotic State.*

To this we can also add *Imagination*, which is the integrating factor which welds belief and expectation into an irresistible force. Indeed this same principle has to be accepted today, no matter whether recovery takes place through the agency of hypnosis, Christian Science or the miracles reported from Lourdes. And this brings us face to face with a truth of the greatest importance: *no psychological cures have ever taken place in the absence of belief.* It was James Braid who finally discarded the terms mesmerism and animal magnetism, and substituted a name of his own invention—hypnotism—which has persisted to the present day.

Subsequent developments originated from the work of Dr Liébeault, in France, who may well be considered the real father of modern hypnotism. He was a modest country practitioner in Nancy who became interested in the phenomena of hypnotism and animal magnetism. Like Braid, he soon refuted the theories of the latter and consequently became the founder of the therapeutics of suggestion. He was certainly the first to demonstrate the curative value of hypnosis on a large scale, for he treated thousands of patients in this way with outstanding success. He accomplished this by waiving his fees altogether if the patient would accept hypnotic treatment in place of more orthodox procedures. In point of fact, so well known did his work become that it came to the attention of Professor Bernheim, a famous neurologist, when he succeeded in curing a chronic case of sciatica which had been under Bernheim's care. Bernheim was so annoyed by the claims which were being made that he determined to visit Liébeault's clinic and expose him as a quack. But he was so amazed at what he saw that he became completely converted and fully accepted Liébeault's views upon the significant part played by suggestion in hypnosis. He rapidly became one of the greatest authorities on the subject, and such was his reputation as a physician throughout Europe that, for the very first time, the medical profession was unable to ignore his opinions and maintain its attitude of hostility. In 1886 he published his famous book, *De La Suggestion*; in it he gave many examples of the curative effects of hypnosis which he fully accepted as being entirely psychical in nature. The work of these two men, following upon that of Braid, laid the foundation upon which the development of modern hypnosis has been erected.

No account of the history of hypnosis, however brief, would be complete without reference to the work of the neurologist, Professor Charcot, and his colleagues at the Salpêtrière Hospital in Paris. Despite his exceptional abilities as a clinician, Charcot seems to have had little understanding of the real nature of hypnosis. He did his utmost to devise scientific tests for it, as a result of which he concluded that hypnosis was a pathological phenomenon similar to hysteria, and consequently the product of an abnormal nervous constitution. Since Charcot used only a limited number of more or less trained subjects, his observations lacked validity and he fell into many errors. Nevertheless, as a result of these findings there followed a bitter struggle between the rival schools of Charcot and Bernheim. Eventually the views of the Nancy School prevailed, the methods and conclusions of Charcot and his followers were exposed as unscientific, and hypnosis came to be considered as a normal manifestation.

Nevertheless many extravagant and unfounded claims were made for hypnosis during this period. The permanency of its results was never checked, largely due to the lack of follow-up studies on patients presumably cured. At this time nothing was known of the defensive value of symptoms and the way in which they often help the individual to adjust to his difficulties. Hypnosis was consequently used merely as a bludgeon to crush the patient's complaints, and it seems probable that failures were far more frequent than cures.

Around 1880 however, Dr Breuer, a Viennese general practitioner, introduced a most important innovation in hypnotic therapy which extended the application of hypnosis far beyond the mere suggesting away of symptoms. He accidentally discovered that when one of his patients was induced to speak freely under hypnosis, she displayed a profound emotional reaction which was followed by the disappearance of many of her symptoms. When Freud's attention was drawn to this case, he joined Breuer in investigating it more fully and succeeded in confirming his results. The importance of this discovery lies in the subsequent change in emphasis in hypnotic therapy *from the direct removal of symptoms to the elimination of their apparent causes*. Indeed, the fact that repressed traumatic experiences can act as the foci of emotional difficulties has attracted more and more attention to the possibilities of hypnotic recall of buried memories. Later on Freud became disappointed in hypnosis since he was unable to induce a sufficiently deep trance state in many of his patients, and subsequently he rejected it altogether in favour of his own discovery of psycho-analysis. This fact, together with the disappointment aroused by the failure of hypnosis to produce a permanent cure of hysteria, nearly succeeded in dealing it a death-blow. However the grave shortage of psychiatrists during the First World War demanded a much abbreviated form of psychotherapy. Hypnotherapy was once again revived and used both for direct symptom-removal and for the restoration of repressed traumatic experiences. War neuroses, in fact, provide the most dramatic examples of how effective hypnosis can be in the dismissal of symptoms through a reliving of the events of a traumatic experience, and the success that was achieved created a wave of enthusiasm for hypnotic methods that has persisted to the present day.

The future of hypnosis is not easy to foretell for, throughout its long history, it has been subject to many ups and downs. But there is little doubt that during recent years hypnotherapy has been slowly gaining ground. The Hypnotism Act of 1952, which strictly limited the conditions under which public demonstrations of hypnosis could be held, has considerably reduced the number of stage performances. Moreover, in 1953 the British Medical Association appointed a Sub-committee of its Psychological Group Committee to enquire into the use of hypnotism in contemporary medicine. It was found that hypnotic phenomena had shed a great deal of light on the role played by the unconscious mind in determining human behaviour, and after issuing a warning against excessive and unjustified claims, the Committee stated that, in its opinion, hypnotism was not only useful but might even be the method of choice in certain psychosomatic and psychoneurotic illnesses. It also thought that it could sometimes play a part in surgery, obstetrics and dentistry as an analgesic and anaesthetic. It should not, however, be regarded as an independent speciality replacing other methods of psychotherapy. Finally, the Committee recommended that hypnotism should be included in the psychiatric courses at medical schools and, possibly, in those for obstetricians and anaesthetists. It felt that there was a need for further organized research into the neuro-physiological and psychological aspects of hypnosis, and indicated certain fields that warranted clinical and laboratory investigation.

This report has already done a great deal to establish a place for hypnotherapy in modern therapeutics, although some of its later recommendations have not yet been fully implemented. None the less, valuable research into new techniques and methods of treatment has been done in recent years, particularly in America, and this is gradually helping hypnosis to emerge from its past atmosphere of mysticism and over-simplification. The history of hypnosis has proved conclusively that it is no miracle-worker, but deprived of exaggerated claims it can still be a valuable therapeutic tool.

CHAPTER 2

The Nature of Hypnosis

Before studying the various techniques for inducing the hypnotic state, it is necessary to learn something about the nature of hypnosis and the important part that is played by suggestion, both in the actual production of the trance and in subsequent therapy. There are many different theories concerning the nature of the hypnotic state, and these are discussed in Chapter 11. Here I propose to deal only with the suggestion theory, since I believe it renders the whole process of hypnotic induction much easier to understand.

The first step is to try to make clear what we understand by suggestion and suggestibility. Definitions are always awkward and seldom complete, but as they are necessary to a proper understanding of the subject I have attempted to provide a simple but viable explanation of these terms.

Suggestion is the process whereby an individual accepts a proposition put to him by another, without having the slightest logical reason for doing so. In a different sense, the term is also used to describe an idea which is presented to the individual for his uncritical acceptance.

Suggestibility is the degree to which an individual is inclined towards the uncritical acceptance of ideas and propositions. In other words, it is a measure of the extent to which an individual will react to what is said to him, without employing his critical faculties.

Perhaps few of us realize that we spend every day of our lives constantly exposed to suggestion of various kinds. Leading articles in the daily newspapers suggest what we should think about politics; attractively dressed shop-windows suggest what we should buy; advertisements in magazines, on poster-hoardings or on television screens suggest to us what cigarettes we should smoke, what beer we should drink or what particular toothpaste we should use. No matter where we go we cannot escape entirely from this barrage of suggestion which tends to influence our daily thoughts and actions, for the most part quite unconsciously. Indeed, the effect of a suggestion may sometimes be much delayed, as the following example will show:

Let us suppose that you are in the habit of using a particular brand of toothpaste. You have used it for years—you are perfectly satisfied with it and you have not the slightest intention of changing it. One day, on your way to work, you see a striking new poster with a very witty caption advertising the latest kind of toothpaste. You cannot help noticing it—you think it is a very clever and attractive advertisement, and there the matter rests. You are not even tempted to try it: you are completely satisfied with the brand you have. Some six months later you go away on holiday, and when you arrive at your destination you find you have forgotten to pack your toothpaste. You call on the local chemist and ask for your usual brand. Since this is out of stock, he offers you several alternatives from which you select the one that you had seen advertised several months ago. Long after you have forgotten the original advertisement, it has still influenced you into buying its particular product.

It is a mistake to think that suggestion is only likely to act upon weak-willed people, or those who are unduly susceptible. Even the strong-willed individual can be influenced by suggestion if it is made in such a way that the person has no idea that he is being influenced. For instance, if I wished to influence a man who held very strong and decided views, I would never try to convert him to my opinions by trying to convince him that his own were wrong. In the course of conversation I should do no more than try to implant a seed of doubt in his mind as to whether the conclusions he was putting forward were, in fact, quite as correct as he supposed. This would certainly not influence him at the time, so I would just let the matter drop and leave what I had said to sink in. Now any idea that is introduced in this way will probably lie latent for a time; but when it eventually takes effect the person will quite probably put forward views in complete agreement with mine, which he will firmly believe to have originated in himself. Through indirect suggestion of this kind, he will not have the slightest suspicion that I have had anything whatever to do with the modification of his views. One of the finest examples of insidious suggestion working in this way is to be found in Shakespeare when the subtle and deadly insinuations of Iago work on the mind of Othello. And here, we discover a very significant and important truth: *the power of suggestion is tremendously enhanced when it acts upon the unconscious rather than on the conscious mind.*

The reason for this we shall presently discover. In view of these facts, it would seem that we are now justified in concluding that Mesmer's cures depended not upon iron rods or magnetic fluids, but upon the implicit belief in recovery that was instilled in the patient's mind because his suggestibility had been greatly increased by the mysterious ritual and ceremonial.

It is now necessary to venture a simple definition of the hypnotic state, which, incomplete though it may be, will still adequately cover many of the observed facts.

Hypnosis is essentially a particular state of mind which is usually induced in one person by another. It is a state of mind in which suggestions are not only more readily accepted than in the waking state, but are also acted upon much more powerfully than would be possible under normal conditions. In other words, the hypnotic state is always accompanied by an increase in the suggestibility of the subject.

The question now arises as to why suggestions should be accepted and acted upon more readily in the hypnotic than in the waking state. Quite briefly, the answer is to be found in the following simple fact: in the hypnotic state, the power of criticism is either fully or partially suppressed.

To understand how this occurs we must first accept the concept of the *unconscious mind.* This postulates that in everyone there is a portion of the mind that is constantly influencing our thoughts and behaviour, the existence of which we are normally unaware. The conscious mind is the part of the mind which thinks, feels and acts in the present. It is the part of the mind which I am using in writing this page, and it is the part of the mind which you are using whilst reading it. The unconscious mind is a much greater part of the mind, and normally we are quite unaware of its existence. It is the seat of all our memories, all our past experiences, and indeed of all that we have ever learned. In this respect it resembles a large filing cabinet to which we can refer in order to refresh our memory whenever we need to do so. Under certain circumstances it can also undertake most of the functions of the conscious mind, with one important exception—the power of criticism.

For the moment, however, let us return to the comparison with the filing cabinet. In it a great deal of information is stored for which you have no immediate use, and which you could not hope to keep in mind. Nevertheless, you know where to put your finger on it whenever it is required. On such occasions you go to the cabinet, you open one of the drawers, you extract the appropriate folder and look at it, thus bringing the necessary information into consciousness. But the filing cabinet itself cannot make use of the information stored in it. Someone has to go to it, extract the required information, and bring it into consciousness before it can be used.

This same process takes place whenever you need to make use of some previous knowledge or experience you have gained. For instance, if I put a proposition to you that you wish to criticize, you have to open the drawer of your unconscious mind and extract the necessary memories and information to bring them back into consciousness. Only then will you be able to criticize what I have said, in the light of your previous knowledge and experience. Perhaps the following example will illustrate the way in which this mechanism works.

Suppose I give you a fountain-pen to hold in your hand, and as you are holding it I suggest to you that it is gradually becoming hotter and hotter and will soon burn your fingers.

Nothing will happen.

In a fraction of a second several thoughts will have flashed through your mind, enabling it to exercise the function of conscious criticism. You will have said to yourself ' Rubbish. No fountain-pen has ever become hot before. Why should this one? Besides, it can't possibly become hot. There's nothing to make it hot.' Notice how you have drawn upon the past experience and knowledge in your unconscious mind in order to criticize the proposition I have made, as a result of which you have been able to reject it completely.

Let us suppose now that I make the same suggestions to a deeply hypnotized subject, who is holding the pen. In the deep hypnotic state, the conscious mind and its power of criticism will have been entirely suppressed. It will be powerless to draw upon the information that is stored in the unconscious mind. The suggestions will consequently enter the individual's unconscious mind which, possessing no power of criticism itself, will be unable to reject them. So the individual will promptly accept the suggestions without reservation. He will believe implicitly that what you tell him is going to happen will be bound to occur. He will thus begin to feel a sensation of heat, his fingers will relax their grip, and the pen will fall to the floor.

The important conclusions to be drawn from these two experiments can be summarized in the following way.

1. The power of criticism is restricted largely to the conscious mind.

2. It is by virtue of this alone that the conscious mind possesses the ability to reject any suggestions that may be made.

3. When suggestions by-pass the conscious mind, as they do under hypnosis, they penetrate directly to the unconscious mind which, being

able to exercise little or no power of criticism, is quite unable to reject them, and the individual is bound to act upon them.

Suggestions are therefore not only more readily accepted, but are also realized to the fullest possible extent during the hypnotic state since direct access is gained to the unconscious part of the mind. We are now able to define certain further principles applicable to the hypnotic state.

1. The response to hypnosis will depend upon the extent to which the power of criticism is suppressed and the power of rejection normally exercised by the conscious mind is removed.

2. The depth of hypnosis in any given case will be directly related to the degree of suppression attained. Slight suppression will result in light hypnosis only: complete suppression will result in deep hypnosis or somnambulism.

3. The more the conscious mind is suppressed, the more the suggestibility of the individual will increase.

Consideration of another simple analogy may help to show more clearly what we try to achieve when we induce the hypnotic state.

If we look at an iceberg we know that we can see only one-eighth of its total bulk above the surface of the waves; seven-eighths is hidden from sight. What we try to do when we start to induce hypnosis is to cause the iceberg to topple over, so that the hidden seven-eighths rises above the surface and the visible one-eighth disappears. In other words, the unconscious mind rises to the surface, becomes more accessible, and eventually assumes temporary control. Moreover, the degree of displacement achieved will correspond roughly with the various stages of hypnosis. If the iceberg only topples over slightly the result will be light hypnosis, and the power of criticism will be somewhat impaired but not to any great extent. If it topples three-quarters of the way, the result will be medium to deep hypnosis; the power of criticism will be much more gravely impaired, and the suggestibility of the subject greatly increased. Even so, it will not be completely abolished. But when the iceberg becomes completely reversed, the result will be very deep hypnosis or somnambulism. In this case the conscious mind will have sunk completely below the surface and will be completely inactive. The unconscious mind will have temporarily assumed control and the power of criticism will be removed altogether.

In trying to induce hypnosis, the main problem is to get the conscious mind out of the way so as to make use of the increased degree of suggestibility that will inevitably follow. Fortunately this is not as formidable a task as it might seem, since the secret lies in a very simple but universal fact.

Even in every-day life, whenever concentration of attention occurs, it induces a tendency towards a splitting of consciousness which renders the unconscious mind much more accessible.

Of the many instances that could be quoted I have selected two hypothetical but typical experiences.

1. I have recently been attending a serious case of pneumonia at number 127 High Street. It has caused me a great deal of anxiety and I have been in the habit of calling at this address at least once or twice a day for the last fortnight. The patient is now convalescent and I have not had to see him today, but intend to call on him tomorrow. As I leave the surgery to set out on my round, a new call is handed to me requesting me to visit number 136 High Street. (Note that it is the same street but a different number.) On my way to this house I pay several other calls. As I leave the last of these and get into the car to drive to High Street, I am feeling both worried and puzzled about the condition of the patient I have just left. My conscious mind is preoccupied with certain important questions. Ought I to obtain another opinion or would it be better to move the patient into hospital? Still pondering over this problem, I drive to High Street. I stop the car and find to my surprise that I am knocking at the door of number 127, the house that I have been in the habit of visiting daily but which I had consciously not intended to visit on this particular occasion.

This is a typical example of concentration of attention. My conscious mind was wholly preoccupied with the serious condition of the last patient I visited. Consequently, splitting of consciousness occurred, as a result of which my unconscious mind temporarily assumed control of my actions and led me to the house that I had been in the habit of visiting daily, instead of the one at which I intended to call.

2. Tomorrow, I have to give a lecture on hypnosis. Since I have not given this particular lecture for some considerable time, I begin to read my lecture notes in order to refresh my memory. I concentrate intently upon these, and become completely absorbed in my task. Whilst I am reading my wife comes to the door and asks me a question. Without looking up I answer her and she goes out again. Presently, she comes in again to tell me that supper is ready. I close my book and go to have my meal, during which she mentions the question she had asked me and the reply I had given. To her astonishment I stoutly deny ever having

said anything of the kind: I have not the slightest recollection of having been questioned or of having replied.

Note the sequence of events. Whilst my conscious mind was completely occupied with my notes I had no wish to be disturbed. Here we have once again concentration of attention. This was naturally followed by splitting of consciousness as a result of which my unconscious mind, which had temporarily assumed control, made me answer quite automatically. Then, when I closed my book and my conscious mind reassumed control, I was completely unaware of what had occurred—hence my loss of memory.

Both the actions and behaviour of a deeply hypnotized subject have been aptly compared with those of a person suffering from absent-mindedness. Now absent-mindedness is a state of mind that comes on suddenly and unexpectedly. It lasts for an indefinite period and then passes off equally suddenly and unexpectedly. In such a fit of absent-mindedness, a man will often start to do a job, and will do it just as efficiently and thoroughly as he would in his normal state of mind. Yet when the fit of absent-mindedness suddenly terminates, he will look at what he is doing and will say, ' Good Heavens, when did I start doing this? ' In its deeper stages, the hypnotic state is extremely similar to this. Indeed one might almost look upon it as a controlled state of absent-mindedness which can be brought on whenever one wishes, which can be prolonged as long as one needs to make use of it, and which can be terminated the moment one has no further use for it.

CHAPTER 3

General Principles Underlying the Induction of Hypnosis

As we have already discovered, the main clue to the successful induction of hypnosis lies in the fixation of attention. The moment you fix your attention intently upon something, your field of consciousness becomes narrowed and your unconscious mind becomes accessible. Suggestions then slip past the conscious mind and enter the unconscious, where they are accepted and acted upon without criticism. Moreover, every suggestion that is accepted and acted upon greatly increases the suggestibility of the subject and facilitates the gradual deepening of the hypnosis. So we can now enumerate certain conditions which are essential to the successful induction of the hypnotic state.

1. Motivation.
2. Removal of doubts and fears.
3. Fixation of attention.
4. Limitation of the field of consciousness.
5. Relaxation and limitation of voluntary movements.
6. Monotony.
7. Suppression of all ideas except those upon which attention is to be concentrated.

We must begin by examining the first two in some detail, since they will often be the determining factors between success and failure.

Motivation

It is normally quite impossible to hypnotize a person against his will, for in order to succeed, he must be neither unwilling nor afraid. He must either want to comply with the suggestions of the hypnotist or must feel that, regardless of his own will, he cannot resist. Indeed the more one can increase the desire of a person to be hypnotized, the more successful the induction is likely to be. Consequently, the most important of all the preliminary steps in the induction of hypnosis is the preparation of the patient's mind to accept it—to fertilize the soil as it were. This is not a difficult task, provided that you set about it systematically. Try to find out whether the subject really wants to be hypnotized— whether he believes in hypnosis and whether he feels it is worth while in order to get rid of his symptoms. Discuss these symptoms with him, and how much inconvenience they are causing him. Point out to him how different life would be and how much more he would be able to enjoy it if he got rid of them. Provided that his case is suitable for treatment by hypnosis, you can tell him quite truthfully that hypnotic treatment is likely to act more powerfully and get him better more quickly than any other method. It is most important that the patient is willing to be hypnotized and believes in the usefulness before you begin an induction.

The Removal of Doubts and Fears

This is another vitally important preliminary step *which must never be omitted* if you wish to ensure a successful induction in the majority of your cases. Many patients are understandably timid, anxious and apprehensive, and will certainly never be able to enter the hypnotic state until their fears have been removed. These fears and anxieties, which can often prove serious obstacles to trance induction, usually fall into two categories:

1. *Fear of failure and over-anxiety to succeed.* The one almost invariably leads to the other, and jointly they can be a source of considerable difficulty. You must remember that many patients who come to you for hypnosis have already tried almost every other method of treatment without success. They have consequently become convinced that hypnosis can offer them a last chance of recovery.

Now this might seem to be a great asset, but unfortunately the patient feels that so much is at stake that the mere possibility of failure appals him, and he consequently becomes over-anxious to succeed. This produces so much mental tension and anxiety that it is impossible for him to relax or even concentrate sufficiently for an induction to be successful. And unless prompt steps are taken to deal with this by offering the strongest reassurances, all attempts at induction will be bound to end in failure.

The patient unconsciously looks upon hypnosis as a test of his ability to perform, and since the neurotic is always afraid of failure, difficulty will be inevitable.

2. *Fear of the hypnotic state itself.* This particular difficulty is much more commonly met. Indeed there is a surprisingly large number of patients who are both afraid and suspicious of what is involved in hypnosis, and who greatly dislike the idea of giving up control. Such doubts and fears as these are almost always due to a complete misconception on the patient's part regarding what is likely to take place in the hypnotic state.

Sometimes the patient will be entirely unaware of his difficulty, for many people are both anxious and willing to submit to hypnosis yet quite unconsciously their minds will entertain these fears. And under these circumstances, the mind will conjure up any excuse or reason for not giving up control. Unconscious resistance such as this may show itself in many different ways. During the actual induction, the patient may seem to be highly amused and even laugh. He may, on the other hand, complain of physical discomfort. Both reactions are evidences of his unconscious resistance to hypnosis and are merely rationalizations, and so it is important to convince him that nothing unnatural is happening and that he will not appear in any way ridiculous.

Occasionally the reverse situation can occur, which emphasizes even more strongly the significance of unconscious attitudes, for an unconscious desire to be hypnotizable may sometimes be stronger than the conscious desire to resist. Under these circumstances, many people who fight against succumbing to a trance are quite unable to stay awake once the induction process is started.

In order to succeed with inductions, all difficulties such as these must be adequately dealt with before you begin. Indeed, the preparation of the patient's mind is the most important stage of all in the successful induction of hypnosis. *Most failures to induce the hypnotic state are due to lack of adequate preparation of the subject, and lack of adequate discussion before induction is attempted.*

This problem presents more difficulties to the dental surgeon than to the doctor, for the dentist who wishes to use hypnosis to secure relaxation or analgesia must necessarily achieve the trance state quickly. He is consequently not able to spend as much time in preparation as the doctor can. Fortunately, in many cases it is not so essential since a considerable number of dental patients are otherwise in good health, and likely to prove more susceptible and less difficult than many of the cases with which the doctor has to deal. But whilst the motivation of such patients for hypnosis is certainly strong, it must not be forgotten that the dentist has his other problems to overcome—fear of visiting the dentist and fear of the hypodermic needle. Effective preparation of the patient, however, need not necessarily be a very lengthy procedure, but none the less time spent upon it is never wasted, and will pay handsome dividends. For this reason, I propose to deal with it in some detail.

The Preparation of the Patient's Mind

There are certain difficulties which occur from time to time, any one of which can seriously interfere with the successful induction of hypnosis.

1. A complete misunderstanding of what is likely to happen during the hypnotic state.
2. Confusion of hypnotic sleep with ordinary sleep.
3. The expectation of amnesia following the trance.
4. The part played by ' will-power ' in inducing the trance.
5. The fear of being dominated by the hypnotist.

One or more of these arise so frequently in patients' minds that it is most important that every one of these points should be adequately dealt with in your preliminary talk, so that the patient knows exactly what to expect. Once this has been accomplished successfully, the induction of hypnosis will offer much less difficulty. Possibly the easiest way to explain them is to describe the procedure that I myself adopt when preparing a patient who has never been hypnotized before.

1. *I begin by asking him what he knows or what he has heard about hypnosis, and what he expects to happen during and after the hypnotic state.* I almost invariably find that, if he knows anything at all, his ideas have been derived from newspaper articles, sensational magazine stories, stage performances or television. More often than not I find that he expects to be completely unconscious during the period of the trance, and to remember nothing at all of what has happened once he is wide awake again. Consequently I explain to him that medical hypnosis is not at all like this, and that hardly any of the things that he expects will, in fact, occur.

2. *I tell him that there is no real resemblance between hypnotic sleep and ordinary sleep.* Although during the induction his eyes will begin to feel more and more tired and will close just as they do when he goes to sleep, yet all the while they are closed he will remain just as wide awake and alert as when they were open. I usually describe this to him in the following words.

When you go to sleep at night and put your head on the pillow, your eyes begin to feel more and more tired until eventually they close. And the moment you fall asleep, you become completely unconscious and unaware of your surroundings until you wake up.

If I were to come into your bedroom and speak quietly to you without waking you up, you would not know I was there and you would not hear a single word I said.

When you go into hypnotic sleep your eyes will begin to feel tired and will close exactly as they do when you go to bed at night. But there will be one important difference.

You will not lose consciousness for a single moment.

You will remain just as alert and wide awake as you were before your eyes closed. You will still know that you are in this room with me. You will be able to hear everything that I say to you. If I ask you a question, you will be able to answer me without waking up.

If you were to become unconscious as you do in ordinary sleep, you would not be able to hear me at all, and *if you couldn't hear what I said, how could I possibly help you?*

Even if you go into the deepest possible trance, you will always hear everything I say, and remain fully aware of everything that is going on.

I then drive this point home by telling the patient that I am going to show him exactly how he can expect to feel when he is in the hypnotic state.

I want you to lie back in the chair and close your eyes for a few moments. Don't open them until I tell you to. Just listen to what I am saying.

Now, you're lying back comfortably in the chair with your eyes closed, and if anyone came into the room they would think that you were fast asleep.

But you know that you're not asleep. You are just as wide awake as you were before you closed your eyes.

You can hear everything that I am saying to you.

If the telephone-bell rang, you would hear it. And if I answered it, you would not be able to help taking a mild interest in what I was saying.

I now tell the patient to open his eyes, and I explain the purpose of what he has just done.

No matter how deeply you go into the hypnotic state, you will always feel much the same as you did then. Except for one slight difference.

If you went into a very deep trance state, you would still remain fully aware of everything that was going on, but you would feel so remote from them that they wouldn't seem to concern you at all. You would still hear the telephone-bell and what I said when I answered it, but it would seem so far away that you wouldn't be the least bit interested in what I was saying.

You may possibly wonder why I consider it necessary to go into this matter in so much detail. The reason is both simple and highly important.

Most people seem to start with the wrong impression in their minds. When they are hypnotized they expect to experience a sort of ' black-out ' during the trance, and after awakening to remember nothing of what has taken place. Although this may not be serious enough to prevent the induction of light hypnosis with spontaneous closure of the eyes, it will often be extremely difficult, if not impossible, to deepen the hypnosis any further. The patient's eyes will close. He will enter the light hypnotic state and he will not try to open them until he is told to do so. But he will fail to respond to any deepening technique. Once he is awakened, he will very often say ' I don't think I've been hypnotized. Nothing actually happened to me. I knew everything that was going on.' And as long as the patient entertains a doubt in his mind as to whether he has actually been hypnotized or not, you will have the greatest difficulty in inducing him into any deeper stage. Indeed, when you try, and fail, he is quite likely to say, ' Just give me some proof that something has happened. If only you can convince me that I have really been hypnotized, I know I shall be able to go deeper.'

Unfortunately he is asking the impossible during these early stages, for only when considerable depth has been achieved can satisfactory proof be afforded. So the awkward situation will probably arise when the patient says, ' Give me some proof that I've been hypnotized. and I'll be able to go deeper.' To which you have to reply, ' You go deeply first, and then I'll be able to give you plenty of proof.' And the result will be a complete deadlock. Indeed the odds are that you will never be able to make much further headway with this particular patient.

If, before attempting induction, you have given the patient a full explanation of what he must expect and what he is likely to feel, this particular difficulty will not occur. Occasionally such a patient will still find it hard to believe that he has really been hypnotized despite all your explanations, but curiously enough if these have been made, his doubts no longer seem to be strong enough to prevent further deepening.

3. *I tell the patient that he need not necessarily expect to forget what has happened during the trance once he is wide awake again.* Since the patient has probably seen demonstrations of hypnotic experiments on television, in which specially trained subjects are used, he will often get the idea that exactly the

same things are going to happen to him if he allows himself to be hypnotized. Most important is the fact that he will certainly expect to have a complete loss of memory for what has occurred during the trance state, and when he finds that he remembers everything that has happened he will be convinced that he has never actually been hypnotized at all. Consequently if you fail to correct his views upon these points, particularly regarding his anticipated loss of memory, you will encounter exactly the same scepticism that we have just discussed and a similar result will be inevitable.

I usually tell the patient that few people are able to achieve such depth, and that for ordinary medical purposes it is certainly not necessary and very seldom desirable. I explain that the subjects he has seen have been specially trained to achieve great depth, in order to be able to take part in experimental work and research. I also point out that in routine medical hypnosis, ' loss of memory ' only rarely occurs, and that I seldom try to induce it since it is hardly ever essential for ordinary treatment purposes. If by chance, however, he should spontaneously forget what has happened during the trance there would still be nothing for him to worry about. It would simply mean that he was an exceptionally good subject, and he would still be able to recollect anything that he particularly wanted to.

4. *I explain to the patient that whilst will-power is most important in the induction of hypnosis, it is in fact his own will-power that plays a significant part and not that of the hypnotist.* There is a widespread impression amongst the general public that if you allow yourself to be hypnotized, you have no choice but to obey implicitly all the hypnotist's commands. That it is his greater will-power that causes you to surrender yours completely with the result that you are bound to carry out his orders quite automatically. This, of course, links up the next difficulty on our list—the fear of being dominated—with the fear of losing control which has already been mentioned.

I tell the patient that if we really believed this to be true, I don't think many of us would be willing to allow ourselves to be hypnotized. I know that I shouldn't.

If hypnosis could only be produced through the stronger will-power of the hypnotist, it would naturally follow that the easiest people to hypnotize would be very weak-willed people. This is certainly not the case, for in actual fact the reverse happens to be true. It is always difficult and sometimes impossible to hypnotize very weak-willed individuals. This is because the weak-willed person cannot concentrate sufficiently and you cannot hold his attention long enough to permit him to enter the hypnotic state. On the other hand, amongst the easiest people in the world to hypnotize are the strong-willed, dogmatic, self-opinionated business men who tend to scare their secretaries and intimidate their executives, always provided that they are willing subjects and anxious to succeed. This is because they can use their will-power to force themselves to concentrate intently upon whatever you wish, thereby greatly increasing their susceptibility.

5. *I assure the patient that he need have no fear whatever of being dominated by the hypnotist, and that he can never be compelled to do or say anything to which he strongly objects.* I explain that if one were to try to compel him to do such a thing it would arouse so much mental conflict in his mind (*I must, but I can't*), that he would either wake up spontaneously or would display so much mental distress and anxiety that there would be no alternative but to awaken him immediately.

I am quite honest with him, and tell him that if he allows me to induce a really deep trance state, there is no doubt that he will feel impelled to carry out my instructions implicitly, but only in so far as he is prepared to do so and yield authority temporarily to me. I should still be unable to compel him to do anything to which he had a rooted objection. I also give him my assurances that apart from the usual steps necessary to induce and deepen hypnosis, nothing further will be done and no questioning undertaken without having previously obtained his consent.

It may seem to you that I have considered this subject of the preparation of the patient's mind prior to induction, at unnecessary length. I can assure you that this is far from being the case. I have done so deliberately because I firmly believe that it is the main key to success, and that more failures result from too hasty and inadequate preparation than from any other cause. The time spent in removing misconceptions, doubts and fears is never wasted. It will not only ensure more rapid and successful inductions, but failure will become much less frequent.

When I have completed my explanations to the patient, I always ask him whether he has any other questions he would like to put to me. If so, by answering them, I am usually able to dispel any last lingering doubts and fears, and thus secure his full co-operation and trust.

I let him see quite clearly that hypnosis is essentially a matter of teamwork between doctor and patient. That the part he plays, however passive it may be, is every bit as important as mine, and that without his co-operation and willingness nothing can be achieved.

Many of these preliminary explanations, however, can be dispensed with in the case of children who, unless excessively timid and nervous, are generally speaking much more easily hypnotized than adults. Children are much less critical and are usually much more amenable to persuasion and suggestion. Here one can rely almost entirely on the ' prestige factor', combined with a sympathetic and understanding approach. Indeed, in most cases, the simplest of explanations calculated to inspire confidence will be found to suffice.

I generally tell young children that I would like to teach them how to go into a special kind of sleep. That although their eyes will begin to feel tired and will close exactly as they do when they go to sleep at night, it will be quite different because they will be able to hear everything that I say, and will even be able to talk to me without waking up. Provided that I have already gained the child's confidence and succeed in arousing its interest, I find that this is usually all that is required.

CHAPTER 4

General Principles of Trance Induction

Depth of Trance and Susceptibility to Hypnosis

It is now generally accepted that 90 per cent of the population can be induced into the hypnotic state by any individual hypnotist, provided that the subject is willing and not afraid. The fact, however, that the remaining 10 per cent will probably fail to respond does not mean that they are unhypnotizable. Some other hypnotist may succeed quite easily with them, although he in turn will encounter another 10 per cent with which he will be unsuccessful. So it is possibly true to say that most people are hypnotizable by someone or other.

Children, particularly teenagers, members of the armed forces, nurses, actors and actresses usually prove to be excellent subjects. This is largely because their training has accustomed them to accept instructions without question. As might be expected, sleep-walkers or natural somnambulists can not only be easily hypnotized but can generally be induced into the deeper stages without difficulty. On the other hand, analytically-minded people, who almost invariably try to work out the whys and wherefores of what is happening to them, are not likely to be easy subjects. Nor are people who are naturally fussy or restless. I think it is probably true to say that hypnosis is much easier to induce and deepen in people who are in good health than in those who are suffering from illnesses, particularly when these are nervous in origin. Yet even in these cases, sufficient depth for successful treatment can usually be obtained with adequate preparation, gradual training, patience and perseverance. Mentally retarded individuals are not good subjects, and it is rarely possible or even profitable to hypnotize the insane.

Different authorities have described over twenty stages of the hypnotic trance, but for practical clinical purposes, these may be conveniently reduced to three:

1. Light hypnosis.
2. Medium-depth hypnosis.
3. Deep hypnosis or somnambulism.

If we adopt these three stages, then the average susceptibility of the general public can be expressed in the following figures.

Ten per cent will probably fail to respond at all. These, however, might still do so in the hands of a different hypnotist.

Ninety per cent will probably achieve the light trance state. Even in this state, anxiety and nervousness can be considerably diminished.

Seventy per cent of these subjects will probably achieve the medium depth trance. At this stage, much more passivity and relaxation can be secured. Some degree of analgesia can often be obtained: dental fillings can sometimes be done with diminished discomfort, and burns dressed with less pain and inconvenience to the patient.

Twenty per cent of these subjects will be able to achieve the deep trance. At this depth, considerable degrees of analgesia can usually be secured.

Now, you must not expect to be able to obtain these figures when you first start using hypnosis. If you do, I am afraid you are likely to be disappointed. You will probably find that a higher percentage of your cases will appear to be unhypnotizable, and that most of the trances you succeed in inducing will be either light or medium. You must not become discouraged by this, however, for practice makes perfect and the percentage of your successes will improve rapidly as you gain experience. Let me offer you a few words of advice. When you first start to practise hypnosis, you are bound to feel rather anxious and unsure of yourself because you are using a method with which you are not familiar. This, in itself, will affect your early results which may seem disappointing. You see, your subjects will be able to sense this uncertainty on your part, possibly from the way you approach them, possibly from the tone of your voice. They will consequently detect the fact that you lack confidence in yourself, and this will prevent them from responding as satisfactorily as they might otherwise have done. This never happens in the case of the experienced hypnotist, for he believes implicitly in his own skill and ability, and thus approaches each case, confident of success.

But even belief in oneself will be useless unless it is based upon real skill, ability and mastery of techniques, and these can only be acquired by constant practice, even in the face of early setbacks. If you happen to be a type that is normally full of self-confidence, you may achieve tremendous initial success. But once one or two dismal failures have dampened this early enthusiasm, the loss of confidence that will inevitably follow will seriously affect your figures and you will fail to maintain your early success.

Remember that medical and dental hypnosis is nothing more than another useful therapeutic instrument, and you should try to adopt the same attitude towards it as you do when you use a hypodermic syringe. Only when you are able to do this will your percentage figures of success fall into the proportions I have already quoted.

So far, in discussing this question of susceptibility, I have deliberately restricted myself to quoting the average figures which are generally published. But I must point out that with patience, and the gradual training of the patient to enter the deeper stages over a period of several sessions, these results can be greatly improved upon. Indeed, in my own experience, there are relatively few patients who cannot be trained in this manner to achieve sufficient depth to enter the hypnotic state immediately upon a given signal, verbal or otherwise. Such depth will be found to be quite sufficient for most clinical purposes. Only when extensive analgesias or hypno-analytical techniques are required is greater depth likely to be necessary.

The General Principles of Trance Induction

The hypnotic state is produced by the constant repetition of a series of monotonous, rhythmical sensory stimuli, which may be visual, auditory or even tactile.

Visual stimuli. Staring at a fixed point, particularly if the eyes are held in a somewhat strained position, rapidly causes retinal fatigue, blurring of vision, and a feeling of tiredness in the eyes. At the same time it induces concentration and a narrowing of attention.

Other visual stimuli such as a swinging pendulum, or rotating, flickering discs and mirrors have also been used to produce the same result. Even a metronome can be employed for the same purpose, and this will simultaneously provide the advantages of both visual and auditory stimulation.

Auditory stimuli. Talking to the subject in a monotonous, rhythmical and persuasive manner also tends to produce the desired state of mind, particularly when repeated suggestions of relaxation are made. The incorporation of certain key words such as *tiredness, heaviness, drowsiness* and *sleep* will greatly accelerate the process. Some hypnotists even reinforce this with the simultaneous use of soft monotonous background music, with a strongly accentuated beat. After all, the effect of the throbbing of primitive tribal drums upon natives is a well-recognized phenomenon, and even today we can observe how easily the teenager is 'sent' by modern dance rhythms.

Tactile stimuli. The gentle stroking of the skin, particularly that of the forehead, seems to exert a strongly soporific and hypnotic influence. Most of us have experienced that soothing feeling of drowsiness that so often occurs whilst we are having a hair-cut or massage. As part of the induction process, this technique can sometimes prove very helpful in children, but is rarely necessary and probably best avoided in adults.

All the various methods of hypnotic induction depend upon the use of one or more of these forms of stimuli to produce sensory fatigue. We need hardly be surprised at their effect when we realize how often people drop off to sleep whilst listening to monotonous lectures or sermons, or even whilst watching television. Indeed, the hypnoidal state can be produced with fatal ease, and can rapidly merge almost imperceptibly into natural sleep. Many motorists experience a dangerous feeling of drowsiness while driving along roads in France, for the lines of tall trees which flank the road for miles cast ladder-like shadows across the highway which induce a feeling of increasing drowsiness.

Now, before you even start upon the induction of hypnosis, there are certain important decisions that you have to make, which may well decide the precise method of induction that you elect to use.

The Type of Approach to Adopt

Basically, there are two ways in which you can approach the induction of hypnosis, and the one which you select must be largely determined by the personality of the patient with whom you are dealing.

1. *Passivity of mind with distraction.* This involves the encouragement of a lethargic attitude in the subject, with a suspension of organized mental activity. *The subject is told to try not to listen to what the hypnotist says.* At the same time, he is given some mental task to perform which will occupy his mind, and distract attention away from the actual process of induction. In this connection, let me remind you of the incident I described on page 15, when I was concentrating upon my lecture notes and failed to notice when I was spoken to, yet answered quite automatically.

If you can get the subject's conscious mind to concentrate intently upon some simple mental task which will distract his attention from the actual process of induction, his unconscious mind will be rendered much more accessible and he will usually enter the hypnotic state much more quickly and easily.

It is just like watching a mother try to spoon-feed her baby for the first time. She carries the spoonful of food to the baby's mouth but he will have none of it, and pushes the spoon away, spilling the food all over the place. Now the wise mother will never try to force the issue. She will pick up the baby's rattle and shake it, and the moment the baby looks up and his attention is distracted to the rattle, into his mouth goes the spoon and down goes the food. Similarly during this type of induction, whilst the subject's mind is distracted from the actual induction process, into his unconscious mind go the sleep suggestions which consequently produce the desired result.

2. *Active participation with attention.* This is the exact reverse of the previous method for the subject is encouraged to pay the closest attention to what is being said, and what is actually taking place. *The subject is told to listen carefully to everything that the hypnotist says.* He is told to concentrate his attention upon everything that is happening, and upon all the feelings that he experiences during the induction.

Each of these methods naturally has its own advantages, and in comparing them, you should bear in mind the following facts.

1. It is much easier to concentrate upon what is happening than it is to make the mind passive, unless some efficient form of distraction technique is simultaneously employed.

2. There is little doubt that passivity combined with distraction not only favours a quicker induction, but also tends to facilitate the further deepening of the trance since the response tends to be more unconscious. I, myself, feel that passivity of mind is probably the better mental state for the induction of hypnosis, but on this point opinions may differ. You should remember, however, that generalizations are dangerous and that ultimately the question should be decided according to the type of mind and personality of the individual subject. In any case, you should be prepared to be versatile, using passivity of mind with distraction at one time, yet turning to active participation with attention at another should this seem to be advisable, particularly if hypnosis is not achieved at the first attempt. In other words, you must always be prepared to vary your method to suit the requirements of the individual subject.

The Manner of Giving and Phrasing Suggestions

It is not very difficult to induce some degree of hypnosis in most patients who are willing, and you must start your induction feeling reasonably confident that you will succeed. This feeling of confidence is bound to reflect itself in your voice and will go a long way towards ensuring success. If, on the other hand, your voice is hesitant or faltering as it certainly will be if you anticipate failure, you will find it extremely difficult to induce even the light trance state.

Although suggestions delivered in a flat, monotonous voice will often prove successful, there is no doubt that their effectiveness can be greatly increased by the proper use of vocal expression which can be varied in many different ways:

1. Alterations in the volume of the voice.
2. Changes in the rate of delivery.
3. The stressing of particular words.
4. Changes in the inflection and modulation of the voice.
5. The insertion of suitable pauses between successive ideas.

Generally speaking, loud tones are best avoided and it is best to speak quietly and monotonously but with definite emphasis. Indeed, in most cases, a slow deliberate rhythmical delivery in an even tone of voice will often prove effective. Sometimes, however, it may be advisable to speak more quickly in order to keep the subject's mind fully occupied. This will forestall criticism by preventing him from concentrating too much upon his own feelings. On other occasions, particularly when suggestions of heaviness, drowsiness or sleepiness are being made, it is better to speak even more slowly and deliberately than usual, prolonging the key words sufficiently to heighten the impression you are trying to convey.

In some instances, a more thorough and effective response is obtained if, in addition to quickening the delivery, increased stress is placed upon critical words. But as soon as the response is obtained, the voice should once again revert to its former flat monotonous tone. This variation seems to call the subject's attention to what is happening, and exercises a powerful effect in reinforcing the idea.

You must, however, exercise great care in your selection of the correct words to be stressed. The importance of this is illustrated in trance induction, where the hypnosis may either be deepened or even accidentally terminated by the tone of voice and emphasis adopted by the hypnotist. If you say to a subject: ' Try to open your eyes. They are tightly closed. You cannot possibly open them ' the effect produced by this suggestion may depend entirely upon the kind of emphasis you use, and where it is placed. If you accidentally lay emphasis upon the word try—' *Try* to open your eyes '—the last part of the suggestion is bound to be more easily resisted, and the subject will probably succeed in forcing his eyes open and waking up. If, on the other hand, you lay emphasis upon the word cannot—' You *cannot* possibly open them '—the subject will probably fail to open his eyes despite the most strenuous efforts to do so, and his hypnosis will deepen.

The acceptance of a suggestion can often be facilitated by raising the voice towards the end of a sentence, thereby conveying increased emphasis and carrying more conviction. Conversely, the lowering of the voice at the end of such phrases as ' deeper and deeper asleep ' seems to heighten their effect considerably. Also, when giving suggestions, it is wise to pause for at least 15 to 20 seconds between successive phrases or ideas. This not only helps to enhance their effect but also tends to avoid confusion in the subject's mind. In fact, whenever time permits the further lengthening of such pauses it will be found to increase their effectiveness to an even greater extent.

During therapeutic sessions, the effect of a suggestion can often be greatly increased if the hypnotist uses his voice in such a way as to express an emotion in keeping with the idea he is trying to convey. The suggestion of disgust, for instance, can be given much more effectively when the hypnotist adopts a tone of voice in keeping with this, although he is not actually experiencing this emotion at the time.

The Emphatic Method of Giving Suggestions

In this method, suggestions are always given in a commanding, authoritative tone of voice, and if you wish to adopt the ' prestige factor ' in inducing hypnosis you will have to give your suggestions as if they were orders. There is no doubt that sometimes this will succeed despite some resistance on the part of the subject. And when it succeeds, it certainly gives more far-reaching and dramatically successful results than any of the milder forms of suggestion.

Only too frequently, however, it awakens a deliberate conflict of will which ultimately defeats the whole object. It also has the grave disadvantage that suggestions cannot be continuously repeated without losing all their force. All your eggs are literally in one basket. Once a suggestion is given, success or failure must follow immediately, and unfortunately failure is much more likely to occur.

The Persuasive Method of Giving Suggestions

In this case, the suggestions are given almost unobtrusively in a quiet persuasive tone of voice. It cannot be denied that this is a much slower method, but it is much more certain, and possesses certain definite advantages. Instead of losing their force, suggestions given in this way actually gain strength through repetition. And since they become persuasions rather than commands they tend to arouse no conscious resistance whatever.

Since I have already stressed the fact that many subjects dislike the idea of being dominated and are afraid of yielding up control, there can be no doubt at all that, if you are interested in hypnotizing as many of your patients as possible, reducing failures to a minimum, this is by far the wisest method to adopt. Nevertheless, you cannot finally determine the precise way in which you are going to give your suggestions until you have considered two important factors—the depth of hypnosis and the personality of your subject.

Whilst in hypnosis the suggestibility of the subject is always increased, the degree to which this occurs will vary with the depth of the trance, and this has to be taken into account when putting your suggestions into words.

In Light Hypnosis

Suggestions should be phrased less positively and with less emphasis than in the deeper stages. Indeed, your approach should be almost entirely persuasive in character.

In Deep Hypnosis

Suggestions can be given more positively and forcefully, but never to the extent that they would appear to the subject as commands. These would not only be resented but would often be followed by a refusal to comply. It is not a difficult matter to phrase positive, direct suggestion in such a way that the subject will not feel that he is being dominated, yet at the same time convey to him your confidence that it will be accepted.

You should also remember the fact that, since your suggestions are always more likely to succeed when they convince the subject that you, yourself, have a firm belief in the idea you are putting forward, such ideas should not only be logical, but should be accompanied whenever possible by sound reasons for their acceptance.

The Personality of the Subject

This must always be taken into account. The helpless, dependent kind of individual who is vainly seeking some authority upon whom he can rely will both expect and respond to a positive approach. In this case, your suggestions should be given authoritatively, emphatically and with the utmost conviction, but even so must never appear in the nature of commands.

Others will resent the slightest semblance of dominance and will fear losing control. They will require a great deal of reassurance, and consequently your delivery should almost resemble a lullaby, slow and deliberate, monotonous, yet with a marked rhythmical beat.

The General Principles and Laws of Suggestion

Before proceeding to study the various methods of trance induction, it is necessary that we should become fully acquainted with certain principles and laws which govern the action of suggestion. These are not only important to our understanding of the techniques of trance induction and deepening, but will also be found to be equally applicable and significant when we come to consider the question of therapeutic suggestion.

1. *You should always couple an effect that you want to produce with one that the subject is actually experiencing at the moment.* This principle should be employed throughout all trance induction and trance deepening procedures.

> As I stroke your arm . . . it is becoming stiff and straight.
> Just as stiff and as rigid as a steel poker.
> *And as your arm becomes stiff and rigid . . . you are falling into a deeper, deeper sleep.*

The subject invariably relates these in his mind, and consequently as he feels his arm becoming stiffer, he tends to fall into an even deeper sleep. Exactly the same thing occurs in the course of therapeutic suggestion.

> Pain is often caused and is always aggravated by tension.
> *As you become more relaxed and less tense . . . you are beginning to feel more comfortable.*

And as your relaxation increases . . . your pain is becoming less and less . . . and presently it will disappear completely.

In this case, the subject has undoubtedly been feeling more and more relaxed as his hypnosis has deepened, and this will certainly have produced a greater feeling of comfort. By relating the suggested disappearance of the pain to these two established facts, he becomes much more readily convinced that this also will presently occur.

2. *It is always much easier to secure the acceptance of a positive suggestion than a purely negative one.* Once again, I am going to quote from the realm of therapeutic suggestion. It is never very profitable to suggest to a patient suffering from headache that his pain is going to disappear. In most cases, it is comparatively easy to produce a feeling of warmth by direct suggestion, particularly if this is accompanied by gentle stroking of the affected part. If the positive suggestion of this increasing warmth is then coupled to the desired negative suggestion of the gradual disappearance of the pain, this is much more likely to occur.

As I stroke your forehead . . . you can feel a feeling of warmth spreading all over your forehead. And as I continue to stroke your head . . . the warmth is increasing and your head is beginning to feel more and more comfortable. All pain and aching is gradually disappearing . . . and in a few moments, your head will feel so warm and comfortable that the headache will have disappeared completely.

3. *It is sometimes easier to secure the acceptance of a suggestion if it is coupled with an appropriate emotion.* In some subjects it is possible to cause the heart to beat more rapidly by direct suggestion alone. If however the subject has the capacity for visual imagery and is induced to picture himself in a terrifying situation that arouses the emotion of fear, this suggestion is much more likely to succeed. In the treatment of alcoholism the suggestion of the loss of desire for drink will be strengthened if the patient is also told that indulgence will arouse strong feelings of nausea and disgust.

There are also three important laws that govern the effectiveness of suggestion.

1. *The law of concentrated attention.* Whenever attention becomes concentrated upon an idea, that idea spontaneously tends to become realized. In the hypnotic state, it is the attention of the unconscious mind that we are trying to enlist, and this is most easily achieved when no conscious

attention is aroused. Suggestions that are made too forcefully or issued as commands tend to defeat this object. It is the fact that television advertisements are repeatedly inserted in the midst of programme material to which we wish to pay conscious attention that impresses them upon our unconscious minds and eventually causes us to buy the advertised products.

2. *The law of reversed effect.* Whenever the state of mind is such that the subject thinks ' I should like to do this—but I cannot ', despite the fact that he may really wish to do so, the harder he tries, the less he is able. We often come across this in everyday life. The patient who suffers from insomnia goes to bed convinced that he is going to be unable to sleep, and thus the harder he tries, the more wide awake he remains. The same difficulty often hinders trance induction. The more actively the subject tries to co-operate, the less he will be able to do so. But the more passive he remains, the more easily he will enter the trance.

On the other hand, you can employ this law to great advantage in phrasing suggestion during the induction and deepening of the trance.

Your arm has become so stiff and straight that it is impossible for me to bend it. *The harder you try to bend it—the stiffer and straighter it will become.*

3. *The law of dominant effect.* This is based upon the fact that a strong emotion always tends to replace a weaker one. The attachment of a strong emotion to a suggestion will always tend to make that suggestion more effective. Notice how the threat of danger will immediately suppress any feelings of pleasure or comfort. The induced emotion of disgust can nullify the pleasure a child gains from biting its nails.

Naturally, great latitude is permissible in the precise wording of suggestions, but the laws must always be observed if satisfactory results are to be obtained.

1. *Suggestions should always be worded in such a way that they are both clear and unambiguous.* The subject must be left in no doubt as to the intention conveyed. Only one interpretation must be possible. Failure to achieve this will often be followed by the most disconcerting and unexpected results. A patient who was terrified to go into the street because of the traffic was once told by a hypnotist that when she left his rooms she would no longer bother about the traffic, and would be able to cross the road without the slightest fear. She obeyed his instructions so literally that she ended up in hospital.

2. *Over-complication should be avoided at all costs. Simplicity is essential.*
Every effort should be made to avoid confusion in the subject's mind.
The more complicated a suggestion is, the more difficult it will be for
the subject to carry it out.

3. *The word ' must ' should never be employed.* There should never be the
slightest suspicion of domination of any kind.

4. *In phrasing suggestions a definite rhythmical pattern should be aimed at,
and repetition is essential.* The same ideas should be re-stated and constantly repeated, over and over again. In framing my own suggestions
I have found that both rhythm and repetition can best be achieved by
using successively several different words or phrases, each with exactly
the same meaning. Certain words are repeated with particular stress
in order to emphasize the rhythm.

> And these same things will continue to happen to you every day . . . and
> you will continue to experience these same feelings, every day . . . *just* as
> strongly . . . *just* as surely . . . *just* as powerfully when you are back home
> again . . . as when you are with me in this room.

If you repeat these suggestions aloud, you will notice that the stressing
of the word ' just ' serves to accentuate the rhythm, like the beat of a
metronome. You will also notice that the choice of the three words—
strongly, surely, powerfully is quite deliberate. The phrases not only ensure repetition, but also express the same basic idea in three different ways.

I am afraid that far too little attention is often paid to this question
of repetition. I am in the habit of repeating post-hypnotic suggestions
at least once before awakening the subject. In some instances it is even
wise to ask him whether he fully understands what has been said, and to
get him to repeat the exact suggestions that have been given.

5. *No matter how deep the trance, no suggestion should ever be given that the
subject might find distasteful or objectionable.* The temperament of each
individual subject should be taken into account. What one person may
readily accept, another may strongly resent and reject. Even in in-
structional courses where post-hypnotic suggestions are given to
demonstrate the phenomena of hypnosis, the utmost care should be taken
to avoid suggesting any action that might cause the subject to feel
embarrassed or to appear ridiculous in the eyes of other people.

Whilst it is true that even in deep hypnosis some subjects may still
be able to resist suggestions of this type, others will feel compelled to
carry them out despite their dislike. In such cases they will quite

justifiably consider that the trust they have placed in the hypnotist has been grossly abused. After all, the deeper the trance, the more powerfully suggestion will be accepted and acted upon. The less the conscious mind is aware of what has been said, the less interference there will be. Naturally the most effective results will occur when post-hypnotic amnesia for the events of the trance can be suggested.

6. *In therapeutic suggestion, the most important and crucial ones should always be left until the end.* Start your treatment with suggestions of minor importance, followed by those of increased importance and finish with those of greatest consequence. The last suggestions of all are likely to be most readily accepted.

7. *Suggestions should always be worded as far as possible to conform with the known habits and thought of the individual.* If this is done, they will usually be complied with as a matter of course, and will be much less prone to arouse conscious criticism.

To sum up, then, it is of primary importance that suggestions should always be given in a tone of quiet conviction, with the utmost self-assurance and confidence in their effectiveness. Weitzenhoffer expresses it in the following terms: 'Within certain limits, a suggestion will be effective in proportion to the degree that the hypnotist believes in its effectiveness, and in the reality of the phenomena it evokes.'

Suggestibility Tests

Since there is a relationship between some kinds of suggestibility and susceptibility to hypnosis, various 'suggestibility tests' have been described which can be applied before attempting trance induction. If successful, they will help to convince the subject that he will be easily hypnotized, and when markedly positive it is likely that the individual will prove to be a good subject. It should be noted, however, that this is not necessarily the case, but it is probably true to say that the subject who resists these suggestions will not prove very susceptible to hypnosis. Many such tests have been described from time to time, but I propose to confine myself to the four that are most commonly employed.

The Postural-sway Test

The subject is asked to stand erect, with his feet together, and his body held perfectly rigid. He is told to fix his eyes upon a spot on the ceiling directly overhead. The hypnotist stands behind the subject with his hands on the subject's shoulders, and tells him to remain perfectly rigid. He then gently rocks the subject backwards and forwards to disturb his balance in the way that suggestion will presently disturb it. The subject is then asked to close his eyes whilst still trying to look at the spot on the ceiling. He is then given the following instructions:

> Try to imagine yourself becoming as stiff as a board . . . your knees stiff . . . and your body perfectly rigid.
> Although your eyes are closed, hold your head up . . . and keep your eyes still looking up.
> You will begin to feel that you are falling backwards . . . that you will feel a force pulling you backwards towards me.
> Don't resist . . . you won't fall to the ground for I shall catch you . . . but you will begin to fall backwards.
> You are falling . . . falling . . . falling.
> Falling backwards . . . falling . . . falling . . . falling.

Usually the subject will start swaying, and as soon as he does so, the suggestions of falling are repeated with increased emphasis and the pressure of the hands removed from the shoulders. You must always watch carefully in order to be sure of catching the subject when he falls, for this can occasionally happen with surprising rapidity.

This test is the one that is most commonly used by stage performers, and can sometimes be usefully employed by lecturers in hypnosis to select suitable subjects from the audience for demonstration purposes.

The Hand-clasp Test

The subject is told to sit in a chair and to hold his arms straight out in front of him at shoulder level. He is to make them as stiff and rigid as possible, and to clasp his hands tightly together. It is useful here for the hypnotist to demonstrate this to him by momentarily pressing his clasped hands firmly together. He is then told:

> Clasp your hands tighter and tighter together . . . and you will feel your fingers gripping more and more firmly.
> And as you do so . . . I want you to picture a heavy metal vice and imagine the jaws becoming screwed tighter and tighter together.
> Now, picture that vice in your mind and concentrate on it . . . and as you do so, you will imagine that your hands are just like the jaws of that vice . . . becoming screwed up . . . tighter and tighter together.
> As I count up to five . . . your hands will become locked together . . . tighter and tighter . . . and when I reach the count of five, they will be so tightly locked together that they will feel just like a solid block of metal . . .

and it will be difficult or impossible for you to separate them. *One . . .
tightly locked . . . Two . . . tighter and tighter . . . Three . . . very, very
tight . . . your hands feel as if they are glued together . . . Four . . . the palms
of your hands are locked tightly together . . . Five . . . they are so tightly locked
that it will be impossible for you to separate them until I count up to three . . .
the harder you try to separate the palms of your hands . . . the tighter your
fingers will press upon the back of your hands . . . and the tighter your hands will
become locked together.*

The Hand-levitation Test

The subject sits at a table with his elbow and forearm resting upon
the surface of the table, palm downwards. The hypnotist places his own
hand on top of the subject's, and tells him:

> As I place my hand on yours, I want you to concentrate upon all the feelings
> you experience in your hand.

(Here, the hypnotist presses lightly, almost imperceptibly upon the
subject's hand.)

> And as you do so . . . you will gradually get the feeling that your hand is
> becoming lighter and lighter . . . as if it has no weight in it at all.
> It's growing lighter and lighter . . . lighter and lighter . . . very, very light
> indeed.

The subject is then asked if he can feel this sensation of lightness. If
he says ' No ', the suggestions are repeated over and over again. If,
on the other hand he says ' Yes ', the hypnotist slightly relaxes the pressure
of his own hand and says:

> Your hand is now feeling so light that it feels as though there is no weight
> in it at all.
> It is getting lighter and lighter . . . so light, in fact, that it is beginning to
> rise up from the table.
> It is coming right up from the table . . . as if it has no weight in it at all.
> Lighter and lighter . . . up . . . and up . . . and up.
> Rising up into the air . . . higher . . . and higher . . . and higher.

(As the hand starts to rise, the hypnotist gradually relaxes the pressure
of his own hand and then removes it entirely.)

The Pendulum Test (Chevreul's pendulum)

An 8-inch circle is drawn on a card with four radii at right angles
to each other. A ring is tied to the end of a thread about 12 inches

long. The subject to be tested is seated at a table with the card immediately in front of him. He holds the thread with his arm extended so that the ring dangles at the other end of the thread about 3 to 4 inches above the centre of the circle. He is told to allow his eyes to travel round and round the circumference of the circle. He is to pay no attention whatever to the ring, which will begin to swing round and round the circle, gaining speed as it does so. The subject is then told to let his eyes travel up and down one of the radii, and as he does so, the ring will change direction and will swing along the line his eyes are traversing.

I have included details of these suggestibility tests because no account of hypnosis would be complete without them. Personally, I find them of very little practical value and never use them at all, nowadays. If a patient badly needs hypnotic treatment, I feel bound to attempt to induce hypnosis no matter how great or little his susceptibility may be, and since this can usually be increased sufficiently by adequate preparation and motivation the need for preliminary testing does not arise.

Final Instructions before Trance Induction

The induction of hypnosis can easily be carried out in an ordinary consulting-room. Either a couch or a comfortable chair may be used. Each has its advantages and disadvantages. Lying upon a couch may become associated in the patient's mind with the act of going to bed, and thus conjure up and encourage the idea of sleep. On the other hand, the nervous and apprehensive patient may feel much happier in a chair. He will feel less helpless since he could spring out of a chair much more easily than he could from a couch. It is purely a matter of individual choice. Personally, I almost invariably use a comfortable chair, sufficiently deep to afford support to the patient's head. The room should be free from glaring lights and steps should be taken to avoid the intrusion of sudden and unexpected noises. Should the patient need to go to the toilet, this should be attended to before the induction begins.

First of all, make your patient as comfortable as possible and see that he is warm. Either seat him in a comfortable arm-chair with his head supported and his legs stretched out in front of him, or let him lie upon a couch with his head on a pillow and relax all his muscles. Curiously enough, most people seem to be more easily hypnotized if they are made to extend the head backwards, as far as is consistent with comfort, during the induction. It seems that in this particular position mental activity is rendered more difficult, so it is a point worthy of notice. Then talk to him in·the following way.

> I am going to begin by telling you three things.
> First, exactly what *you* have to do.
> Secondly, exactly what I shall be doing.
> And finally, exactly what you may expect to happen and how you will feel. Because of this, nothing will take you by surprise, and you will know exactly how you are going on.

Now what you actually describe to him will, of course, vary according to the particular method of induction you propose to use. But never omit this step, for it will make your task very much easier. Finally, remember to put his mind at rest concerning the only remaining thing that may possibly cause him any doubt or uncertainty as to what has happened.

> As soon as your eyes have closed on their own, you will be in the lightest form of hypnotic sleep.
> You will have not the slightest desire to open them, and will not do so until you hear me count up to *seven*.
> At this stage, you could open them if you wanted to, and what is more I couldn't stop you. Even if I were to tell you that you couldn't, you would be able to open them and defy me.
> In actual fact, you won't open them until I tell you to, for the simple reason that you won't want to.

You will be surprised at the number of people who cannot believe that they have been hypnotized, just because they felt convinced that they could have opened their eyes at any moment. And once this doubt has been allowed to enter their minds, you will have great difficulty in deepening the hypnosis any further.

Before we proceed to consider the various methods of trance induction, let us remind ourselves of the sequence of events through which this, and trance deepening are achieved.

1. All trance-induction methods aim at a gradual restriction of consciousness, by limiting sensory impressions.

2. This is achieved by fixation of attention, either on a material object or upon a group of limited ideas.

3. This sensory restriction is reinforced by a rhythmic, monotonous repetition of suggestions.

4. With each suggestion that is accepted and acted upon, the suggestibility of the subject becomes progressively increased, sometimes to an enormous extent. Conversely, each suggestion that is rejected markedly diminishes the subject's suggestibility.

Most of the methods of induction used nowadays depend upon verbal suggestion which is usually, but not invariably, combined with some form of eye-fixation. The latter is certainly not essential but has the great advantage of producing a ' physiological tiredness of the eyes '. When you do use eye-fixation and you suggest to the subject that his eyes are gradually becoming tired and his eyelids heavier and heavier, this is actually true. His eyes are becoming tired, but he believes that the tiredness is caused by the suggestions you are making, and does not realize that initially it is due to the fact that you are holding his eyes in a strained position. He consequently accepts these suggestions with the result that his suggestibility becomes increased. Thus his eyes become progressively more and more tired and eventually close.

Eye-fixation Techniques

The subject is told to fix his eyes upon some object held above his head and slightly to the rear, about eight inches above his line of sight. He is told to continue to stare at it, and not to let his eyes wander from it for a single moment. I usually tell him that this in itself will not produce hypnosis, but will enable him to fix his attention. As I have already mentioned, the induction will be rendered much easier if care is taken to see that his head is extended backwards.

Alternatively, he may be instructed to pick a spot upon the ceiling of his own choice, still slightly to the rear, and stare upwards and backwards at it without allowing his eyes to stray. And in another method of induction he may be told to gaze into the eyes of the hypnotist.

CHAPTER 5

Methods of Trance Induction by Eye-fixation

So many different techniques have been described for the induction of hypnosis that it would be impossible to discuss them all, nor is it necessary to do so. For our purposes, only a relatively small number need consideration and these I have included in the following list:

1. Eye-fixation with verbal suggestion.
2. Progressive relaxation.
3. Eye-fixation with progressive relaxation.
4. Eye-fixation with distraction.
5. Direct eye-gaze method.
6. Erickson's hand-levitation method.
7. Erickson's confusional technique.
8. Whitlow's carotid artery pressure method.
9. The use of drugs as an adjunct to hypnosis.

Of these methods, the two which are likely to prove the easiest and most satisfactory when first starting hypnosis are eye-fixation with progressive relaxation and eye-fixation with distraction, and these will consequently be described in considerable detail.

Eye-fixation with Verbal Suggestion

The subject either lies flat on a couch with his head supported by a pillow, or sits back comfortably in an arm-chair. He is instructed to look upwards and backwards and to fix his eyes upon a spot on the ceiling of his own choice. Alternatively, he can be told to stare at the tip of a pencil held about eight inches above his eyes and slightly behind him. No matter what fixation point is selected, he must stare at it continuously. Should his eyes wander, his attention must immediately be called to the fact. This fixation of attention tends to diminish all other interests and external stimulations. Whilst he is staring at the selected spot or object, verbal suggestions are made to him quietly and monotonously.

Summary of Method. The subject is told to let himself relax completely . . . to breathe quietly, in and out . . . that as he does so, he will feel that his eyelids are becoming heavier and heavier . . . that as they do so, he will want to blink . . . that he will let them blink as much as they like . . . that his eyes are becoming very, very tired . . . that the blinks are becoming slower and bigger . . . that as they do so, his eyes will feel that they want to close . . . that presently they will close on their own, and he will go to sleep. These suggestions are continued slowly, rhythmically and monotonously until the eyes are observed to flicker and close, and the subject sinks into a light hypnotic sleep.

A Typical Induction Routine

Let yourself relax . . . as much as possible.
Breathe quietly . . . in and out.
Let yourself go . . . quite limp and slack.
And gradually, you will feel that your eyes are becoming very, very tired.
Your eyelids are feeling heavier and heavier.
So heavy . . . that presently they will want to blink.
As soon as they want to blink . . . just let them blink as much as they like.
Let everything happen . . . just as it wants to happen.
Don't try to make anything happen . . . don't try to stop it happening.
Just let everything please itself.

You see . . . your eyelids are beginning to blink already.
Very soon . . . those blinks will become slower and bigger.
And your eyelids will feel so very, very heavy and tired . . . that they will want to close.
Already, your eyes are becoming a bit watery . . . you're feeling very, very drowsy . . . and your eyes are feeling so very, very heavy and tired . . . that they are wanting to close.
As soon as your eyes feel that they want to close . . . just let them close, on their own . . . and you will fall into a deep, deep sleep.

(Should the subject's eyes begin to water a little, you should immediately call his attention to the fact, and the moment the blinks become slower and bigger, your suggestions should be given much more positively and emphatically.)

You see . . . your eyes are wanting to close . . . *now*.
Just let them go . . . they're closing now . . . closing . . . closing tighter and tighter . . . tighter and tighter.
Go to sleep!

(The moment this suggestion is made, the subject's eyes usually close immediately, and remain closed. He has then entered the light hypnotic state.)

Progressive Relaxation

This method depends upon the induction of passivity of mind, without employing any accompanying distraction technique. It is usually preferable to have the subject lying upon a couch, flat on his back, with his head supported by a pillow. Notice that no fixation point is specifically used. In this case, fixation of attention is directed towards a limited group of ideas.

Summary of method. The subject is told to think of a pleasant, peaceful scene . . . to imagine himself lying on the sea-shore, sun-bathing . . . that as he does so, he is to let all his muscles go limp and slack . . . first, his calf muscles . . . then his thighs . . . that as they relax, he will feel a feeling of heaviness in his legs . . . that he is becoming drowsier and drowsier . . . that the relaxation is spreading over his whole body . . . his chest . . . his body . . . and his stomach . . . his neck . . . his shoulders . . . and his arms . . . that as it does so, he is feeling drowsier and drowsier . . . that his eyelids are becoming heavier and heavier . . . that his eyes are wanting to close . . . that presently they will close, and he will go to sleep.

A Typical Induction Routine

As you are lying on the couch . . . I want you to think of a pleasant, peaceful scene.
Just picture yourself lying on the sea-shore . . . sun-bathing.
You can feel the soft, warm sand . . . you can see the blue sky . . . and you can feel the warmth of the sun on your body.
I want you to let all the muscles of your body go quite limp and slack.
First, the muscles of your feet, and ankles.
Let them relax . . . let them go . . . limp and slack.
Now, the muscles of your calves.
Let them go . . . limp and slack . . . allow them to relax.
Now, the muscles of your thighs.
Let them relax . . . let them go . . . limp and slack.
And, already you can feel a feeling of heaviness in your legs.
Your legs are beginning to feel as heavy as lead.
Let your legs go . . . heavy as lead . . . let them relax completely.
And as you do so . . . you are becoming drowsier and drowsier.
You feel completely at peace . . . your mind is calm and contented.

You are really enjoying this very pleasant, relaxed, drowsy feeling.
And now, that feeling of relaxation is spreading upwards over your whole body.
Let your stomach muscles relax . . . let them go . . . limp and slack.
Now, the muscles of your chest . . . your body . . . and your back.
Let them go limp and slack . . . allow them to relax.
And you can feel a feeling of heaviness in your body . . . as though your body is feeling just as heavy as lead . . . as if it is wanting to sink down . . . deeper and deeper into the soft, warm sand.
Just let your body go . . . heavy as lead.
Let it sink comfortably . . . into the sand . . . and as it does so . . . you are feeling drowsier and drowsier.
Your eyelids are becoming heavier and heavier . . . and your eyes, more and more tired.
Presently, they will want to close.
As soon as you feel they are wanting to close . . . just let them go . . . and they will close, entirely on their own.
Just let yourself relax . . . more and more completely.
You can feel the heat of the sun on your body.
You are feeling warm and comfortable . . . completely at peace.
And that pleasant feeling of relaxation is now spreading into your neck . . . your shoulders . . . and your arms.
Let your neck muscles relax . . . let them go . . . limp and slack.
Now, the muscles of your shoulders . . . let them go limp and slack . . . allow them to relax.
Now, the muscles of your arms . . . let them relax . . . let them go limp and slack.
And you can feel a feeling of heaviness in your arms.
As if your arms are becoming just as heavy as lead.
Just let your arms go . . . heavy as lead . . . let them relax completely.
And as you do so . . . your eyes are becoming more and more tired.
So tired that they are wanting to close.
Just let them close . . . on their own.
Closing now . . . closing . . . closing tighter and tighter.
Go to sleep !

As the relaxation gradually spreads over the subject's body, you will see his eyelids beginning to flutter, first spasmodically and then more rapidly, and as soon as his eyes have closed, he has entered into a light trance state. Should his eyes close, as they sometimes will, before you have completed the full relaxation suggestions, call his attention to the fact that he has fallen asleep, and carry on with the routine suggestions until the relaxation of the whole body is complete.

Eye-fixation with Progressive Relaxation

This is a most useful method of inducing hypnosis, and one of the two that you should master thoroughly before attempting any of the more advanced techniques. It is a method that depends upon concentration of attention since the subject listens intently, throughout the induction, to what the hypnotist is saying.

He either lies on a couch or sits in a comfortable chair, and is told to select a spot on the ceiling, slightly to the rear, so that he is looking upwards and backwards at it. He fixes his eyes upon this spot, and must not allow them to wander from it for a single moment. If they do, his attention must immediately be called to the fact.

Summary of method. The subject is told to allow himself to relax completely . . . that he can feel a feeling of heaviness in his feet and ankles . . . in his legs and thighs . . . that his ankles, feet and legs are beginning to feel completely and utterly relaxed . . . that this feeling of relaxation is stealing over his chest and body . . . that as it does so, his eyelids are becoming very, very heavy . . . his eyes, very, very tired . . . that the muscles of his neck . . . his shoulders . . . and his arms are becoming more and more relaxed . . . that he is feeling drowsier and drowsier . . . that his arms are feeling heavier and heavier . . . and that his eyelids are becoming so very, very heavy and tired that they are wanting to close.

These suggestions are repeated monotonously, over and over again, until the subject's eyes are seen to flicker and close, and he sinks into a light hypnotic sleep. The hypnosis is then deepened by the induction of arm-levitation.

Deepening by arm-levitation. The subject is told to concentrate upon the sensations he will experience in his arm . . . that his arm is beginning to feel lighter and lighter . . . as if there is no weight in it at all . . . that it feels as if it wants to rise up in the air . . . entirely of its own accord . . . that it feels lighter and lighter . . . and that as it does so, his sleep is becoming deeper and deeper . . . That it feels as though a balloon were tied to his wrist . . . causing it to float up into the air . . . light as a feather . . . and that as it floats up into the air . . . his sleep is becoming deeper and deeper. The moment the slightest upward movement of the fingers is observed, the subject's attention must immediately be called to the fact, and the suggestions repeated with increased emphasis. As the arm rises higher and higher in the air, he should be told that his sleep is becoming deeper and deeper.

Once a satisfactory result has been obtained, suggestions of gradually increasing heaviness are made until the arm sinks down again. The suggestions of increasing heaviness and downward movement of the arm are constantly related to the further deepening of the sleep. By this time, the subject has probably entered a medium-depth trance. Should the arm fail to rise and no upward movement occurs, lift it up gently by the coat-sleeve two or three inches above the arm of the chair, continuing your suggestions of increasing lightness. Not infrequently, such a voluntary movement can be converted into an involuntary response in this way. Should this fail, however, after the suggestions have been continued for about five minutes, the subject will have failed to go deeper and will have remained in a light trance state. In this case, it would be wise for you to try to deepen the trance by the induction of ' arm-heaviness ' (instructions for which will be found on page 78). This may quite often prove successful.

Finally, an attempt may be made to establish the depth of trance by testing for the degree of analgesia that can be obtained.

A Typical Induction Routine

Lie back comfortably in the chair.
Choose a spot on the ceiling, slightly behind you . . . and look upwards and backwards at it.
Keep your eyes fixed on that spot on the ceiling.
Let yourself go . . . limp and slack.
Let all the muscles of your body relax completely.
Breathe quietly . . . in . . . and out.
Now I want you to concentrate upon your feet and ankles.
Let them relax . . . let them go . . . limp and slack.
And you will begin to feel a feeling of heaviness in your feet.
As though they are becoming just as heavy as lead.
As if they are wanting to sink down into the carpet.
Keep your eyes fixed on that spot on the ceiling.
And as you stare at it . . . you will find that your eyelids are becoming heavier and heavier . . . so that presently they will want to close.
As soon as they feel they want to close . . . just let them close.
Let yourself go completely.
Let the muscles of your calves and thighs go quite limp and relaxed.
Let them relax . . . let them go . . . limp and slack.
And as they do so . . . your eyes are beginning to feel more and more tired.
They are becoming a bit watery.
Soon, they will feel so heavy that they will want to close.

As soon as they feel they want to close . . . just let them close . . . entirely on their own.

Let yourself go completely.

Give yourself up completely to this very pleasant . . . relaxed . . . drowsy . . . comfortable feeling.

Let your whole body go limp and slack . . . heavy as lead.

First, the muscles of your stomach . . . let them relax . . . let them go . . . limp and slack.

Now, the muscles of your chest . . . your body . . . and your back.

Let them go . . . limp and slack . . . let them relax completely.

And you can feel a feeling of heaviness in your body.

As though your whole body is becoming just as heavy as lead.

As if it is wanting to sink down . . . deeper and deeper . . . into the chair.

Just let your body go . . . heavy as lead.

Let it sink back comfortably . . . deeper and deeper into the chair.

And as it does so . . . your eyelids are feeling even heavier and heavier.

So very, very heavy . . . that they are wanting to close.

As soon as they feel they want to close . . . just let them close.

And now, that feeling of relaxation is spreading into the muscles of your neck . . . your shoulders . . . and your arms.

Let your neck muscles relax . . . let them go . . . limp and slack.

Now the muscles of your shoulders . . . your arms . . . let them go . . . limp and slack . . . allow them to relax completely.

And as they do so . . . you will feel a feeling of heaviness in your arms.

As though your arms are becoming just as heavy as lead.

Let your arms go . . . heavy as lead.

Let them relax completely.

And as you do so . . . your eyelids are feeling so very, very heavy . . . your eyes so very, very tired . . . that they are wanting to close.

Wanting to close, now . . . closing . . . closing tighter and tighter.

Go to sleep !

The subject has now entered the light hypnotic state. Should his eyes close, as they may well do, at an earlier stage, it is important to carry on with the relaxation suggestions until they are complete, relating these to further deepening of the sleep.

Deepening by arm-levitation

Let yourself relax completely . . . and breathe quietly . . . in . . . and out.

And as you do so . . . you will gradually sink into a deeper, deeper sleep.

And as you sink into this deeper, deeper sleep . . . I want you to concentrate upon the sensations you can feel in your left hand and arm.

You will feel that your left hand is gradually becoming lighter and lighter.

It feels just as though your wrist were tied to a balloon . . . as if it is gradually becoming pulled up . . . higher and higher . . . away from the chair.

It is wanting to rise up . . . into the air . . . towards the ceiling.

Let it rise . . . higher and higher.

Just like a cork . . . floating on water.

And, as it floats up . . . into the air . . . your whole body is feeling more and more relaxed . . . heavier and heavier . . . and you are slowly sinking into a deeper, deeper sleep.

Your left hand is feeling even lighter and lighter.

Rising up into the air . . . as if it were being pulled up towards the ceiling.

Lighter and lighter . . . light as a feather.

Breathe deeply . . . and let yourself relax completely.

And as your hand feels lighter and lighter . . . and rises higher and higher into the air . . . your body is feeling heavier and heavier . . . and you are falling into a deeper, deeper sleep.

Now, your whole arm, from the shoulder to the wrist, is becoming lighter and lighter.

It is leaving the chair . . . and floating upwards . . . into the air.

Up it comes . . . into the air . . . higher and higher.

Let it rise . . . higher and higher . . . higher and higher.

It is slowly floating up . . . into the air . . . and as it does so . . . you are falling into a deeper, deeper sleep.

Further deepening by arm-heaviness

And now you will feel that your arm is becoming heavier and heavier again.

Heavier and heavier . . . just like a lead weight.

It is slowly sinking downwards . . . on to the chair again.

Let it go . . . heavy as lead . . . let it sink down . . . further and further.

And as it does so . . . you are falling into an even deeper sleep.

Deeper and deeper . . . deeper and deeper asleep.

Your arm is feeling heavier and heavier . . . heavy as lead.

It is sinking down, now . . . on to the chair.

And as it does so . . . you are falling into a deeper, deeper sleep.

The moment your arm touches the chair . . . you will be in a very, very deep sleep indeed.

At this point, the subject has probably entered a medium-depth trance, possibly a deep one. Since, even in medium-depth some degree of analgesia can often be obtained, the next step in determining whether the subject has actually gone deeper than this is to test for analgesia and the extent to which this can be secured.

Determination of depth by testing for analgesia. A hypodermic needle is produced and both the subject's sleeves are rolled up to expose his arms.

I want you to concentrate upon your left arm and hand.
Just notice the sensations that you feel in your left arm and hand.
As you do so . . . it is beginning to feel cold and numb . . . as if it is sur-
rounded with ice.
Just picture your arm and hand . . . being packed round with ice.
It is gradually becoming more and more cold and numb . . . as if the
feeling is going out of it completely.
Colder and colder . . . more and more numb and insensitive.
So cold, in fact . . . so completely numb and insensitive . . . that all the
feeling has gone out of it . . . and you will be able to feel no pain whatever.
Your left arm and hand are now so cold, numb and insensitive . . . so cold,
numb and insensitive . . . that you will not be able to feel any pain in them
at all.

First of all, the right arm (the one upon which the subject has *not*
been told to concentrate) is pricked with the needle and the subject
usually flinches. The left arm is then pricked. If the subject neither
moves nor flinches and shows no response, then some degree of analgesia
has been produced and a medium trance at least achieved. In this case,
firmer pricking without eliciting any further response will establish the
extent of the analgesia.

If the analgesia is complete, it will be possible to push the needle
deliberately right through the skin, without the slightest evidence of
pain being felt. In this case, a fairly deep trance has been secured.

If, on the other hand, the subject shows that he has felt pain, either the
suggestions of analgesia must be continued, or should these fail to produce
any result, an attempt will have to be made to deepen the trance by
other means.

If, despite these measures, pain is still obviously felt, then no analgesia
has been produced and the subject may have achieved no more than a
light trance.

Once testing has been completed, you must *never* forget to remove the
analgesia before awakening the subject.

Your left hand and arm are now becoming quite normal again.
They are feeling warmer . . . the numbness is passing off . . . and the feeling
is coming back into your hand and arm.
The sensation is returning . . . you will be able to feel pain quite normally
again.
Your left hand and arm are now quite normal.

Awakening the Subject

Now, in a few moments . . . when I count up to *seven* . . . you will open your eyes and be wide awake again.

You will feel much better for this deep, refreshing sleep.

You will feel completely relaxed . . . both mentally and physically . . . quite calm and composed . . . without the slightest feeling of drowsiness or tiredness.

And, next time . . . you will not only be able to go into this sleep much more quickly and easily . . . but you will be able to go much more deeply.

Each time, in fact . . . your sleep will become deeper and deeper.

One . . . two . . . three . . . four . . . five . . . six . . . seven !

CHAPTER 6

Induction by Eye-fixation (continued)

Eye-fixation with Distraction

This is a method of induction that I have both used and taught successfully over a period of 25 years. It is both reliable and quick, and provided that the subject's mind has been adequately prepared, it rarely takes more than 2 to 3 minutes at the outside to secure spontaneous eye-closure.

The principle upon which it depends is the exact reverse of that which is involved in the last method that we considered, since passivity of mind is aimed at through the distraction of the subject's mind from the actual process of induction. This is achieved by giving him a simple mental task to perform which will fully occupy his conscious mind, thereby rendering his unconscious mind more accessible. Whilst he is occupied with this task, verbal suggestions of increasing tiredness and heaviness of his eyelids are quietly made, but he is instructed to try *not* to listen to what the hypnotist is saying. He will still hear what is said, but will do his best to ignore it and concentrate entirely upon the mental task that has been imposed.

After prolonged trial of many different ways of securing the necessary distraction, I have found that the most effective mental task is a modification of the counting method first used by Loewenfeld towards the end of the last century. He used to ask his subjects to start counting from 1 to 100, slowly and rhythmically. He proceded this by a short period of eye-fixation, but although he followed it with verbal suggestions, he never attempted to induce either tiredness or closure of the eyes. He aimed solely at a general feeling of restfulness and drowsiness.

I make use of the same principle but in an entirely different way. I ask my subjects to start counting backward from 300, slowly and rhythmically until they hear me tell them to stop. They are not to count out aloud. They are just to continue counting mentally to themselves. I tell them that they need not be accurate in the count. For instance, if they make a mistake in the count, and having reached, say

277, they accidentally follow it with 275, they are not to bother to correct the mistake but to carry on with 274. The important thing is to keep the count going regularly and monotonously, just like the beat of a metronome. I have deliberately fixed the starting point at 300 and reversed the count, since this calls for rather more concentration than counting forwards from 1 to 100. The latter method, however, I often find useful in the case of younger children.

If you wish to test the purpose achieved by this count, just close your eyes and start counting slowly backward to yourself, and go on counting backward from 300 for a minute or two. Then ask yourself this simple question: ' Whilst you were counting, how many other different things were you thinking about? ' Not many, I'll be bound. And even if you did happen to be one of those rare individuals who could simultaneously think of other things as well, the solution would still be quite easy. I should simply tell you to start at 300 and subtract 7's consecutively from it until I told you to stop. I think you will agree that it would be most exceptional if you were able to pay attention to many other things whilst you were doing that. So far, I have never had to adopt this course since I have found the backward count from 300 to be invariably successful. Whenever the conscious mind is distracted in this way, the unconscious mind always becomes more accessible. Suggestion is accepted more readily and is consequently acted upon more quickly and more effectively.

Summary of method. The subject lies back comfortably in a suitable arm-chair with his head supported, and is told to relax as much as possible. I prefer to sit on his left-hand side, slightly to the rear and almost out of his sight. I hold a pencil or pen about eight inches above his line of vision, in such a way that he is compelled to stare upwards and slightly backwards at it. This is just sufficient to hold his eyes in a somewhat strained position. Whilst gazing at the tip of the pencil or pen, he is instructed to start counting backward, mentally, from 300, and to continue until he is told to stop. Whilst he is occupied with the count, he is quietly told that his eyes are beginning to feel very, very tired . . . that his eyelids are becoming heavier and heavier . . . that presently they will want to blink . . . that he will let them blink as much as they like . . . and that as they do so . . . his eyes will become heavier and heavier . . . and that they will want to close . . . entirely on their own.

I watch his eyes very closely, and the moment I see them reacting to these suggestions and starting to show signs of closing, I tell him to go to sleep. Upon receiving this suggestion, which is given firmly and emphatically, the eyes usually close immediately and remain closed, and the subject enters the light hypnotic state.

Deepening by Arm-heaviness

I usually start the deepening process with a sequence of progressive relaxation. This, however, is not an essential feature of this particular technique and can easily be omitted if so desired. I, myself, regard it as a valuable addition. But, instead of attempting arm-levitation as the first stage in deepening the hypnosis, I prefer to effect this by inducing a feeling of arm-heaviness. I place the subject's left arm upon the arm of the chair, and stroke it gently from the shoulder to the wrist.

He is then told that his arm is becoming heavier and heavier . . . that he can feel it pressing down more heavily on the arm of the chair . . . that this feeling of heaviness is increasing with every stroke of the hand . . . that, in a few moments, his arm will feel so very, very heavy that when it is picked up by the wrist . . . and then released . . . it will drop limply back into his lap . . . just like a heavy weight . . . and that as it drops limply back on to his lap . . . he will fall into a deeper, deeper sleep.

As I tell him that his arm is pressing down more heavily upon the arm of the chair, I imperceptibly increase the pressure of my hand as it strokes his arm. Provided that this is done in such a way that the subject fails to notice it, it greatly adds force to the suggestion.

Once his arm has been picked up by the wrist and released so that it has fallen limply on to his lap, the heaviness is removed by stroking his arm again and suggesting that it is becoming quite normal.

A Typical Induction Routine

I want you to lie back comfortably in the chair.
Look upwards and backwards at the tip of the pencil.
Can you see it ? Good !
Don't let your eyes wander from it for a single moment.
Now start counting slowly backwards from 300.
Mentally, to yourself . . . not out loud.
Keep on counting . . . slowly and rhythmically . . . and go on counting until I tell you to stop.
Try not to listen to me . . . any more than you can help.
You'll still hear everything that I say . . . but try not to listen.
Just stick to your counting.

Let yourself go, completely . . . limp and slack.
Breathe quietly . . . in . . . and out.
And, whilst you're breathing quietly . . . in . . . and out . . . you can feel
that your eyes are becoming very, very tired.
They may feel a little watery . . . the pencil may begin to look a little blurred.
Already your eyelids are beginning to feel very, very heavy and tired.
Presently they will want to blink.
As soon as they start to blink . . . just let them blink as much as they like.
You see ! They're starting to blink, now.
Just let everything happen . . . exactly as it wants to happen.
Don't try to make it happen . . . don't try to stop it happening.
Just let everything please itself.
And presently, your blinks will become slower . . . and bigger.
As they do so . . . your eyes will become more and more tired.
So tired that you feel they are wanting to close.
As soon as they feel they want to close . . . let them go . . . just let them
close . . . entirely on their own.

You must watch the subject's eyes carefully, throughout this induction.
Timing is of the greatest possible importance. For instance, as soon as
you notice that the individual blinks are almost shutting the eyes, you
should call the subject's attention to it immediately, and continue your
induction in a more authoritative tone:

Your eyelids are becoming heavier and heavier.
They're wanting to close, now.
Let them close . . . closing tighter and tighter . . . tighter and tighter.
Go to sleep !

If this last suggestion has been timed correctly, the subject's eyes will
close immediately, and will remain closed.

Sleep very, very deeply . . . relax completely . . . give yourself up com-
pletely to this very pleasant, relaxed, drowsy feeling.
Stop counting, now.
Just sleep . . . very, very deeply indeed.

Occasionally, it seems to be almost impossible to induce anything more
than the faintest flickering of the eyelids which obstinately decline to
blink. It seems that no downward movement whatever can be initiated
in them to facilitate their final closure.

In such cases, I continue my suggestions for about a couple of minutes
and watch for a fixed, rather distant 'far-away' look to appear in the
subject's eyes. As soon as I detect this, I separate the first and second

fingers of my left hand and bring them towards the subject's eyes, which then close instinctively. As they do, I say to him firmly ' Go to sleep! ' and his eyes invariably remain closed.

Before deepening the hypnosis by the induction of limb-heaviness, I now prefer to produce complete relaxation of the whole body, stage by stage, continually relating each set of suggestions to the gradual deepening of the sleep. Not only is this relaxation more easily and thoroughly obtained in the light hypnotic than in the waking state, but there is no doubt that as it becomes progressively more complete, the subject does tend to sink into a deeper sleep.

Deepening by Progressive Relaxation

Now a feeling of complete relaxation is gradually stealing over your whole body.
Let the muscles of your feet and ankles relax completely.
Let them go . . . limp and slack.
Now, your calf muscles.
Let them go limp and slack . . . allow them to relax.
Now, the muscles of your thighs.
Let them relax . . . let them go . . . limp and slack.
And as the muscles of your legs and thighs become completely limp and relaxed . . . you can feel a feeling of heaviness in your legs.
As though your legs are becoming just as heavy as lead.
Just let your legs go . . . heavy as lead.
Let them relax completely.
And as they do so . . . your sleep is becoming deeper and deeper.
That feeling of relaxation is now spreading upwards . . . over your whole body.
Let your stomach muscles relax . . . let them go . . . limp and slack.
Now, the muscles of your chest . . . your body . . . and your back.
Let them all go . . . limp and slack . . . allow them to relax.
And as you do so . . . you can feel a feeling of heaviness in your body . . . as though your body is becoming just as heavy as lead.
As if it is wanting to sink down . . . deeper and deeper . . . into the chair.
Just let your body go . . . heavy as lead.
Let it sink back comfortably . . . deeper and deeper . . . into the chair.
And as it does so . . . you are gradually falling into a deeper, deeper sleep.
Just give yourself up completely . . . to this very pleasant . . . relaxed . . . drowsy feeling.
And now, this feeling of relaxation is spreading into the muscles of your neck . . . your shoulders . . . and your arms.

Let your neck muscles relax . . . particularly the muscles at the back of your neck.
Let them relax . . . let them go . . . limp and slack.
Now, your shoulder muscles.
Let them go limp and slack . . . allow them to relax.
Now, the muscles of your arms.
Let them relax . . . let them go limp and slack.
And as you do so . . . you can feel a feeling of heaviness in your arms.
As though your arms are becoming as heavy as lead.
Let your arms go . . . heavy as lead.
And as you do so . . . your sleep is becoming deeper . . . deeper . . . deeper.
And as this feeling of complete relaxation spreads . . . and deepens over your whole body . . . you have fallen into a very, very deep sleep indeed.
You are so deeply asleep . . . *that everything I tell you that is going to happen . . . will happen . . . exactly as I tell you.*
And every feeling that I tell you that you will experience . . . you will experience . . . exactly as I tell you.
Now, sleep very, very deeply.
Deeper and deeper asleep . . . deeper and deeper asleep.

By now, the subject should be firmly established in the hypnotic state and further deepening techniques can be employed.

Deepening by Induction of Arm-heaviness

I am now going to place your arm on the arm of the chair.
And I am going to stroke it gently . . . from the shoulder to the wrist.
And as I stroke it . . . you will begin to feel a feeling of heaviness in your arm.
That feeling of heaviness is increasing . . . with every stroke of my hand.
Your arm is beginning to feel heavier . . . and heavier . . . just as heavy as lead.
You can feel it pressing down more firmly on the arm of the chair.

(As you say this, you should imperceptibly increase the pressure of your own hand, as you stroke his arm.)

And in a few moments . . . your arm will feel so very, very heavy . . . *that, when I pick it up by the wrist . . . and let it go . . . it will drop limply back on to your lap . . . just like a lead weight.*
And as it drops limply back . . . on to your lap . . . you will fall into a deeper, deeper sleep.

Now, lift up the subject's arm by the wrist, and release it. It will drop back heavily on to his knees. Replace it on the arm of the chair, and *proceed to restore it to normal by removing the induced feeling of heaviness.* This emphasizes a most important rule which you must never fail to observe when you are practising hypnosis: *during hypnosis, no matter what effect you produce, whether it be limb-heaviness, limb-rigidity or analgesia—particularly the latter—you must never forget to remove it again and restore normality before you awaken the subject.*

> You have now fallen into a much deeper sleep.
> And, as I stroke your arm in the opposite direction . . . you will notice that all feelings of heaviness are leaving your arm.
> It is coming back to normal . . . and now feels just the same as your other arm.
> And as it does so . . . your sleep is becoming even deeper . . . and deeper.

This concludes the first stage of the deepening process.

If you consider the prospects are favourable you can now proceed to deepen the hypnosis further, or you may find it best to defer this until the next session. I usually make this decision by watching carefully the extent and ease with which the subject has complied with these suggestions. If the results have been easily obtained I proceed with further deepening techniques, such as the induction of graded responses, which will be described in a later chapter. On the other hand, if any difficulty has been experienced I awaken the subject, having given him the post-hypnotic suggestion that on the next occasion he will be able to go to sleep even more quickly and deeply.

Awakening the Subject

> In a few moments . . . when I count up to *seven* . . . you will open your eyes and be wide-awake again.
> You will wake up feeling wonderfully better for this deep, refreshing sleep. You will feel completely relaxed . . . both mentally and physically . . . quite calm and composed . . . without the slightest feeling of drowsiness or tiredness.
> And next time . . . you will not only be able to go into this sleep much more quickly and easily . . . but you will also be able to go much more deeply.
> Each time, in fact . . . your sleep will become deeper and deeper.
> One . . . two . . . three . . . four . . . five . . . six . . . seven !

After awakening the subject, I always discuss with him the sensations that he has actually experienced during the induction. This not only enables me to set his mind at rest concerning any doubts he may have entertained, but also informs me of any feelings he may have experienced other than those that I had suggested. I note these carefully in order to incorporate them as additional suggestions during his next induction. This process is known as the feed-back method, and can often greatly facilitate the induction and deepening of hypnosis.

The Advantages and Disadvantages of the Eye-fixation with Progressive Relaxation and the Eye-fixation with Distraction Methods of Trance Induction

Although many different methods of trance induction have been described, you will probably find that when you first start using hypnosis, these two methods are likely to be the most useful to adopt as standard-ized procedures. Indeed, you should make yourself competent in both of these, since it is always a mistake to become restricted to one particular method. Both have their advantages and disadvantages, and the choice of which you decide to use as your standard method must ultimately depend upon your own individual preference and experience. No single method can ever be described or even recommended as the best method of inducing hypnosis since results will vary considerably in the hands of different operators. The most important thing is to understand the principles underlying the various methods of trance induction and to make your choice in any individual case with due regard to the two following considerations:

1. The method must suit your own personality.
2. It must also suit the personality of your subject.

But remember, no matter what method you finally evolve as your favourite technique, you must still be prepared to vary it when occasion demands. You will certainly fail with many of your patients if, so to speak, hypnosis is ' bought off the peg ', ready-made. On the other hand, few patients will present great difficulty provided that the hypnosis is tailored to suit their individual requirements.

After 25 years experience, it is hardly surprising that my own prefer-ence should be for the eye-fixation-distraction method of induction, followed by the deepening techniques which will be described later, which I have gradually developed and modified throughout this period. But whilst I use this in the great majority of my cases, there are still times when I should fail completely if I were not prepared to vary it. There is not the slightest doubt in my mind that whenever you have to deal with a very nervous, anxious and apprehensive patient, the eye-fixation-progressive relaxation method is a much better approach to the initial induction of hypnosis. I, myself, always adopt it under these particular circumstances. I also find it useful occasionally as a means of introducing hypnosis to the patient who would otherwise be too terrified to accept the idea of medical hypnosis as a form of treatment. In such cases I say nothing to the patient, but having obtained the relatives' permission to try hypnosis, I proceed to teach the full relaxation technique only. I give no suggestions whatever of eye-tiredness or eye-closure but when the eyelids start to flicker, as they almost invariably do, I quietly tell the patient that if the eyes feel that they want to close to let them close. When I subsequently reveal the fact that a very light hypnotic state has actually occurred, the patient is always so reassured that there is no further difficulty in proceeding with orthodox hypnotic treatment. But even when I use this method, once the eyes have closed, I never begin the deepening process by attempting to secure arm-levitation. I much prefer to proceed with my own standardized deepening routine, by the induction of graded responses starting with arm-heaviness. You will notice how the most useful features of one or two different methods can be advantageously combined in this way to suit individual circumstances.

My own reasons for feeling that the eye-fixation-distraction method offers certain material advantages in the majority of cases can be briefly summarized as follows:

1. It saves time. It is a rapid and efficient method of induction, spontaneous eye closure usually being obtained within 2 to 3 minutes. The subject enters the hypnotic state almost before he is aware of the fact. Light hypnosis always seems to be induced more quickly and easily when the subject does not have to concentrate his attention upon the suggestions that are being made. His conscious mind is distracted away from the actual induction process by the counting technique. He is consequently much less critical towards what is being said, and is thus prone to accept suggestion much more rapidly and readily.

2. In the first stage of deepening the hypnosis, it is much easier to induce a feeling of arm-heaviness since the natural tendency for the arm to fall, owing to the force of gravity, greatly augments the strength of the suggestion. Arm-levitation is not as certain to succeed and sometimes cannot be produced at all. Failure is always a set-back, and temporarily at least diminishes the subject's susceptibility to alternative deepening procedures. Even when it succeeds, since the arm has to rise in opposition

to the force of gravity, it is only natural that the effect should take longer to occur. It must be admitted, however, that when arm-levitation does succeed it certainly goes a long way towards convincing the subject that he has actually been hypnotized, since something has occurred that is quite out of keeping with his normal experience, and the increase in depth that follows is usually greater. Despite this obvious advantage, it seems to me that since an equivalent depth can generally be achieved without difficulty as a result of subsequent techniques, the induction of arm-heaviness, which is not only more likely to succeed but is also more quickly and more readily secured, has much to commend it.

3. The complete unpredictability of the occurrence and extent of induced analgesia, in my opinion, renders it unsuitable as a test of depth in the course of routine inductions. Sometimes considerable degrees of analgesia can be obtained in medium-depth hypnosis, on other occasions no analgesia at all can be produced until deep hypnosis or even somnambulism has occurred. I have seen a complete somnambule in whom no significant amount of analgesia whatever could be obtained, despite the fact that every other conceivable phenomenon could readily be elicited. Consequently, there is always the danger that, if this particular test fails, the susceptibility of many subjects will become diminished to such an extent that they will find it difficult, if not impossible to achieve the depth which otherwise they might have attained.

The Direct Eye-gaze Method

This is a method of induction which I consider to be useful only under certain special circumstances. Whilst it undoubtedly tends to produce a rather deeper form of hypnosis which facilitates further deepening, in my opinion it is far too authoritative, and for this reason alone I would never recommend its use as a routine procedure. It relies far too much upon the prestige factor and the subject is bound to feel that he is being dominated by the hypnotist, both undesirable features which are best avoided.

I reserve it for the rare occasions when the subject's reactions to other methods of induction indicate clearly that his personality is only likely to respond to a dominant approach. On the other hand, if I come across a subject who finds it impossible to accept the fact that he has really been hypnotized, which fortunately seldom happens, I occasionally resort to it in the form of a challenge, the subject being told to resist the sleep suggestions as long as he can, and that the harder he tries to keep his eyes open—the more quickly they will close. Whilst this never fails to carry conviction, I would not advise you to try it until you have gained a great deal of confidence and experience.

Summary of method. The hypnotist sits in front of the subject and leans slightly forward. He holds the subject's hands, and tells him to gaze into his eyes from a distance of approximately two feet. Since this involves the slight risk that the hypnotist, if unduly susceptible himself, might be the first to succumb, it is usually advisable not to stare directly into the subject's eyes, but to gaze at the bridge of his nose. He will be quite unable to detect the difference.

During the induction, should the hypnotist's own eyes become tired, or should he feel the least bit drowsy himself, he should deliberately close the subject's eyes with his fingers whilst simultaneously closing his own, in order to give them a brief rest. It is quite safe to do this because the subject will never realize that it is not an essential part of the technique. After a few moments, the hypnotist can open the subject's eyes again and resume his fixed stare. Whilst the subject's eyes are held unwaveringly in this manner, the same type of verbal suggestions of relaxation, drowsiness, heaviness of the eyelids and eye-closure are made, as in the techniques already described.

This is not a particularly difficult method of induction, but its success depends upon one's ability to maintain an unblinking stare long enough to cause the subject's eyes to close. The eyes can be trained for this technique by gazing fixedly at the tip of a pencil held about 18 inches in front of the eyes. Practice will greatly increase the length of time they can be kept open before they start to water or blink.

CHAPTER 7

Erickson's Hand-levitation and Other Methods of Induction: Drug Induction

Erickson's Hand-levitation Method

This procedure was originally devised by Erickson in 1923, whilst experimenting with suggestions conducive to automatic writing as an indirect technique of trance induction for naïve subjects. Although successful, it proved to be too slow and laborious an induction technique in most instances. It was consequently suggested to the subject that, instead of writing, the pencil-point would merely move up and down on the paper, or from side to side. Erickson quickly realized that the pencil and paper were superfluous and that the ideo-motor activity was the primary consideration, and succeeded in inducing a somnambulistic trance by substituting a simple ' hand-levitation ' technique.

The following full description and analysis of hypnosis by means of hand-levitation is that given by Wolberg in his book, *Medical Hypnosis*, Vol. 1. It is probably one of the best of the induction techniques, since it not only permits the subject himself to play a greater part in the actual induction, but also allows him to take his own time in falling asleep.

Summary of method. The subject is told to sit back comfortably in a chair and to rest his hands, palms downwards, upon his thighs. He is then told to gaze fixedly at his hands and to concentrate his attention upon the sensations he can feel in them. He is told that although his hands seem to be motionless some movement is still present. Very soon, he is told, one of his fingers or his thumbs will twitch; as soon as this occurs his attention is drawn to the fact, and he is told that the spaces between his fingers will gradually widen and that his fingers will slowly but surely begin to separate. When this is seen to occur the suggestions are changed to those of gradually increasing lightness in the fingers and hand. He is told that his fingers are beginning to rise up from his leg—that they are slowly floating upwards—that his hand and arm are floating up into the air—upwards—upwards—upwards. Then, when his hand and arm have risen to the level of his face, he is told that his hand is changing direction and that it is now being attracted towards his face. As his hand approaches his face he is told that he is beginning to feel very, very drowsy, that his eyelids are becoming very, very tired—heavier and heavier—and that as soon as his hand touches his face his eyes will close and he will fall into a deep, deep sleep.

His hypnosis can then be further deepened by any of the standard techniques.

A Typical Induction Routine

I want you to sit comfortably in the chair.
Let yourself relax.
Place your hands, palms downward, upon your thighs.
Fix your eyes upon your hands . . . and keep watching them . . . very, very closely.
And whilst you are relaxing like this . . . you will notice that certain things are happening . . . that you had not noticed before.
I will point them out to you.
Now, I want you to concentrate upon all the sensations and feelings that you notice in your hands . . . no matter what they may be.
It may be that you will feel the texture of the material of your trousers . . . as your hands rest upon your thighs.
You may feel the warmth of your hand on your leg . . . or you may feel a certain amount of tingling in your hand.
No matter what your sensations may be . . . I want you to observe them closely.
Keep watching your hand.
It seems to be quite still . . . and resting in one position.
Yet some movement is there . . . although it is not yet noticeable.
Keep watching your hand.
Don't let your attention wander from it.
Just wait to see what movement is going to show itself.

The subject's attention is now firmly fixed upon his hand, and he is curious about what is going to happen. Sensations such as anyone might normally feel have been suggested to him as possibilities. No attempt has been made to force any suggestion on him: what he observes he considers to be a product of his own experience.

The idea is to induce him to respond to the suggestions of the hypnotist as if they, too, are parts of his own experience. A subtle attempt is being made to establish a link in his mind between his own sensations and the words spoken to him. In this way, at a later stage, this linkage will cause words or commands to tend to produce further sensations or actions.

Unless there is any conscious resistance on the subject's part, a slight twitching or jerking will occur in one of the fingers, or in the hand. As soon as this happens, the subject's attention must be drawn to the fact and he must be told that the movement will probably increase. Any other movement of the legs or body, or any alteration in the breathing should also be commented upon. This linking of the subject's reactions with the remarks of the hypnotist causes an association between the two to be formed in the subject's mind.

> It will be interesting to see which of your fingers moves first.
> It may be any finger . . . or it may even be your thumb.
> But one of the fingers is going to twitch or move.
> You don't know which one . . . or even in which hand.
> Neither do I . . . but keep watching . . . and you will find that one of them will move.
> Possibly in your right hand.
> See! The thumb twitched and moved . . . just as I said.
> And now you will notice that a very interesting thing is beginning to happen.
> You will notice that the spaces between your fingers are gradually beginning to widen.
> The fingers will move slowly apart . . . and you'll see that the spaces will become wider and wider.
> Your fingers are slowly moving apart . . . wider . . . wider . . . wider.
> The spaces are slowly becoming wider . . . wider . . . wider.

This is the first suggestion to which the subject is expected to respond. If the fingers do move apart, it is because the subject is beginning to respond to suggestion. The hypnotist continues to talk, however, as if it were something that had taken place in the natural course of events.

> Now, I want you to watch carefully what is taking place.
> Your fingers will want to rise up slowly from off your thigh.
> As if they want to lift up . . . higher . . . higher . . . higher.

(The subject's forefinger starts to move upward slightly.)

> You see!
> Already your forefinger is beginning to lift up.
> As it does so . . . all the other fingers will want to follow.
> Up . . . and up . . . and up.
> Rising up slowly into the air.

(The other fingers begin to rise.)

As the other fingers lift . . . your whole hand is beginning to feel lighter
and lighter.
So light . . . that your whole hand will slowly rise into the air.
As if it feels just as light as a feather . . . just like a feather.
As if a balloon is slowly lifting it up in the air.
Lifting . . . lifting . . . up . . . and up . . . and up.
Pulling it up . . . higher . . . higher . . . higher.
Your hand is becoming lighter and lighter.
Very, very light indeed.

(The hand starts to rise.)

As you watch your hand rise . . . you will feel that your whole arm is
beginning to feel lighter and lighter.
It is wanting to rise up in the air.
Notice how your arm is lifting up into the air . . . up . . . and up . . . and
up . . . a little higher . . . and higher . . . and higher.

(The arm has now lifted about six inches above the thigh, and the subject
is gazing at it intently.)

Keep watching your hand and arm . . . as it rises into the air.
And as it does so . . . you will begin to feel drowsy and tired.
Notice how drowsy and tired your eyes are becoming.
As your arm continues to rise . . . you will feel more and more tired and
relaxed . . . very, very sleepy . . . very, very sleepy indeed.
Your eyes will become heavier and heavier . . . and your eyelids will want
to close.
As your arm rises . . . higher and higher . . . you will want to feel more
and more relaxed.
You will want to enjoy this very, very pleasant . . . relaxed . . . sleepy
feeling.
Just let yourself go.
Give yourself up entirely to this very, very comfortable . . . relaxed . . .
drowsy feeling.

Notice how as the subject carries out one suggestion, his response
is used to reinforce and facilitate the next suggestion. As his arm rises,
it is suggested by inference that he will become drowsy because his arm
is rising. This is yet another example of the important principle of
coupling, which we have already considered (p. 35).

Your arm is lifting up . . . and up . . . and up.
Higher . . . and higher . . . and higher.

And you are feeling very, very drowsy indeed.
Your eyelids are becoming heavier . . . and heavier.
Your breathing is becoming slower . . . and deeper.
Breathe slowly and deeply . . . in . . . and out . . . in . . . and out.

(The subject's arm is now stretched out straight in front of him. His eyes are beginning to blink, and his breathing is deep and regular.)

As you keep watching your hand and arm . . . you are feeling more and more drowsy . . . and relaxed.
And now you will notice that your hand is changing its direction.
The elbow is beginning to bend . . . and your hand is beginning to move . . . closer and closer to your face.
Your hand feels as though it were being strongly attracted to your face.
Your hand is moving . . . slowly but surely . . . towards your face.
And as it becomes closer and closer . . . you are feeling drowsier and drowsier . . . and you will fall into a very deep sleep.
Closer and closer . . . drowsier and drowsier . . . sleepier and sleepier.
Although you are becoming sleepier and sleepier . . . you must not go to sleep until your hand touches your face.
But when your hand touches your face . . . you will fall immediately into a deep, deep sleep.

The subject is being asked to choose his own pace in falling asleep, consequently when his hand touches his face and his eyes do close, he is perfectly satisfied that he is, in fact, asleep. Constant coupling of the hand-levitation and sleepiness techniques causes them to continue to reinforce each other.

When the subject does finally close his eyes, he will have entered a trance in the production of which he, himself, will have participated. He will thus be much less likely to deny that he has been in a trance.

Your hand is now changing its direction.
It is moving closer and closer to your face.
Your eyelids are feeling heavier and heavier.
You are becoming sleepier . . . and sleepier . . . and sleepier.

(The subject's hand is now approaching his face, and his eyelids are blinking more rapidly.)

Your eyes are becoming heavier . . . and heavier.
Your hand is moving closer and closer towards your face.
You are becoming drowsier . . . and drowsier . . . more and more tired.
Your eyes are wanting to close now . . . closing . . . closing.
When your hand touches your face . . . they will close immediately.

You will fall into a very, very deep sleep.
Drowsier . . . and drowsier . . . very, very sleepy . . . very, very tired.
Your eyelids are beginning to feel just as heavy as lead.
Your hand is moving closer and closer to your face.
Closer . . . and closer . . . closer to your face.
The moment it touches your face . . . you will fall into a very, very deep sleep.

(The subject's hand touches his face, and his eyes close.)

Go to sleep ! Go to sleep ! Sleep very, very deeply !
And as you sleep . . . you will feel very, very tired . . . and relaxed.
Let yourself go . . . Let yourself relax completely.
Think of nothing but sleep . . . *deep, deep sleep !*

Notes on the hand-levitation method. You should notice that no attempt whatever is made in the early stages to force any suggestions upon the subject. Sensations that almost anyone might experience are suggested to him as possibilities. Consequently, as he observes them, he looks upon them as a product of his own experience, and this renders him much more likely to respond to the suggestions of the hypnotist as if they, too, are parts of his own experience.

The first real suggestion is made when he is told that his fingers are beginning to separate, and if they do, then he is definitely responding to suggestion. When he is told that as his hand approaches his face he will become drowsier and drowsier, he is actually being requested to choose his own pace in falling asleep. Thus when his hand eventually touches his face, he will feel himself to be asleep to his own complete satisfaction, and will then be much less likely to deny the fact that he has been hypnotized.

There is little doubt that the subject hypnotized for the first time by this method will usually achieve depth hypnosis much more easily than he would, had any other method of induction been used. The method, however, has the grave disadvantage of being much more difficult and time-consuming than any of the usual methods. Once started, it must be persevered with until the arm eventually rises, even if this takes an hour or more to achieve. Moreover, it is exceedingly likely to fail unless the hypnotist has had wide technical experience. It is definitely a method for the expert, and in his hands it can prove to be one of the most valuable of all methods, since when successful it lends itself admirably to the more advanced analytical techniques. The serious student of hypnosis, however, would be well-advised to avoid it until he has gained considerable experience and confidence, for failure would almost inevitably render the subject much more difficult to hypnotize by any alternative procedure.

Erickson's Confusional Technique

This procedure can be extremely useful in circumventing unconscious resistance in a subject who consciously wishes to be hypnotized. It can also be used to induce hypnosis when the subject is unaware that hypnosis is even contemplated. The method was originally designed and employed for the purposes of ' age-regression ', but was later found to be applicable to the induction of hypnosis and other hypnotic phenomena. Its main object is to set up a situation in which the subject is never sure whether he is actually co-operating or not, and under these circumstances his defences become ineffective. It is primarily a verbal technique which is based upon three main devices:

1. *A play upon words.* The following example is quoted by Erickson: ' Write right right, not rite or write.' This can be easily understood by the reader but not by the listener, who consequently struggles in vain to find some meaning in it. Before he can reject it, a further statement is made to engage his attention. Similarly, two words with opposite meanings can be correctly used to describe the same object—' If you lose your left hand in an accident, your right [hand] is left.'

2. *Alterations in the tenses.* This keeps the subject constantly trying to discover the intended meaning. For example—' Today *is* today, but it *was* yesterday's future, even as it *will be* tomorrow's *was*.'

Here, it will be noticed that the past, the present and the future are all used in connection with the reality of today.

3. *The employment of irrelevancies.* Each of these, taken out of context, appears to be a sound and sensible communication. Taken in context, they are confusing, distracting and inhibiting, and lead to a growing desire and need on the part of the subject to receive some communication which he can easily understand, and to which he can respond.

When using confusional techniques, the operator must maintain a casual but interested attitude and must speak seriously and intently, as if he expects the subject to understand exactly what is being said. The tenses must be carefully and constantly shifted, and a ready flow of language maintained. The subject should be given a little time to respond, but never quite sufficient for him to react fully before the next idea is presented. He consequently becomes so confused and frustrated that he feels a growing need for a clear-cut communication to which he can respond. Confusion techniques are prolonged and highly complex procedures, but once mastered they can lead to easy and rapid trance induction under the most unfavourable circumstances. A great deal of skill and experience is required, and they are not to be recommended to the beginner (Erickson gives a fascinating account of them in the *American Journal of Clinical Hypnosis*). If they are used in conjunction with hand-levitation, the operator makes a series of contradictory statements in such a way that the subject feels that something meaningful and precise is being said. But he is still given insufficient time to realize how illogical the suggestions are:

> Your right hand is rising into the air . . . and your left hand is pressing down on the arm of the chair.
> Let your left hand rise into the air . . . and your right hand press down on the arm of the chair.
> Both hands are pressing down on the arms of the chair.
> One hand is now lifting up into the air . . . and the other is pressing down on the arm of the chair.
> Your right hand is rising into the air . . . and your left hand is pressing down on the arm of the chair . . . (Original suggestion.)

Confused by these rapidly conflicting instructions, in sheer desperation the subject is likely to accept and carry out the first positive suggestion that will enable him to escape from his dilemma.

Whitlow's Carotid Artery Pressure Method

This rapid method of induction was first described by Dr Joseph Whitlow. With the subject's head supported by the left hand, the right finger and thumb press upon the vagus nerve and carotid artery in each side of the neck; at the same time suggestions are made that the eyes will close and the subject will go to sleep. The pressure, which must never be maintained for longer than 10 to 15 seconds, is released as soon as the subject relaxes, and he remains in a state of hypnosis.

Dr Whitlow claims to have hypnotized scores of patients successfully by this method, which is also popular with stage hypnotists because of its rapid and dramatic effect. Quite rightly, however, it has never received professional approval or support in this country, for serious risks and dangers can easily be involved. Brain damage from lack of blood, or even death, could occur if the pressure on the vagi and carotids were maintained too long.

The Use of Drugs as an Adjunct to Hypnosis

Many drugs have been tried to facilitate the induction or deepening of hypnosis in difficult subjects, but the results seem to be both variable and unpredictable. The intravenous barbiturates appeared promising since they are often used to secure the release of emotional material. Their action in this respect, however, may or may not be related to hypnosis which can be used on its own to produce similar abreactions. Intravenous thiopentone (Pentothal) is occasionally helpful, but is more often disappointing; this is unfortunate since only short-acting drugs of this type can be safely given to out-patients. The oral administration of amylobarbitone sodium (Sodium-Amytal), 6 to 9 grains, or pentobarbitone sodium (Nembutal), 3 grains, about 30 minutes prior to the induction of hypnosis can sometimes be of assistance; but these are long-acting drugs and sufficient time must be allowed after their use for the subject to sleep off their effects. It has recently been reported, however, that the administration of Tabs Valium, 2 mg or 5 mg three times on the day preceding treatment, followed by one 5 mg tablet half an hour before attending the dental surgery, seems to facilitate the induction of hypnosis in the agitated and apprehensive dental patient.

CHAPTER 8

Deepening the Trance State

The precise depth of trance which any individual subject attains after three or four successive inductions, and after all methods of deepening have been attempted, is likely to remain fairly constant. Once having reached this depth, the subject does not tend to vary or fluctuate much unless he becomes emotionally disturbed. Consequently, if after several sessions the subject has only succeeded in entering a light trance state, it is most unlikely that further training in hypnosis will convert him into a deep-trance subject. There are, of course, exceptions to this rule, but for ordinary medical and dental purposes it may be taken to be generally applicable.

After the first successful induction, when the subject's eyes have closed and he has entered a light hypnotic state, the next object is to gradually deepen the trance as much as possible. There are many ways of achieving this, but I propose to confine myself only to descriptions of those that are likely to prove most useful in routine clinical practice.

Methods of Deepening the Trance

1. By direct suggestion.
2. By relation of depth to performance.
3. By counting and breathing techniques.
4. By the induction of graded responses.
5. By 'visualization' techniques (*see* Chapter 9).
6. By Vogt's 'fractionation' method (*see* Chapter 9).
7. By the 'dissociation' method (*see* Chapter 9).

Of these methods, only the first five will normally need to be employed as routine procedures. Vogt's method can occasionally prove extremely useful in refractory cases, but the dissociation method is not altogether devoid of risk and is probably best left to the psychiatrist. The first two methods particularly have already been incorporated in most of the typical trance inductions that have been described.

1. Deepening by Direct Suggestion

During the course of trance induction it is continually suggested to the subject, over and over again, that he is falling into a deeper and deeper sleep. Indeed, the repetition at intervals of the words 'Deeper and deeper asleep' and 'Very, very deeply asleep' have a strong influence in eliciting the desired response. Post-hypnotic suggestion, with which the subject will comply after being awakened, can also be made to play an important part.

> Next time . . . you will not only fall asleep more quickly . . . but you will also fall into a deeper, deeper sleep . . . much deeper than this one.

It is always wise to give this particular suggestion at the end of each session, before awakening the subject.

2. Deepening by the Relation of Depth to Performance

The subject is repeatedly told to relate the performance of something that is actually happening to him during the hypnotic state to further deepening of the trance. Similarly, any feeling that he is experiencing can be similarly related to an increase in depth.

> As your arm falls limply back on to your lap . . . you are falling into a deeper, deeper sleep.
> As your hand floats upwards into the air . . . your sleep is becoming deeper and deeper.
> As you feel more and more relaxed . . . so you are falling into a deeper, deeper sleep.

I have already pointed out the importance of coupling in this way the suggestion of something that you want to happen with something that is actually happening at the time.

3. Deepening by the Use of Counting and Breathing Techniques

The efficiency of these particular methods of deepening can be greatly heightened if you first explain to the subject the reason why his depth is going to increase.

> Although none of us normally realize it, each time we breathe out in everyday life, we tend to relax. Perhaps you would like to try this for yourself. Take a deep breath . . . fill your chest . . . and hold it until I tell you to 'Let go'.
> Now I want you to notice the tension in your chest-muscles . . . the tension in

your shoulders and upper arms.   And I want you to pay particular
attention to how . . . the moment I say ' *Let go* ' . . . all that tension disappears
immediately . . . and you tend to sag limply down into the chair.
Now . . . ' *Let go* '.

The subject invariably finds this simple demonstration most convincing
and it greatly facilitates the procedures you are intending to employ.

There are a number of variations in the use of counting and breathing
techniques and although a simple count alone is often considered to be
sufficient, as a routine procedure I prefer a combination of the two, in
which the subject is told that, as the hypnotist counts slowly from one
to five, he will take five very deep breaths, and that each time he breathes
out—slowly and deliberately—he will feel himself becoming more and
more deeply relaxed and falling into a deeper, deeper sleep.

I am going to count slowly up to *five* . . . and as I do so . . . you will take
five very deep breaths.
And with each deep breath that you take . . . each time you breathe out . . .
you will become more and more relaxed . . . and your sleep will become
deeper and deeper.
One . . . Deep, deep breath . . . more and more deeply relaxed . . . deeper
and deeper asleep.
Two . . . Very deep breath . . . deeper and deeper relaxed . . . sleep becoming
deeper and deeper.
Three . . . Deeper and deeper breath . . . more and more deeply relaxed . . .
more and more deeply asleep.
Four . . . Very, very deep breath . . . deeper and deeper relaxed . . . sleep
becoming even deeper and deeper.
Five . . . Very, very deep breath indeed . . . very, very deeply relaxed . . .
very, very deeply asleep.

Not only is this an efficient method of deepening the trance, but the
extent to which the subject's respiratory efforts are increased affords a
useful guide to the extent to which he is responding to suggestion.
This procedure can often be followed most effectively by a modification
of the suggestions given to the subject in the first place, as follows:

Once again . . . I want you to take one very deep breath . . . fill your chest . . .
and hold it until I say . . . ' *Let go* '.
Then . . . let your breath out *as quickly as possible* . . . and as you do so . . .
you will feel yourself sagging limply back into the chair . . . and you will
become twice as deeply relaxed as you are now . . . twice as deeply asleep.
Now, take that very deep breath . . . fill your chest . . . *Hold it* . . . (15

seconds pause) . . . *Hold it* . . . (15 seconds pause) . . . *Hold it* . . . (20 to 30 seconds pause) *Let go.*

Hardly ever does this fail to achieve a significant deepening of the trance, and in many cases you will observe the subject slumping down into the chair and his head sagging either sideways or forwards, indicating a considerable increase in relaxation and consequent deepening of the trance. The subject who has been instructed in auto-hypnosis (pages 181-182) can easily be taught to deepen his self-induced trance by employing the same technique, only in this case he is instructed to take the same deep breath but *to hold it as long as he can, then to let it out as quickly as possible.*

4. Deepening by the Induction of Graded Responses

This method involves deepening the hypnosis by the application of a series of graduated tests, each being a little more difficult than the last. A successful response to each of these in turn will progressively increase the subject's suggestibility and pave the way for the next.

There are seven main responses that can be suggested consecutively, each of which is rather more complicated and difficult to elicit than the preceding one, and the subject who responds successively to each of these has certainly achieved a medium trance state, and often a deep or even somnambulistic trance. In my experience, it has proved to be one of the most valuable and satisfactory methods of progressively deepening the trance. Of these seven tests, however, I rarely employ the two which involve a direct challenge, which always tends to re-awaken conscious activity.

1. The induction of limb heaviness.
2. The induction of limb catalepsy.
3. The induction of lid catalepsy.
4. The induction of limb rigidity.
5. The inhibition of voluntary movements.
6. The induction of automatic movements.
7. Dream induction.

1. *The Induction of Limb Heaviness*

The subject's arm is placed upon the arm of the chair and is stroked gently from the shoulder to the wrist. He is told that it is gradually feeling heavier and heavier, and that presently, when it is picked up by the wrist and then released, it will drop limply back on to his lap just like a lead weight.

I am now going to place your arm on the arm of the chair.
And I am going to stroke it gently . . . from the shoulder to the wrist.
And as I stroke it . . . you will begin to feel a feeling of heaviness in your arm.
That feeling of heaviness is increasing . . . with every stroke of my hand.
Your arm is beginning to feel heavier . . . and heavier . . . just as heavy as lead.
You can feel it pressing down more firmly on the arm of the chair.

(As you say this, you should imperceptibly increase the pressure of your own hand, as you stroke his arm.)

And in a few moments . . . your arm will feel so very, very heavy . . . *that when I pick it up by the wrist . . . and let it go . . . it will drop limply back on to your lap . . . just like a lead weight.*
And as it drops limply back . . . on to your lap . . . you will fall into a deeper, deeper sleep.

The subject's arm is then lifted up by the wrist and released—it will drop back heavily on to his knees. His arm should then be replaced on the arm of the chair and restored to normality by gently stroking it in the opposite direction.

You have now fallen into a much deeper sleep.
And as I stroke your arm in the opposite direction . . . you will notice that all feelings of heaviness are now leaving your arm.
It is coming back to normal . . . and feels just the same as your other arm.
And as it does so . . . your sleep is becoming even deeper, and deeper.

This restoration to normality is an important step which must never, under any circumstances, be forgotten.

2. *The Induction of Limb Catalepsy*

The subject's arm is raised above his head and he is told that all sensations of heaviness are leaving it and that it is becoming lighter and lighter as if there were no weight in it at all. He is told that when his arm is released it will no longer want to drop on his lap, but will remain just where it is without him having to make the slightest effort to keep it there.

Your arm no longer feels heavy.
In fact . . . it is beginning to feel lighter and lighter.
Just as light as a feather . . . as if there is no weight in it at all.
And when I release your wrist . . . your arm will no longer want to drop

down . . . on to your lap.
It will want to remain just where it is . . . exactly where I leave it.
It will no longer want to fall . . . it will remain just where it is . . . without your having to make the slightest effort to keep it there.

When the subject's wrist is released, his arm will remain poised in the air. This catalepsy can be checked by picking up his other arm which, without any further suggestion, will probably remain in any position in which it is placed. Even should it tend to fall, one or two slight jerks in an upward direction will usually prove quite sufficient to anchor it. This, of course, is an example of non-verbal suggestion.

Both arms are then replaced on the arms of the chair and restored to normal.

Your arms are both becoming quite normal again.
That feeling of lightness and weightlessness has disappeared completely . . . and your arms are now quite normal.
And you have fallen into a much, much deeper sleep.

Instead of checking the catalepsy by using the other arm, still further deepening may be secured by suggesting that the raised arm is gradually becoming heavier and heavier, and that as it slowly sinks back on to the arm of the chair the subject is falling into a deeper, deeper sleep.

Your arm is now becoming heavier and heavier.
And as it becomes heavier . . . and heavier . . . it is gradually sinking down on to the arm of the chair.
And, the moment your arm touches the arm of the chair . . . you will fall into a deeper, deeper sleep.

These suggestions are continued until the arm is seen to sink on to the arm of the chair. Normality is then restored in the manner just described.

3. *The Induction of Lid Catalepsy*
Whilst the success of this response will usually facilitate further deepening procedures, failure, which is quite likely to occur, will undoubtedly make these much more difficult. Lid catalepsy is most unpredictable. In good subjects, it can be one of the earliest and most convincing signs of hypnosis to be elicited, and can often be successfully induced immediately after eye closure. The subject naturally accepts this as proof that something has actually occurred, his susceptibility consequently increases and he will much more readily accept suggestions of further deepening of his hypnosis. It should be pointed out, however,

that in subjects of this calibre, the phenomenon is rarely likely to be essential to the successful induction of greater depth. In other cases it will be found impossible to secure this response until the subject has already entered a deep trance, and failure to do so at an earlier stage will inevitably diminish the subject's suggestibility and render further deepening difficult, if not impossible. This is a grave disadvantage which, in my opinion, renders it quite unsuitable as a routine procedure since the direct challenge that is involved invariably re-awakens some degree of conscious activity. I use it only when I am satisfied that further depth will only be obtained after I have convinced the subject of the genuineness of his hypnosis by establishing my authority. This, of course, can only be done by successfully challenging his ability to perform a certain action in defiance of my command.

The subject is told that his eyes are so tightly closed that the eyelids feel that they are glued together . . . that it will be impossible for him to open them . . . no matter how hard he tries, until he is told to do so . . . and that the harder he tries to open them—the tighter they will close. Notice how this last statement turns the efforts of the subject to resist the suggestion against himself, and helps to defeat any attempts that he may make. It is also useful, as this command is given, to press one hand firmly upon the subject's forehead. This seems to greatly increase its force.

> Your eyes are now so tightly closed . . . that the eyelids feel as though they are firmly glued together.
> So tightly closed . . . so firmly glued together . . . that it will be impossible for you to open them, until I tell you to do so.
> *The harder you try to open them . . . the tighter they will close!*

(Now, press your hand firmly upon the subject's forehead.)

> *It is impossible for you to open your eyes!*
> *You cannot possibly open them!*
> *The harder you try . . . the harder they will close!*
> Now try to open your eyes.
> You see! You *cannot* possibly open them!

Should the subject show signs of being able to open his eyes, say to him quickly, ' Open them, now! You notice how difficult it was. Next time, it will be even more difficult.' Always try to get him to admit that he did feel some difficulty. The effectiveness of this procedure may often be increased if you begin by pressing one finger-tip gently on the top of his head. Then say to him:

I want you to imagine that you have a sore spot . . . just where my finger is resting on your head.

With your eyes still closed . . . I want you to roll them upwards behind the closed lids . . . and look firmly, upwards and backwards at that sore spot. Don't let your eyes wander from it for a moment . . . and you will find that your eyes are now so tightly closed . . . etc.

If you try this for yourself in the waking state, you will find how difficult it is for you to open your eyes as long as you keep looking upward and backward. That is because the eye-muscles are being held in such a position that it is practically impossible for them to lift the lids. The subject, of course, attributes his inability solely to the effect of hypnotic suggestion.

As an alternative and more 'permissive' method of securing lid catalepsy, you can instruct the subject to *pretend* that his eye-lids are so tightly closed that as long as he continues to pretend, he will allow them to become so completely relaxed that he will find it quite impossible to open them.

I want you to pretend that your eyes are so tightly closed that you cannot possibly open them.

And as long as you continue to pretend . . . you will keep relaxing your eye-muscles more and more . . . deeper and deeper.

Let all those muscles around your eyes relax more . . . and more . . . and more . . . until they are so completely relaxed that as long as you keep on pretending that you cannot open them . . . *it will be impossible for you to do so.* When you try . . . you'll find that they just won't respond.

They just *won't* open.

If you do manage to open them . . . it will simply mean that you have stopped pretending . . . and have not allowed those muscles of your eyes to relax completely. What I want you to do . . . is to get them so relaxed that they just won't open. After all . . . a relaxed muscle cannot contract . . . so, as long as you keep on pretending . . . and really have those eye-muscles relaxed . . . they just can't open. So, go on pretending . . . and relax them more and more.

And the moment you're sure that you have them so relaxed that they won't open . . . I want you to test them for yourself.

You see . . . you can wrinkle your forehead . . . you can lift your eye-brows . . . *but you just cannot open your eyes.*

More often than not, these suggestions will act in the waking state, so one need hardly be surprised that they are frequently effective under hypnosis and facilitate deepening of the trance.

4. *The Induction of Limb Rigidity*

The subject's arm is extended horizontally at shoulder level, and he is told to hold it out, stiff and rigid, with the palm facing the ceiling. His arm is then stroked gently from the shoulder to the wrist, and he is told that it is becoming stiffer and straighter and more and more rigid, that it is feeling just as stiff and rigid as a steel poker, so that it cannot possibly be bent at the elbow, until the count of three.

As I stroke your arm . . . you will feel that it is becoming much stiffer and straighter.
The stiffness is increasing . . . with every stroke of my hand.
You can feel all the muscles tightening up . . . pulling your arm out . . . stiffer and straighter . . . with every stroke of my hand . . . until it is beginning to feel just as stiff and rigid as a steel poker . . . from the shoulder to the wrist.

Now, I want you to concentrate on a steel poker.
Picture a steel poker in your mind.
And as you do so . . . you will feel that your arm has become just as stiff and rigid as that steel poker.
As if the elbow joint is firmly locked.
As if there is no elbow joint there at all.
So that it will be impossible for me to bend your arm at the elbow . . . until I count up to ' three '.
The harder I try to bend it . . . the stiffer, and more rigid it will become.
But, the moment I count ' three ' . . . all the stiffness will pass away immediately . . . your arm will bend quite easily . . . and, as it does so . . . you will fall immediately into a deeper, deeper sleep.
Stiff and straight . . . just like that steel poker !

At this point, you will usually find that the arm is so stiff and rigid that you will be quite unable to bend it, even if you apply considerable force. Having tested it, count up to three, and you will notice that the stiffness passes off quite suddenly, sometimes with a distinct jerk. You can do a great deal to ensure the success of this response by seeing that the arm is being held absolutely stiff and rigid in the first place, before you begin to stroke it and suggest increased stiffness and rigidity. It is also important to see that the palm of the hand faces upwards towards the ceiling. Some authorities, Weitzenhoffer for example, always use a direct challenge to the subject after inducing arm rigidity, on the grounds that if the trance is not deep enough to make this suggestion effective it would be better to start all over again, preferably using a different method. I have not found the necessity for this. Possibly the precise wording of the suggestion—'It will be impossible for *me* to bend it'—acts as a disguised challenge, for subsequent testing certainly convinces the subject that it cannot be bent, and further deepening techniques are usually successful, sometimes to the extent of producing somnambulism. Avoiding a direct challenge in this way not only diminishes the risk of failure, but also prevents unnecessary re-activation of the subject's conscious mind.

5. *The Inhibition of Voluntary Movements*

As in the case of lid catalepsy, the success of this response in deepening hypnosis is dependent upon a direct challenge to the subject. For the reasons already stated, I feel that it is as well to avoid its use as a routine deepening procedure, and to reserve it for special circumstances only.

As the state of hypnosis becomes deeper, the subject becomes more and more susceptible to suggestions that he will lose control over various groups of voluntary muscles. Small isolated groups will tend to be affected at first, but eventually the whole body may become involved.

Many different tests have been devised of which the hand-clasp test (p. 40) is probably the most useful and convenient.

> I want you to hold your arms straight out in front of you.
> Hold them as stiff and rigid as you can, and clasp your hands together.
> Interlock your fingers, and keep them tightly locked together.
> Tighter and tighter.

(At this point, it is helpful to press the subject's clasped hands firmly together.)

> As you clasp your hands tighter and tighter together . . . you will feel your fingers gripping more and more firmly.
> And as they do so . . . I want you to picture a heavy metal vice.
> Imagine you can see the jaws of that vice . . . being screwed tighter and tighter together.
> Now, picture that vice clearly in your mind . . . and concentrate on it.
> And as you do so . . . just imagine that your hands represent the jaws of that vice . . . that they are slowly becoming screwed up . . . tighter and tighter together.
> As I count up to *five* . . . your hands are becoming locked together . . . tighter and tighter . . . and when I reach the count of *five* . . . they will be so tightly locked . . . that they will feel just like a solid block of metal . . . and it will be quite impossible for you to separate them.
> One . . . tightly locked . . . two . . . tighter and tighter . . . three . . . very, very tight . . . four . . . the palms of your hands are locked tightly together . . .

five . . . they are so tightly locked that it will be impossible for you to separate them until I count up to 'three' . . . the harder you try to separate the palms of your hands . . . the tighter your fingers will press upon the back of your hands . . . and the tighter your hands will become locked together.

Various other suggestions can be made. The subject may be given something to hold in his hand and told that he will be unable to drop it. He may be told that he will be unable to pronounce certain words, or that his body muscles have become so limp and relaxed that he will find it impossible to get up out of his chair. Tests of this kind have been extremely popular with stage hypnotists.

6. *The Induction of Automatic Movements*

The production of automatic movements always signifies a rather deeper stage of hypnosis. The subject's arm is placed upon the arm of the chair. It is then grasped by the wrist, and the fore-arm raised into a vertical position, the elbow remaining supported by the arm of the chair. The hand and fore-arm are then slowly moved, backwards and forwards.

As I move your arm slowly . . . backwards and forwards . . . backwards and forwards . . . I want you to imagine that the centre of a piece of cord is tied around your wrist . . . and that someone at each end of the cord is pulling your arm . . . first backwards . . . then forwards.
Now, picture that piece of cord, tied round your wrist . . . pulling your arm slowly . . . backwards . . . and forwards.
And as you do so . . . you will find that, in a few moments, when I release your wrist . . . it will feel as if that piece of cord is still tied to your wrist . . . still pulling your arm . . . backwards and forwards.
And your arm will go on moving . . . entirely on its own . . . backwards and forwards . . . backwards and forwards . . . until I tell you to stop.
You won't try to make it move!
You won't try to stop it moving!
You will just let it please itself . . . and it will go on moving on its own . . . quite automatically . . . backwards and forwards . . . backwards and forwards . . . until I tell you to stop.
Backwards and forwards . . . backwards and forwards . . . backwards and forwards.

(At this point, the subject's wrist is released, and his arm continues to move automatically, backwards and forwards until he is told to stop.)

Now, stop!
Put your arm back . . . on to your lap . . . and as you do so . . . you are

falling into an even deeper, deeper sleep.
Sleep . . . very, very deeply!

As the subject's arm moves backwards and forwards, I find it useful to tell him that his sleep is becoming ' deeper, deeper, deeper '—timing this so that the word deeper is repeated on each alternate forward movement of his arm.

Another method of eliciting this phenomenon is to grasp the subject's wrists and bend his elbows, bringing his fore-arms and hands horizontally in front of his body. Then rotate his hands and wrists around each other in a circular movement, and tell him that when you release his wrists, his hands will continue to revolve around each other . . . quite automatically . . . faster and faster . . . until you tell him to stop. And that as they do so . . . his sleep is becoming deeper . . . deeper . . . deeper. This is a most useful technique whenever conditions are such that you have to undertake trance induction with the subject sitting in an upright chair, without any arms upon which to rest his elbows.

7. Dream Induction

In this particular technique, the subject is told that presently he is going to dream, and that he will dream that he is performing whatever action he is instructed to dream about. The particular action that is suggested should always be made as simple and natural as possible. For instance a woman can be told that she will be able to picture herself tidying her hair, or removing an ear-ring. A man can be told that he is straightening his tie, brushing his hair or doing up or undoing a button on his coat or jacket.

When these instructions have been given and the suggestion made to the subject that he will dream, he is told to *show* the hypnotist exactly what he is dreaming about. If a successful response is obtained, the subject's hands will move slowly upwards and he will actually carry out the suggested action.

You are now so deeply asleep . . . that everything that I tell you that is going to happen . . . *will* happen . . . *exactly* as I tell you.
And every feeling I tell you that you will experience . . . you will experience . . . *exactly* as I tell you.
Moreover, every single instruction that I give you . . . you will carry out faithfully.
Just as your arm felt heavy . . . when I told you it would feel heavy.
Just as your arm felt stiff . . . when I told you it would feel stiff.

Just as your arm moved on its own . . . when I told you it would move on its own.

So . . . everything else I tell you that is going to happen . . . *will* happen . . . *exactly* as I tell you.

Every feeling I tell you that you will experience . . . you *will* experience . . . *exactly* as I tell you.

And every single instruction that I give you . . . you will obey faithfully.

You are now so deeply asleep . . . that, in a few moments . . . when I tell you to dream . . . *you will dream !*

And you will dream that you are performing whatever simple action I tell you to dream about.

You will be able to picture yourself . . . quite clearly . . . and see yourself . . . quite vividly . . . in your own mind . . . carrying out whatever action I have told you to dream about.

Just as you pictured that steel poker . . . in your mind . . . when your arm went stiff.

Just as you pictured that piece of cord, tied round your wrist . . . when your arm moved on its own.

So . . . you will be able to picture yourself in your dream . . . equally vividly and clearly . . . performing whatever simple action that I tell you to dream about.

Now . . . you are going to dream . . . that you are straightening your tie.

You are going to dream . . . that you are straightening your tie.

Now dream ! Dream ! Dream !

(Pause)

Now . . . show me what you are dreaming !
Show me, now !
Show me what you are dreaming !

When this test succeeds the subject's hands will be seen to move slowly upwards and he will actually carry out the suggested action. Sometimes there is a delay, and if so, just watch his hands carefully. The slightest movement of them betrays an impulse to comply with the suggestion, in which case the repetition, once or twice in a more authoritative tone, of the instruction to show what he is dreaming, will usually secure the desired response. If he still fails to comply, he should be asked whether he is dreaming, and if not, why he thinks he is unable to dream.

I can remember a female subject who had responded extremely well to all the previous deepening routines, yet dream induction seemed to fail completely. I had told her to dream that she was in the bathroom at home, washing her hands. When she failed to respond, I asked her whether she was dreaming, and she said no. I then asked her why she wasn't dreaming, and was somewhat taken aback by her reply that she hadn't got a bathroom at home. A subsequent suggestion that she would dream that she was knitting elicited an immediate response, and she knitted away furiously. Obviously, one has to be careful not to unwittingly impose impossible conditions.

In my experience, the main value of this particular deepening technique lies in the fact that, whenever it succeeds, the subject will never fail to accept the post-hypnotic suggestion that, in future, he will always enter the hypnotic state immediately upon word of command. This is known as post-hypnotic conditioning.

5. Deepening by the Use of ' Visualization ' Techniques

These can prove extremely effective, but before you use them it is always wise to test your subject's capacity for visual imagery. People vary in this respect, and if they do not possess this ability it is a waste of time attempting such procedures. Testing can be done quite quickly and easily in the following manner:

> I am going to test your powers of imagination, so whilst you are lying comfortably relaxed in the chair, I want you to imagine that you can see a pair of shoes. Just visualize them . . . and try to picture them quite clearly in your mind's eye.
>
> Tell me . . . what colour are those shoes ?
> What are they made of ?
> What kind of heels have they ?
> Do they fasten up at all . . . and if so . . . how ?

Notice that you do not ask the subject whether he can visualize the shoes. You ask him ' *What colour are they?* ' so that if he responds, there is no doubt that he is picturing them. Otherwise, he would be unable to answer this question. If he has little or no difficulty in describing these shoes, you can feel confident that he possesses a sufficient capacity for visual imagery for you to proceed with one or other of the visualization techniques.

1. The ' *Descending Lift or Elevator* ' Method of *Trance-deepening*

In all visualization methods it is not generally realized that the effectiveness is greatly increased if the therapist suggests that he, himself, is accompanying the subject as he descends.

> I want you to imagine that we are standing together on the fifth floor of a large department store . . . and that we are just stepping into the lift . . . to descend to street level.

And, as we go down . . . and as the lift gates open and close as we arrive at each floor . . . you will become more and more deeply relaxed . . . and your sleep will become deeper and deeper.

The gates are closing now . . . and we are beginning to sink slowly downwards.

The lift stops at the fourth floor . . . several people get out . . . two more get in . . . the gates close again . . . and already you are becoming more and more deeply relaxed . . . more and more deeply asleep.

And as we sink to the third floor . . . and stop, whilst the gates open and close again . . . you are relaxing more and more . . . and your sleep becoming deeper and deeper.

We slowly sink down to the second floor . . . one or two people get out and several get in . . . and as they do so . . . you are feeling much more deeply relaxed . . . much more deeply asleep.

Down once again to the first floor . . . the gates open and close . . . but nobody gets out or in. Already you have become still more deeply relaxed . . . and your sleep still deeper and deeper. Deeper and deeper asleep . . . deeper and deeper asleep.

Down further and further . . . until the lift stops at last at street-level. The gates open . . . and everybody gets out.

But we do not get out.

We decide to go still deeper . . . and descend to the basement.

The lift gates close again . . . and down we go . . . down and down . . . deeper and deeper . . . and as we arrive at the basement . . . you are feeling twice as deeply and comfortably relaxed . . . twice as deeply asleep.

The total unexpectedness of this last stage—the journey down to the basement—takes the subject completely by surprise, and usually succeeds in producing even greater depth.

Instead of employing the visualization of a lift or elevator, the subject may be told to picture himself descending upon an escalator in a similar manner. As a preliminary, however, it is prudent to find out whether or not the subject has undergone such an actual experience in the past.

2. *The ' Descending Stair-case' Method of Trance-deepening*

Many different versions of this exist, but the one I am going to describe, I have found to be most effective since it is combined with a counting and breathing technique.

I want you to picture us standing together on a terrace, overlooking a beautiful garden. There are five wide steps leading down to a smaller terrace . . . and then another five, down to the garden itself.

We are going down those steps into the garden . . . and I will count each step as we go down.

As we go down each step . . . you will take one very deep breath . . . and as you breathe out . . . you will become more and more deeply relaxed . . . more and more deeply asleep.

Now, just picture us standing at the top of the first flight of steps . . . and as soon as you have done so . . . please lift up one hand.

One . . . Down the first step . . . deep, deep breath . . . deeply relaxed . . . deeper and deeper asleep.

Two . . . Down the second step . . . deep, deep breath . . . very deeply relaxed . . . sleep becoming deeper and deeper.

Three . . . Down the third step . . . deep, deep breath . . . more and more deeply relaxed . . . more and more deeply asleep.

Four . . . Down the fourth step . . . deep, deep breath . . . very, very deeply relaxed . . . sleep becoming still deeper and deeper.

Five . . . Down the fifth step, and on to the small terrace . . . deep, deep breath . . . very, very deeply relaxed . . . very, very deeply asleep indeed.

And as we pause on the terrace . . . you will notice a stone pedestal supporting a bowl of flowers. You will probably like to stop and look at them . . . or even smell them.

Tell me . . . what colour are those flowers ?

(The subject says ' Red.')

What kind of flowers are they ?

(The subject says ' Gladioli.')

Describe anything else you can see on the terrace.

That's fine. Now we'll go down the second flight of steps into the garden.

One . . . Down the first step . . . deep, deep, breath . . . deeply relaxed . . . deeper and deeper asleep.

Two . . . Down the second step . . . deep, deep breath . . . very deeply relaxed . . . sleep becoming deeper and deeper.

Three . . . Down the third step . . . deep, deep breath . . . more and more deeply relaxed . . . more and more deeply asleep.

Four . . . Down the fourth step . . . deep, deep breath . . . very, very deeply relaxed . . . sleep becoming still deeper and deeper.

Five . . . Down the last step and into the garden . . . deep, deep breath . . . very, very deeply relaxed . . . very, very deeply asleep indeed.

It is surprising how many subjects are able to hallucinate as they proceed down the steps, and this certainly adds materially to the depth of trance achieved. If your subject has responded well, provided that you first take the precaution of finding out whether he likes dogs or cats, you might even proceed as follows:

As we step into the garden . . . you will notice a dog lying at the foot of the steps. It is wagging its tail . . . looking up at you . . . hoping that you'll pat it. Just pat it . . . if you feel you'd like to.

I want you to really enjoy this wonderful feeling of relaxation and comfort in your whole body . . . it feels so comfortable that you are not paying any attention to it at all. In fact, your body is sleeping . . . more and more deeply . . . whilst your mind remains wide-awake and alert.

Sleep deeply . . . sleep soundly . . . sleep continuously.

Deep . . . deep . . . profound sleep.

CHAPTER 9

Other Methods of Trance Deepening

No account of trance-deepening procedures would be complete without reference to Vogt's fractionation method and the dissociation method, both of which can prove extremely useful under certain circumstances.

6. Deepening by Vogt's Fractionation Method

This method is reputed to be one of the most effective methods of inducing very deep trance states, and it is claimed that it will often succeed when every other method has failed. It is certainly an excellent way of handling difficult subjects who, having entered a light hypnotic state, upon awakening express grave doubts as to whether they have actually been hypnotized at all.

The essential feature of this method is the repeated hypnotizing and awakening of the subject in rapid succession, several times in the course of each of the first few sessions. The theory is that each hypnotization renders the subject more suggestible, and thus favours the induction of a deeper state at each successive attempt. I have found that one of the most effective ways of using it is that described by Weitzenhoffer, which forms the basis of the routine that I generally employ:

I am now going to waken you up by counting up to *seven*.
After I have done so . . . although your eyes will be open . . . whilst I am talking to you . . . you will begin to feel very, very drowsy and sleepy again. You will find it harder and harder to keep your eyes open . . . and to stay awake.
Your eyes will feel very, very heavy . . . the eyelids will feel heavier and heavier . . . and will begin to blink.
You will not be able to stop them blinking.
And as they blink . . . you will find it more and more difficult to keep them open.
They will want to close . . . you will not be able to stop them from closing.
Every moment . . . as I go on talking . . . you will feel drowsier and drowsier . . . sleepier and sleepier.

> Your eyes will close . . . and you will fall into a deep, deep sleep.
> You will be in a much deeper sleep than you are now!
> I am going to count slowly up to *seven*.
> As I do so . . . you will open your eyes and wake up.
> But you will feel very, very drowsy . . . very, very sleepy.
> Your eyes will feel so heavy . . . so very, very tired . . . that you will not be able to keep them open for long.
> They will start to blink . . . you will be unable to stop them from blinking.
> And as they do so . . . your eyes will feel so very, very tired that they will close . . . and you will fall into a much, much deeper sleep!

After being awakened, the subject's eyes will either start to blink, or he may seem to remain sleepy with his eyes half-closed. He should be asked what is the matter with his eyes, and may even say that he feels sleepy. Sometimes, however, he will seem to be puzzled and say that he doesn't know, or that the light is troubling his eyes. A simple comment at this point, to the effect that he is feeling sleepy and that it is difficult for him to keep his eyes open, will often suffice to start him blinking or even closing his eyes. This must be followed up immediately:

> You see! Your eyes *are* feeling heavier and heavier!
> You *are* feeling very, very drowsy . . . and sleepy.
> Your eyes are closing . . . and you are falling into a deeper, deeper sleep.
> *Go to sleep!*

Sometimes, this will be unnecessary since the eyes will not only start to blink but will also close entirely on their own. In this case, the above suggestions should be modified accordingly.

> You see! Your eyes *have* closed on their own.
> Sleep very, very deeply . . . very, very deeply.
> Deeper and deeper asleep . . . deeper and deeper asleep!

Alternatively, just as his eyes seem about to close, you can say to him authoritatively:

> *Sleep!*
> *Sleep . . . very, very deeply . . . very, very deeply!*
> *Deeper and deeper asleep . . . deeper and deeper asleep!*
> *Go to sleep . . . very, very deeply!*

Although the trance may now be further deepened by any of the usual procedures, this is not often done since the method in itself is designed to effect further deepening. Nevertheless, I find it useful to deepen it further by using the counting and breathing technique before awakening the subject and repeating the procedure.   This I do on several occasions during each of the first few sessions.

Subsequent procedures.   Before being awakened, the subject can be told that whenever you either suggest sleep or even mention the word sleep, his eyes will close and he will fall into a deep sleep from which he will not awaken until told to do so.

Tell him that when you count up to seven, he will open his eyes and wake up.   But as soon as you begin to talk to him, no matter what you are saying, his eyelids will begin to feel heavier and heavier . . . he will feel drowsier and sleepier . . . and that the moment he hears you mention the word sleep, or anything to do with sleep, he will be quite unable to resist the urge to close his eyes and fall into a deep, deep sleep.

When successful, and the trance has been deepened by a few more suggestions, Weitzenhoffer advises the use of the lid catalepsy and the limb rigidity techniques, but avoiding the use of challenges in the following manner:

> Your eyes are now so tightly closed . . . that they feel as if the eyelids are firmly glued together.
> So tightly glued together . . . that it will be impossible for you to open your eyes.
> Even if you tried . . . you would find it quite impossible to open them.
> *But you will have no wish to try !*
> You are just relaxing . . . more and more completely . . . and sinking into a deeper, deeper sleep.

Alternatively, after you have stiffened the subject's arm, and made it rigid, you can say:

> You cannot bend your arm, now!
> It is so stiff and rigid . . . it is quite impossible for you to bend it.
> Even if you tried . . . you would find it impossible to bend it.
> *But you will have no wish to try !*
> The moment I count *three* . . . your arm muscles will relax . . . the stiffness will pass off again . . . and your arm will bend quite easily.
> And as it does so . . . you will fall into a deeper, deeper sleep.

This technique is continued until the subject goes to sleep both quickly and easily.   The time it takes to achieve this will vary with the type of subject with whom you are dealing, and how long you are prepared to spend with him at each session.   But once he has reached this stage, you can proceed as follows:

From now on . . . whenever you hear me say ' *Go to sleep* ' . . . your eyes will close immediately . . . and you will fall into a sleep . . . just as deep as this one.

You should repeat this instruction twice, firmly, and with conviction. Then awaken the subject, and in a few seconds' time, in an authoritative tone of voice tell him to go to sleep:

Go to sleep ! Sleep deeply ! Very, very deeply !

If his eyes fail to close immediately, these suggestions should be repeated with even greater emphasis. Should they still remain open, you should extend your first and second fingers and bring them slowly towards his eyes, thus causing them to close instinctively. As they do so, repeat the above suggestions even more emphatically. This procedure should be rehearsed over and over again until the subject's eyes close immediately, whenever he is instructed to go to sleep.

Some hypnotists prefer to employ a shortened version of this technique. They simply tell the subject that each time he falls asleep, his sleep will become deeper and deeper. They then proceed to hypnotize him and awaken him several times in rapid succession, until he enters the hypnotic state as soon as the induction is started.

The Feed-back technique. This is a variation of Vogt's method which can sometimes be extremely effective. It often succeeds with subjects who experience difficulty in achieving depth. The subject is asked to describe the exact sensations that he felt as he went into the light hypnotic state. Such sensations will be found to vary greatly in different subjects. The hypnotist takes careful note of each successive sensation, and the exact order in which they were actually experienced. During the next induction, suggestions are then made that the subject is going to feel each sensation that he did on the previous occasion, in the exact order in which they originally occurred.

This feed-back technique has certain definite advantages. It avoids the suggestion of experiences that the subject may never have felt, or those to which he may have either an unconscious or even conscious resistance. Since the events suggested to him are those which have actually happened already, they are much more likely to happen again.

7. Deepening by the Dissociation Method
This depends upon the production of a fantasy in the subject's mind that he is actually watching someone else being induced into a deep

hypnotic sleep. Since he begins by thus ' dissociating ' himself from what is taking place, his own resistances are not aroused. The description of what is occurring, however, gradually induces him to identify himself with the supposed subject, and he begins to feel that the phenomena are actually happening to himself. He is able to allow this to happen because his resistances never become activated.

> I want you to imagine that you are standing outside a consulting-room door.
> You are beginning to feel quite strange . . . and as you grasp the handle of the door . . . and slowly open it . . . this feeling of strangeness is increasing.
> As you walk into the room . . . you feel as though you are a complete stranger.
> There is a doctor in the room, who is dealing with a patient.
> The doctor is wearing . . .

(Here you describe roughly what you, yourself, are wearing.)

> The patient is wearing . . .

(Here you describe what your subject is actually wearing.)

> Now, watch the doctor . . . and notice what is happening to the patient with him.
> He is talking to the patient . . . and as he does so . . . something very curious is happening.
> See how the patient's right hand and arm are starting to float up into the air.
> His right hand is floating up . . . and up . . . and up.
> Now, his whole arm is floating up . . . and up . . . and up.
> And as it does so . . . you can see that he is falling into a deeper, deeper sleep.

(During this description, your subject's own arm usually starts to rise, as he identifies himself with the patient.)

This is an extremely powerful method of producing a deep trance state, since it depends upon what is called dissociation or temporary splitting of the subject's mind. It could be very dangerous in a person with a schizoid personality, in whom even under normal conditions the mind possesses a strong tendency to split. Such a person might interpret this procedure as giving your full approval to the splitting process, and you might consequently find it difficult if not impossible to achieve re-integration when you awakened him.

The Management of the Trance in Resistant Subjects

Although in the average case when the subject is willing and co-operative the induction of hypnosis is comparatively easy to achieve, you will from time to time encounter cases in which you will experience varying degrees of difficulty. Whenever this occurs, it is most important to try to discover the nature of the difficulty with which you are confronted. For instance, if a subject fails to enter a trance state at all during the first hypnotic session, there is always some reason for this, and until you have discovered and dealt with it adequately, further attempts at induction will probably prove equally unsuccessful. It may be that the technique you have adopted will have to be modified to suit the needs of this particular subject, but even this cannot properly be decided until the nature of the difficulty is known.

The best way of approaching this problem is to question the subject closely as to the precise sensations he experienced during the induction, and any difficulties that he may have felt. It is surprising how much valuable information can often be obtained from this simple measure alone. Even when the subject is unconscious of the real reason for his failure, talking it over with him will often afford you the necessary clue. Sometimes you will find that the method of induction you have tried has not suited his personality, in which case you must study this carefully in order to choose the one most likely to fulfil his requirements. This is not as difficult a task as it might seem, provided that you are well acquainted with various kinds of difficulty that most commonly arise.

1. Over-anxiety and fear of failure.
2. Fear of the hypnotic state itself.
3. Inadequate preparation before induction.
4. Defiance of authority.
5. Fluctuating attention.
6. Need to prove superiority.
7. Physical discomfort.
8. Dislike of the method of induction employed.

1. Over-anxiety and Fear of Failure

This is a very common source of difficulty. Indeed, over-anxiety to succeed with hypnosis is almost bound to interfere with successful induction. It is nearly always present to some extent in the patient who seeks psychological help and advice. Such patients have usually undergone many other kinds of treatment, none of which have succeeded in affording them the relief that they seek. Finally, as a last resort, they turn to hypnosis with the conviction that this alone is capable of solving their problems. They consequently attach so much importance to their need to enter the trance successfully that the mere possibility of failure appals them, and the over-anxiety produced in this way is often quite sufficient in itself to prevent them from achieving even the light trance state.

You will also meet the patient who, because of a strong inferiority complex, regards hypnosis as yet another test of his ability to perform. Since such a person is always convinced of his own inadequacy, failure is almost inevitable.

The only way of dealing with this situation is to give the patient the strongest possible reassurance and encouragement before proceeding with any further attempts at induction.

You should tell him that it is not in the least important that he should succeed at the first attempt. I usually remind him of what happened when he first learned to ride a bicycle. During his first lesson it was impossible for him to go on his own without somebody supporting him by holding the saddle. On the next occasion, he found himself able to keep his balance, unsupported, for a few yards at a time and to proceed in a rather unsteady manner. Then, with each subsequent lesson, his control over his balance improved until he was able to manage on his own, without the need of any support at all. I tell him that he can be taught to enter the hypnotic state in easy stages in exactly the same way, so that there is actually nothing for him to worry about. I also explain that deep hypnosis is neither necessary nor even desirable for most treatment purposes. Such relatively simple measures as these will often enable him to relax sufficiently to respond to future attempts at induction.

2. Fear of the Hypnotic State Itself

It sometimes happens that whilst the subject may be ' consciously ' anxious and willing to be hypnotized, he may also be ' unconsciously ' afraid of succumbing to the trance. When this is so, his ' unconscious ' fear is usually that of ' losing control ', and the mental conflict that consequently arises in his mind is quite sufficient to prevent him from entering the hypnotic state at all.

Now, this fear of losing control is much more common than you might imagine, and can manifest itself in two ways.

1. *If the subject's anxiety on this score is great* he will be quite unable to enter even the lightest hypnotic state.

2. *If he is only moderately worried* he may be able to achieve the light trance, but further deepening will usually prove impossible.

Obviously, the more you can allay his anxiety and his fears, the deeper the trance you will be likely to obtain. This particular difficulty, however, arises much less frequently when the subject's mind has been properly prepared before induction.

Not only should you give the subject the reassurance he requires regarding his fears, but you should also promise him that *nothing will be done without his prior knowledge and consent.* It is also useful to stress the fact *that it will be impossible to obtain any effect that he, himself, is unwilling to produce.*

Another excellent way of overcoming this fear of losing control is to prove to the patient that he can awaken himself from the trance at any moment he chooses. Tell him that once he has entered the trance state and you are giving him suggestions, he is to select any moment he likes, and deliberately awaken himself by counting up to ' seven ' . . . that the moment he reaches the count of ' seven,' his eyes will open and he will be wide-awake again. Once he has put this to the test, you assure him that he will always be able to awaken himself immediately at any moment he feels uneasy, even before his treatment is completed. This simple procedure usually affords him all the reassurance he needs.

3. Inadequate Preparation before Induction

Most of the difficulties encountered in trance induction will be greatly lessened, if not entirely removed, if the subject's mind has been fully prepared before any attempt is made (*see* pp. 20–21). Many of the difficulties that arise in the induction of hypnosis are due to far too little importance being given to the preparatory talk.

Just occasionally, a subject will say to you when he has been awakened:

As you told me—I could hear everything that you said.
At one stage, however, I thought I might have gone to sleep—but something seemed to stop me.

Now this is very important and should not be overlooked, for it shows that he could have gone deeper. He didn't—simply because at the last minute he became afraid of losing control. In such a case, full discussion may not only shed a great deal of light upon his difficulties, but he may even be able to suggest possible ways of overcoming them.

4. Defiance of Authority

Sometimes a subject will admit the fact that, during the induction of hypnosis, he experiences an irresistible impulse to oppose everything that is being suggested. Questioning will often reveal that this is a life-long trait in his character and that even as a schoolboy he strongly resented authority. Curiously enough, ventilation and discussion of these feelings will often succeed in increasing his susceptibility. You should point out to him that hypnosis is essentially a matter of team-work, that without his full co-operation nothing can be achieved, and that you seek to exercise no more authority over him than he is willing to grant in order to treat his condition successfully.

5. Fluctuation of Attention

This is a difficulty that is encountered from time to time during the induction of hypnosis. It usually occurs in the subject who has, what is aptly called, a ' grasshopper ' mind. His power of concentration is poor, and his mind cannot remain fixed upon one idea, or his attention held for long enough to permit the induction to become successful. It flits incessantly from one subject to another.

The best way of dealing with this, by far, is to use a modified counting technique. This probably explains why this particular difficulty is much less frequently encountered when the eye-fixation-distraction method of induction is used.

The following modification is the one which I have found to be most satisfactory:

> I want you to start counting slowly, to yourself . . . and to go on counting until you hear me tell you to stop.
> When you say . . . *one* . . . Close your eyes!
> When you say . . . *two* . . . Open your eyes!
> When you say . . . *three* . . . Close your eyes!
> When you say . . . *four* . . . Open your eyes.

As the subject counts to himself, he opens and shuts his eyes deliberately with each alternate count. Whilst he is doing this he is quietly told how sleepy he is becoming, that his eyes are becoming more and more tired and his eyelids heavier and heavier, that presently they will want to remain closed and he will fall into a deep, deep sleep.

6. Need to Prove Superiority

From time to time, you will come across a subject to whom the mere induction of hypnosis seems to represent a challenge to his ability to perform. I have found that this particular resistance is often linked with one that we have already considered, namely defiance of authority, for once again a few simple questions will often reveal the fact that all his life the subject has resented taking orders from anyone. This is most important for if there is the slightest hint of dominance in the course of induction failure will be inevitable.

In dealing with such subjects it is necessary to emphasize, even to over-emphasize, the importance of the part that they themselves play in the actual induction of hypnosis. At the same time every possible step should be taken to increase their motivation and pride of achievement. You should tell them that it is only very intelligent people who make good hypnotic subjects, since a considerable degree of concentration and co-operation is required. Since, under most circumstances, the subject unconsciously tends to feel that he is the better man, this puts him upon his mettle and offers him the chance to prove it. For this reason alone, it is necessary to frame your suggestions in such a way as to challenge his ability to perform well. They should also succeed in conveying to him the impression that every effect that is produced has actually been achieved by his own efforts.

Hold your arm out . . . stiff and straight . . . palm facing the ceiling.
Now, I want you to tell yourself . . . that your arm is becoming stiffer and straighter . . . just like a steel poker.
This needs a great deal of concentration . . . but you can do it quite easily . . . if you want to.
Just concentrate upon letting your arm go stiff and straight.
You want it to become so stiff . . . so straight . . . so rigid . . . that it will be quite impossible for *me* to bend it at the elbow.
If you concentrate enough upon wanting this to happen . . . it *will* happen . . . it *will* become stiff and straight . . . so rigid . . . that I shall be quite unable to bend it at the elbow . . . until I ask you to count *three*.
But . . . the moment you count *three* . . . your arm will bend quite easily again . . . and your sleep will become much, much deeper.

7. Physical Discomfort

Physical discomfort can greatly hinder the successful induction of hypnosis, therefore the subject should always be made as comfortable as possible. He should visit the toilet before settling down on the couch or chair. Draughts should be avoided, and he should be kept warm and, if necessary, given a rug. Loud and unexpected noises should be avoided if possible. Care should be taken to see that he is not holding his head and neck in a position of undue strain when he is asked to look upwards and backwards. Sometimes the subject himself when awakened will remark that he was not comfortable and that this prevented him from going to sleep, or that he felt quite shivery and cold or that his neck felt strained.

You must bear in mind, however, that these simple explanations are not always founded upon fact. They are often pure rationalizations of the real reason for failure, which is to be found in unconscious anxiety.

Be that as it may, you should always take prompt steps to correct anything that seems to be worrying the subject—real or imaginary. At the next induction he should be seated in a chair, provided with a travelling-rug or given a pillow for his head, for any measures taken to rectify his complaints will afford him considerable reassurance. He is bound to feel that he himself is helping in the induction and is thereby retaining some measure of control over the situation.

8. Dislike of the Method Employed

Sometimes a subject dislikes the method of induction or he may dislike something in the actual phrasing of your suggestions. For instance, some subjects occasionally object to the word *sleepy*. If so, you should discard it completely and substitute the words *tiredness* and *drowsiness* only, during the next induction. Similarly, when the phrase *you are sinking into a deeper, deeper sleep* has been used, a subject has been known to complain that upon the word *sinking*, he invariably experienced a most uncomfortable sinking sensation in the pit of his stomach. In this case, the mere substitution of the word *falling* will be quite sufficient to remove this discomfort, and also reassure the subject that nothing will be forced upon him. Whenever it is the actual induction method that the subject dislikes, you should always adopt an alternative procedure at your next attempt at induction.

Just occasionally a subject may say: ' I could see you sitting there all the time and it distracted my attention. I found that the light was worrying me as well.' Although this may seem both unimportant and irrelevant, don't forget to sit behind him next time and see that he has his back to the light. It is remarkable to what extent such simple precautions as these can help in the induction and deepening of the hypnotic trance.

Difficulties in Terminating the Trance

Once the trance state has been induced and deepened, it is most unlikely that you will experience any difficulty in awakening your subject, although this has been known to occur. In this connection, you should remember that whilst it is generally assumed that the trance can always be terminated by simple suggestion to this effect, this is not necessarily the case. This assumption depends entirely upon the old idea that the hypnotized subject was completely passive, under the control of the hypnotist and subject only to his will. This, of course, is absolutely untrue for the trance situation in reality is nothing more or less than a relationship between two individuals, each of whom must be regarded as a person in his own right. Consequently, if you do come across a subject who declines to awaken when you instruct him to do so, you should bear in mind the fact that he has some reason, conscious or unconscious, for not complying with the suggestion. There seem to be three main reasons for a subject's refusal to awaken:

1. *It may be a defensive reaction.* The subject may have experienced so much pleasure and peace that he wishes the trance to continue and is reluctant to awaken to face reality again. On the other hand, it can be the unconscious means of expressing hostility or resentment toward the hypnotist. The subject may feel that he is not being treated as he would like, or may resent certain things that have occurred during his treatment.

2. *It may be due to a misconception as to what should occur.* I once had a patient who told me he had never been hypnotized before, who went into a somnambulistic trance and obstinately declined to awaken when told to do so. When I questioned him as to why he didn't wake up, he told me he couldn't since the *last time he was hypnotized*, he had to sleep it off for an hour or so. Further questioning elicited the fact that he had not in fact been hypnotized, but had undergone a drug-induced abreaction (Thiopentone). I explained to him that he had had no drug injected into his arm this time and that consequently there was no reason why he should not awaken immediately when told to do so. Subsequently he woke up with no further difficulty.

3. *It may be due to a post-hypnotic suggestion he dislikes.* In this case, he will avoid the necessity of complying with it by the simple expedient of

remaining in the trance. Questioning will soon reveal the cause of the trouble, and the offending suggestion can be promptly withdrawn.

If the subject's dislike is not sufficiently strong to prevent him from awakening, he may still unconsciously express his resentment by feeling discomfort such as headache or dizziness once he is awake. Should this occur in a case in which a post-hypnotic suggestion has been given, re-hypnotize the subject immediately and withdraw the suggestion, avoiding any necessity for compliance.

If a subject fails to awaken from his trance when instructed to do so, the golden rule is to ask him why he is unable to wake up. In the majority of cases this will give you the necessary clue as to how to proceed. In other cases it may even help to ask the subject himself what to do in order to awaken him. In most instances, this will be quite sufficient to resolve the difficulty.

Erickson meets this situation with some of the specialized hypno-therapeutic techniques, making use of the patient's behaviour pattern in order to solve the problem. He often manipulates the time-factor, projecting the patient well into the future, bringing him back to a less distant but still future time, taking him still further into the future and returning him closer to the present, eventually encouraging the patient to awaken at his correct age. In an obsessional case, he will induce in the patient a compulsive need to sleep for a stated period whilst simultaneously implanting an obsessional doubt as to whether they will be able to accomplish this. As a result of this, the trance is usually terminated within a few minutes.

CHAPTER 10

A Comprehensive System of Trance Induction and Trance Deepening Leading to Post-hypnotic Conditioning

I have found this method to be most consistently successful in securing adequate depth for all ordinary clinical purposes; only when complete analgesia or hypno-analytical techniques are required is greater depth likely to be necessary. Provided that the subject's mind has been fully prepared beforehand failure to produce a trance hardly ever occurs, and only rarely does the subject fail to become conditioned to enter the hypnotic state in future immediately it is suggested that he should do so. In a reasonably good subject, the whole routine can be successfully completed in a single period of about twenty minutes. In less responsive cases the same result can easily be obtained if the subject is trained more gradually over two or three consecutive sessions.

The eye-fixation distraction method is used for the initial induction, and the trance is gradually deepened by progressive relaxation, the induction of graded responses and a counting and breathing technique. Although the following description necessarily involves a great deal of repetition, this will probably prove more convenient than otherwise, since it is a verbatim account of the full routine which I employ in the majority of my cases. But whilst I seldom fail to teach my subjects to enter the hypnotic state upon a given signal, verbal or otherwise, by the use of this method, I am fully aware that other psychological factors are also involved, such as belief, confidence, personality, experience and even possibly reputation. Nevertheless, I have been greatly encouraged by the fact that most of my medical and dental colleagues who have been introduced to this technique and have tested it thoroughly in their own practices have not only confirmed many of the advantages described, but have subsequently incorporated it into their own routines.

As I have already stated, no single method can ever be said to be the best method of inducing and deepening hypnosis. Each aspiring operator must gradually evolve the one best suited to his own personality, and this may well incorporate features characteristic of a number of different techniques.

A Complete Routine for the Induction of Hypnosis, Trance Deepening and Post-hypnotic Conditioning

Preliminary Induction

I want you to lie back comfortably in the chair.
Look upwards and backwards at the tip of the pencil.
Can you just see it? Good!
Don't let your eyes wander from it for a single moment.
Now start counting slowly backwards, from 300.
Mentally, to yourself . . . not out loud.
Keep on counting . . . slowly and rhythmically . . . and go on counting until you hear me tell you to stop.
Try not to listen to me . . . any more than you can help.
You'll still hear everything I say . . . but try not to listen.
Just stick to your counting.
Let yourself go completely . . . limp and slack.
Breathe quietly . . . in . . . and out.
And whilst you're breathing quietly . . . in . . . and out . . . you can feel that your eyes are becoming very, very tired.
They may feel a little watery . . . the pencil may begin to look a little blurred.
Already, your eyelids are beginning to feel very, very heavy and tired.
Presently, they will want to blink.
As soon as they start to blink . . . just let them blink as much as they like.
You see! They're starting to blink, now.
Just let everything happen . . . exactly as it wants to happen.
Don't try to make it happen . . . don't try to stop it happening.
Just let everything please itself.
Presently, your blinks will become slower . . . and bigger.
And as they do so . . . your eyes will become more and more tired.
The eyelids . . . heavier . . . and heavier.
So heavy . . . that they feel they are wanting to close.
As soon as they feel they want to close . . . let them go . . . just let them close . . . entirely on their own.
They're wanting to close, now . . . let them go . . . closing tighter and tighter . . . tighter and tighter.
Go to sleep!

Sleep very, very deeply.
Relax completely . . . and give yourself up completely to this very pleasant
. . . relaxed . . . drowsy feeling.
Stop counting, now.
Just sleep . . . very, very deeply indeed.

Deepening by Progressive Relaxation

Now, a feeling of complete relaxation is gradually stealing over your
whole body.
Let the muscles of your feet and ankles relax completely.
Let them go . . . limp and slack.
Now, your calf muscles.
Let them go limp and slack . . . allow them to relax.
Now, the muscles of your thighs.
Let them relax . . . let them go . . . limp and slack.
And as the muscles of your legs and thighs become completely limp and
relaxed . . . you can feel a feeling of heaviness in your legs.
As though your legs are becoming just as heavy as lead.
Let your legs go . . . heavy as lead.
Let them relax completely.
And as they do so . . . your sleep is gradually becoming deeper and deeper.
That feeling of relaxation is now spreading upwards . . . over your whole
body.
Let your stomach muscles relax . . . let them go . . . limp and slack.
Now, the muscles of your chest . . . your body . . . and your back.
Let them all go . . . limp and slack . . . allow them to relax.
And, as you do so . . . you can feel a feeling of heaviness in your body . . .
as though your body is becoming just as heavy as lead.
As if it is wanting to sink down . . . deeper and deeper . . . into the chair.
Just let your body go . . . heavy as lead.
Let it sink back comfortably . . . deeper and deeper . . . into the chair.
And as it does so . . . you are falling, slowly but surely, into a deeper,
deeper sleep.
Just give yourself up completely . . . to this very pleasant . . . relaxed . .
drowsy . . . comfortable feeling.
And now, this feeling of relaxation is spreading into the muscles of your
neck . . . your shoulders . . . and your arms.
Let your neck muscles relax . . . particularly the muscles at the back of your
neck.
Let them relax . . . let them go . . . limp and slack.
Now, your shoulder muscles.
Let them go limp and slack . . . allow them to relax.
Now, the muscles of your arms.

Let them relax . . . let them go . . . limp and slack.
And as you do so . . . you can feel a feeling of heaviness in your arms.
As though your arms are beginning to feel just as heavy as lead.
Let your arms go . . . heavy as lead.
And as you do so . . . your sleep is becoming deeper . . . deeper . . . deeper.
And as this feeling of complete relaxation spreads . . . and deepens . . . over
your whole body . . . you have fallen into a very, very deep sleep indeed.
*You are so deeply asleep, in fact . . . that everything that I tell you that is going
to happen . . . will happen . . . exactly as I tell you.*
*And every feeling that I tell you that you will experience . . . you will experience
. . . exactly as I tell you.*
Now, sleep . . . very, very deeply.
Deeper and deeper asleep . . . deeper and deeper asleep.

Deepening by the Induction of Arm-heaviness

I am now going to place your arm on the arm of the chair.
And I am going to stroke it gently . . . from the shoulder to the wrist.
And, as I stroke it . . . you will begin to feel a feeling of heaviness in your
arm.
That feeling of heaviness is increasing . . . with every stroke of my hand.
Your arm is beginning to feel heavier . . . and heavier . . . just as heavy as
lead.
You can feel it pressing down more firmly upon the arm of the chair.

(As you say this, imperceptibly increase the pressure of your own
hand as you stroke his arm.)

*And in a few moments . . . your arm will feel so very, very heavy . . . that, when
I pick it up by the wrist . . . and let it go . . . it will drop back on to your lap
. . . just like a lead weight.*
*And as it drops limply back . . . on to your lap . . . you will fall into a deeper,
deeper sleep.*

This response is now tested, following which the arm is restored to
normal.

You have now fallen into a much deeper sleep.
And, as I stroke your arm in the opposite direction . . . you will notice that
all feelings of heaviness are now leaving your arm.
It is coming back to normal . . . and now feels just the same as your other
arm.
All that feeling of heaviness has passed away completely . . . and your sleep
has become even deeper . . . and deeper.

Deepening by the Induction of Arm-catalepsy
(This is not an essential step, and often omitted.)

As your arm rests upon the arm of the chair . . . I am going to stroke it again.
This time . . . instead of feeling heavier . . . it will begin to feel lighter and lighter.
Just as light as a feather . . . as if there is no weight in it at all.
Lighter and lighter . . . lighter and lighter.
So light, in fact . . . that when I take it by the wrist . . . and lift it above your head . . . it will no longer want to drop down on to your lap when I release your wrist.
It will want to remain just where it is . . . exactly where I have left it.
When I release your wrist . . . your arm will no longer want to fall . . . it will remain just where it is . . . without your having to make the slightest effort to keep it there.

When the response is positive, the gradual restoration of the arm to normal may be used as an additional deepening technique.

As I am talking to you . . . your arm is gradually feeling heavier and heavier.
Heavier and heavier . . . heavier and heavier.
So very, very heavy . . . that it is beginning to sink down . . . slowly but surely . . . on to the arm of the chair.
And as it slowly sinks down on to the chair . . . your sleep is becoming deeper and deeper.
And, the moment your arm touches the arm of the chair . . . you will fall into a much, much deeper sleep.
Heavier and heavier . . . down and down . . . deeper and deeper asleep.
Very, very deeply asleep, indeed!

Once again the arm must be restored to normality.

As I gently stroke your arm . . . it is gradually coming back to normal.
All that feeling of lightness and weightlessness is leaving it . . . and it is now feeling just the same as your other arm.
And your sleep has become deeper . . . and deeper.

Deepening by the Induction of Limb-rigidity

Now, I want you to hold your arm out . . . level with your shoulder . . . stiff and straight . . . with the palm facing the ceiling.
And as I stroke your arm . . . you will feel that it is becoming much stiffer and straighter.
That stiffness is increasing . . . with every stroke of my hand.
You can feel all the muscles tightening up . . . pulling your arm out . . .

stiffer and straighter . . . with every stroke of my hand . . . until it is begin-
ning to feel just as stiff and rigid as a steel poker . . . from the shoulder to
the wrist.
Now, I want you to concentrate on a steel poker.
Picture a steel poker in your mind.
And as you do so . . . you will feel that your arm has become just as stiff
and rigid as that steel poker.
As if the elbow joint is firmly locked.
As if there is no elbow joint there at all.
*So that it will be impossible for me to bend your arm at the elbow . . . until I
count up to ' three '.*
*The harder I try to bend it . . . the stiffer and straighter . . . and more rigid it
will become.*
*But, the moment I count ' three ' . . . all the stiffness will pass away immediately
. . . your arm will bend quite easily . . . and as it does so, you will fall immediately
into a deeper, deeper sleep.*
Stiff and straight !   Just like that steel poker !
One . . . two . . . three !

Deepening by the Induction of Automatic Movements

Now, place your elbow on the arm of the chair . . . and hold your arm
upwards, with the fingers pointing towards the ceiling.
And I'm going to take it by the wrist . . . and move it slowly . . . backwards
and forwards . . . backwards and forwards.
And as I do so . . . I want you to imagine that the centre of a piece of cord
is tied round your wrist . . . and that someone at each end of the cord is
pulling your arm . . . first, backwards . . . then forwards.
Just picture that piece of cord, tied round your wrist . . . pulling your arm
slowly . . . backwards . . . and forwards . . . backwards . . . and forwards.
And as you do so . . . you will find that when I release your wrist . . . it
will feel as if that piece of cord is still tied to your wrist . . . still pulling
your arm . . . backwards . . . and forwards . . . backwards and forwards.
And your arm will go on moving . . . entirely on its own . . . backwards
and forwards . . . backwards and forwards . . . until I tell you to stop.
You won't try to make it move!
You won't try to stop it moving!
You will just let it please itself . . . and it will go on moving on its own
. . . quite automatically . . . backwards . . . and forwards . . . backwards
. . . and forwards . . . until I tell you to stop.
*Backwards . . . and forwards . . . backwards . . . and forwards . . . backwards
. . . and forwards !*

When the arm is moving freely, tell the subject that his sleep is becoming deeper and deeper, timing this so that you repeat the word deeper on each alternate forward movement of his arm.

> Now, stop!
> Put your arm back . . . on to your lap . . . and as you do so . . . you are falling into an even deeper, deeper sleep.
> *Sleep! Very, very deeply!*

At this point, the subject is certainly in a medium, and possibly a deeper stage of hypnosis. Further deepening is now effected by the use of a counting and breathing technique.

Deepening by a Counting and Breathing Technique

> In a few moments . . . I am going to count slowly up to *five* . . . and as I do so . . . you will take *five very deep breaths.*
> And with each breath that you take . . . each time you breathe out . . . you will become more and more relaxed . . . and your sleep will become deeper and deeper.
> *One* . . . Deep, deep breath . . . more and more deeply relaxed . . . deeper and deeper asleep.
> *Two* . . . Very deep breath . . . deeper and deeper relaxed . . . sleep becoming deeper and deeper.
> *Three* . . . Deeper and deeper breath . . . more and more deeply relaxed . . . more and more deeply asleep.
> *Four* . . . Very, very deep breath . . . deeper and deeper relaxed . . . sleep becoming even deeper and deeper.
> *Five* . . . Very, very deep breath indeed . . . very, very deeply relaxed . . . very, very deeply asleep.
> And I would now like you to take one very deep breath . . . fill your chest . . . and hold it until I say . . . ' *Let go* '.
> Then, *let that breath out as quickly as possible* . . . and as you do so . . . you will feel yourself sagging limply back into the chair . . . and you will become twice as deeply relaxed as you are now . . . twice as deeply asleep.
> Now take that very deep breath . . . fill your chest . . . and *Hold it* . . . (15 seconds pause) . . . *Hold it* . . . (15 seconds pause) . . . *Hold it* . . . (15 to 20 seconds pause) *Let go!*
> Sleep very, very deeply . . . deeper and deeper asleep . . . deeper and deeper asleep.

By now, the subject is usually in a sufficiently deep sleep to permit post-hypnotic conditioning to be attempted with a considerable chance of success.

The Induction of Post-hypnotic Conditioning

You are now so deeply asleep . . . that everything that I tell you that is going to happen . . . *will* happen . . . *exactly* as I tell you.

Every feeling . . . that I tell you that you will experience . . . you *will* experience . . . *exactly* as I tell you.

And every instruction that I give you . . . you will carry out faithfully.

Now . . . in a few moments . . . I shall waken you up by counting up to ' seven '.

You will wake up . . . feeling wonderfully better for this long sleep.

And after you have wakened up . . . I shall talk to you for a minute or two.

Then, I shall ask you to lie back in the chair . . . and look straight into my eyes.

Whilst you are looking at me . . . I shall say :

Go to sleep !

And the moment you hear me say . . . ' Go to sleep ' . . . your eyes will close immediately . . . and you will fall immediately into a sleep, just as deep as this one.

This instruction should be repeated at least once, quietly and firmly.

In a few moments . . . I am going to wake you up by counting up to ' seven '.

And after you have wakened up . . . I shall talk to you for a minute or two.

Then, I shall ask you to lie back in the chair . . . and look straight into my eyes.

Whilst you are looking at me . . . I shall say :

Go to sleep !

And the moment you hear me say . . . ' Go to sleep ' . . . your eyes will close immediately . . . and you will fall immediately into a sleep, just as deep as this one !

The subject is then awakened.

In a few moments . . . when I count up to ' seven ' . . . you will open your eyes . . . and be wide awake again.

You will wake up feeling wonderfully better for this long sleep.

You will wake up feeling completely relaxed . . . mentally and physically . . . feeling quite calm and composed.

One . . . two . . . three . . . four . . . five . . . six . . . seven !

As soon as he is awake, I usually ask him a few questions about his own feelings during the hypnosis, and briefly discuss his reactions. Then, I ask him to lie back in the chair . . . and look straight into my eyes.

Whilst he is doing this, I say to him, firmly:

Go to sleep !

and usually his eyes close immediately, and he sinks into a deep hypnotic sleep.

Occasionally, if there is some delay and the subject's eyes do not close immediately, I repeat the suggestion much more firmly and authoritatively, once or twice if necessary, with the result that the eyes generally close without more ado.

After awakening him again, I explain that the only reason that his eyes failed to close immediately lay in the fact that he just could not believe that such a thing could possibly happen. I point out to him that, despite his doubts, it did actually happen, and that when I tell him to go to sleep again, in a few moments' time—on this occasion he will find that his eyes will close without delay. This usually proves to be the case, but if the reactions are still inclined to be sluggish, a few more rapid rehearsals will generally produce the desired result. I then proceed to consolidate this conditioning for all future occasions.

From now on . . . you will never have to look at the pencil again.

From now on . . . *whenever you want me to give you treatment* . . . all I shall have to do is to ask you to lie back comfortably in the chair . . . and look straight at me.

Whilst you are looking at me . . . I shall say :

Go to sleep !

And from now on . . . whenever you hear me say . . . ' *Go to sleep* ' . . . your eyes will always close immediately . . . and you will always fall immediately into a sleep . . . just as deep as this one.

It doesn't matter whether it is *tomorrow* . . . *next week* . . . *next month* . . . or even *next year.*

From now on . . . whenever you hear me say . . . ' *Go to sleep* ' . . . your eyes will always close immediately . . . and you will always fall immediately into a sleep . . . just as deep as this one.

And that is exactly what is going to happen when you come to see me next. After our preliminary chat . . . as soon as you are ready for treatment . . . I shall ask you to lie back comfortably in the chair . . . and look straight at me.

Whilst you are looking at me . . . I shall say :

Go to sleep !

And next time . . . and, indeed, on every future occasion when you want me to give you treatment . . . the moment you hear me say . . . ' *Go to sleep* ' . . . your eyes will close immediately . . . and you will fall immediately into a sleep . . . just as deep as this one.

I then finally awaken the subject.

In a few moments . . . when I count ' *seven* ' . . . you will open your eyes and be wide awake again . . . feeling wonderfully better for this long sleep. You will wake up . . . feeling really fit and well . . . feeling completely relaxed . . . mentally and physically . . . feeling quite calm and composed . . . and feeling much more confidence . . . both in yourself . . . and in the future.

One . . . *two* . . . *three* . . . *four* . . . *five* . . . *six* . . . *seven !*

In this routine there are one or two points that are worth noting. Although the subject certainly falls asleep immediately he is told to do so, the procedure is not as dominating as it might appear. The subject has been given some choice in the matter since the conditions under which he will respond have been precisely specified. The phrase *whenever you want me to give you treatment* allows him to select the occasions upon which he will be ready to comply with the suggestion, and this feeling of independence is furthered by the phrases *whenever you lie back comfortably in the chair* and *look straight at me*, which also define the limited conditions under which he will respond. The freedom thus allowed seems to afford a great deal of reassurance, and does a lot to ensure wholehearted co-operation.

Should the first attempt at post-hypnotic conditioning fail, I take no further steps until the next session. I then repeat the whole induction and deepening procedures as before, but with the addition of dream induction before trying again. In my experience, whenever a positive response is obtained to this technique, the post-hypnotic conditioning routine can be suggested with every expectation of success. Although this has already been described, I propose to repeat it here for the sake of convenience.

Deepening by Dream Induction

You are now so deeply asleep . . . that everything that I tell you that is going to happen . . . *will* happen . . . *exactly* as I tell you.

And every feeling I tell you that you will experience . . . you *will* experience . . . *exactly* as I tell you.

Moreover, every single instruction that I give you . . . you will carry out faithfully.

Just as your arm felt heavy . . . when I told you it would feel heavy . . .

Just as your arm felt stiff . . . when I told you it would feel stiff . . .

Just as your arm moved on its own . . . when I told you it would move on its own ;

So . . . everything else that I tell you that is going to happen . . . *will* happen
. . . *exactly* as I tell you.
Every feeling I tell you that you will experience . . . you *will* experience
. . . *exactly* as I tell you.
And every single instruction that I give you . . . you will obey faithfully.
You are now so deeply asleep . . . that, in a few moments . . . when I tell
you to dream . . . *you will dream !*
And you will dream that you are performing whatever simple action I tell
you to dream about.
You will be able to picture yourself quite clearly . . . and see yourself quite
vividly . . . in your own mind . . . carrying out whatever action I have told
you to dream about.
Just as you pictured that steel poker . . . in your mind . . . when your arm
went stiff.
Just as you pictured that piece of cord . . . tied round your wrist . . . when
your arm moved on its own.
So . . . you will be able to picture yourself . . . in your dream . . . equally
vividly and clearly . . . performing whatever simple action that I tell you
to dream about.
Now, you are going to dream that you are straightening your tie !
You are going to dream that you are straightening your tie !
Now, dream ! Dream ! Dream !
Now . . . show me what you are dreaming
Show me, now !
Show me what you are dreaming !

In a positive response, the subject's hands will move slowly upwards and
will perform the action that has been suggested.

Stop dreaming, now.
Just let yourself relax completely . . . and you are falling into a deeper,
deeper sleep.

Except under special circumstances I adopt this as my standard method
of inducing and deepening hypnosis. I have always found it to be quick,
reliable and efficient. Even with a subject who has never been hypnotized
before, provided that his mind has been properly prepared, it rarely
takes more than 2 to 3 minutes to secure spontaneous closing of the eyes
and the light hypnotic state. And as already mentioned, in a good
subject the whole induction and deepening routine, including post-
hypnotic conditioning, can be completed in a single session of approximately 20 minutes' duration. Even more difficult subjects can still be
trained to go to sleep immediately it is suggested that they should do so,

if they are gradually trained over several consecutive sessions.

I tell my patients that although nearly everyone is capable of being hypnotized, the susceptibility of different individuals varies a great deal. If they happen to be good subjects, they will probably enter the deep hypnotic state during the first induction; if not, they can still be taught to achieve sufficient depth for treatment purposes in the course of two or three consultations. I hardly ever attempt to induce hypnosis during the first interview.

1st Session. I get to know my patient, take his case-history, and try to obtain his confidence. I decide whether his case is suitable for hypnotherapy or whether some alternative form of treatment is more appropriate. If considered suitable, I discuss the question of hypnosis with him, explain it to him fully, correct his ideas, banish his doubts and fears, and generally prepare his mind to accept it.

2nd Session. I begin by asking him whether he has any questions to put to me, arising from our previous discussion. If so, I proceed to answer them in order to dispel any last lingering doubts. I then explain to the patient exactly what he has to do, what I have to do, and exactly what he may expect to happen. I then induce light hypnosis, and deepen it by the use of progressive relaxation and limb-heaviness and, occasionally, limb catalepsy.

3rd Session. I discuss with him his reactions to the previous session and try to correct any misconceptions he may still hold. I induce and deepen his hypnosis as before, following on with limb rigidity and terminating with automatic movement.

4th Session. Once again, his reactions are thoroughly ventilated and discussed. I then repeat the whole induction and deepening procedure in full, with the addition of the counting and breathing technique, followed by post-hypnotic conditioning. This is usually successful and the subject subsequently enters the hypnotic state immediately, whenever he is instructed to do so. Should any difficulty arise the whole process is repeated at the next session, any further attempt at conditioning being preceded by dream induction.

With this system of gradual training, I hardly ever encounter a patient, even those suffering from neuroses, who cannot be taught to enter the hypnotic state immediately the appropriate suggestion or signal is given. The scheme just described, however, is far from being rigid. For instance, I watch carefully the way the subject reacts to each phase of the induction and deepening process, and if his responses indicate a considerable degree of susceptibility, I often proceed to the stage of automatic movement during the first actual hypnotic session. Indeed, whenever the subject is really susceptible, I can complete the entire conditioning routine in a single session.

Although I use this scheme daily, I do not suggest that it will prove ideal in everybody's hands, or that it should be adopted in its entirety. Anyone who wishes to succeed with hypnosis must formulate his own individual technique through painstaking trial and error, but it is hoped that my experience with this routine may afford some assistance to those who are trying to develop their own particular methods.

PART TWO

THE THEORIES AND PHENOMENA
OF HYPNOSIS

CHAPTER 11

The Theories and Phenomena of Hypnosis

In Chapter 2, when I attempted to give an explanation of the nature of hypnosis, I deliberately over-simplified the question in order to render it as intelligible as possible. I consequently explained it solely in terms of suggestion and dissociation, but also pointed out at the time that there were many other theories of the hypnotic state to be considered, and it is the more important of these which must now engage our attention. There are nine principal theories:

1. Charcot's 'pathological' theory.
2. The 'physical' theory.
3. The 'modified sleep' theory.
4. The 'conditioned reflex' theory.
5. The 'dissociation' theory.
6. The 'suggestion' theory.
7. The 'role-playing' theory.
8. The 'psycho-analytic' theory.
9. Meares' theory of 'atavistic regression'.

1. Charcot's Pathological Theory

Charcot, who trained as a neurologist, formed the opinion that hypnosis was a pathological condition similar to hysteria, and considered it to be the product of an abnormal nervous constitution. There seems to be little truth in this since at least 90 per cent of ordinary people can be hypnotized and obviously it is ridiculous to suppose that most of the population is markedly hysterical.

Even if Charcot's opinion is held to apply to deep-trance subjects only it is still difficult to justify, for it is often extremely difficult to hypnotize a hysterical person at all, let alone to induce a deep trance. Moreover, it has been found that a much higher proportion of deep-trance subjects is obtained from healthy volunteers than from those who are psychologically disturbed.

More recently, Eysenck devised a method of assessing hysterical personality traits and tested a random group of persons for both hysteria and hypnotizability. He failed to obtain any correlation whatever between the two, but did succeed in establishing a close connection between hypnotizability and suggestibility. Few people today are prepared to accept Charcot's theory.

2. The Physical Theory

This theory maintains that hypnosis is a purely physical phenomenon which is accompanied by biochemical or electrical changes in the cerebral cortex and central nervous system. Despite the fact that it is claimed that such changes can be detected and measured, little evidence exists that they actually occur.

3. The Modified Sleep Theory

It has frequently been suggested that hypnosis is a modified kind of sleep, but this is certainly not likely to be true. In natural sleep consciousness or awareness is entirely suspended, whereas in hypnosis it is definitely present no matter what the depth may be.

It has also been found that physiological estimations performed in the two states fail to establish the slightest similarity. In natural sleep, there is usually a fall in blood-pressure, a slowing of the heart rate, a reduction in urinary secretion and a diminution or abolition of certain reflexes; all these can be measured with accuracy. In hypnotic sleep, no matter how long the trance state is maintained, none of these differences occur and the blood chemistry remains unaltered.

Yet another proof that hypnosis and sleep are far from being identical is found in the fact that either condition can change into the other. It is possible to whisper suggestions softly, over and over again, to a person in natural sleep until he begins to respond to the suggestion that he will raise his arm without awakening. When he complies with this suggestion, he has passed from the sleeping state into a state of hypnosis. Conversely, a subject may sometimes pass from the hypnotic state into normal sleep. This has been known to occur as a means of avoiding the need for carrying out a suggestion that the subject has found objectionable. Quite apart from this, however, it can happen in the natural course of events. If a hypnotist were to collapse and die just after completing the induction of a deep trance state, no serious consequences would follow. The subject would eventually fall into a normal sleep. from which he would awaken in the ordinary way after a period of time which might vary from perhaps 15 minutes to 12 hours, depending upon how tired he happened to be at the time.

So although the reactions of the subject during the average induction process closely resemble those of the early stages of normal sleep, the state of hypnosis itself is in no way related to sleep. In fact, hypnosis is often used in the treatment of insomnia, in which case the patient can be hypnotized and left in the hypnotic state until it eventually merges into normal sleep. Indeed, he can even be taught self-hypnosis to do this for himself whenever the need arises.

4. The Conditioned Reflex Theory

This theory is based upon the work of Pavlov and the East European scientists who have adapted and developed reflex psychology. It will be remembered that Pavlov rang a bell before each occasion on which a dog was given food, and after a number of occasions upon each of which feeding was preceded by the ringing of the bell, saliva would flow whenever the bell was rung even though no food was offered. This process was called *conditioning*. Pavlov also found that de-conditioning could be effected if a small unpleasant electric shock was administered when the bell was rung. It should be noted, however, that both conditioning and de-conditioning require the process to be repeated on many consecutive occasions.

Explained in these terms, hypnosis is considered to be a physiological state produced by a life-time of conditioning, in the course of which certain words tend to act like Pavlov's bell in causing effects due to long association. For instance, when the word *sleep* is mentioned to a subject, he immediately associates this with feelings of tiredness, heaviness and drowsiness. He will thus come to associate the word *sleep* with such words as *heavy*, *tired*, *drowsy* and *relaxed*, and the constant repetition of these words during induction produces a state which the subject has become conditioned to associate with such words.

There can be no doubt whatever that conditioning does play an important part in the induction of hypnosis, and it has been shown that people who are capable of establishing conditioned reflexes easily are usually good hypnotic subjects. But it is far from being the whole story. In the first place, the theory assumes that the states of hypnosis and normal sleep are similar, and as we have just seen this is certainly not the case. Secondly, an even more convincing argument against hypnosis being solely a conditioned process lies in the fact that de-conditioning has always involved a slow, repetitive procedure, the length of time required depending largely upon the time taken to achieve the original conditioning. In the hypnotic state, however, de-conditioning can be effected immediately upon word of command. Thirdly, to regard hypnosis as being a conditioned reflex takes no account of the fact that people have often been hypnotized by rotating discs, mirrors or metronomes, none of which could have been associated by previous conditioning with the idea of the hypnotic trance.

5. The Dissociation Theory

This theory was originally formulated by Pierre Janet, who worked at the Salpêtrière Clinic and believed, as did Charcot, in the close association between hysteria and hypnosis. He eventually concluded that hysteria was caused by a splitting of the mind into two parts and that hypnosis represented the same splitting process, artificially induced.

This concept of splitting of consciousness has proved to be a very valuable one, and has entered into medicine under the technical term *dissociation*. For many years, this theory of dissociation was considered to be the key to hypnosis, the depth of which was held to be directly related to the degree of dissociation achieved. In many ways it is an attractive theory and as in the case of the conditioned reflex, there is probably a great deal of truth in it. But whilst it explains some of the phenomena of hypnosis, it fails to account for many others. Undoubtedly the tendency to dissociate can be greatly increased by suggestion, but this does not necessarily prove that hypnosis and dissociation are one and the same thing.

I have already indicated the part dissociation probably plays in the induction of hypnosis (p. 15) when I compared the mind to an iceberg, and the development of the hypnotic state to the gradual toppling over of the iceberg. Simple though this explanation may be, it does not seem entirely unreasonable since there is little doubt that the unconscious mind not only becomes more accessible, but is much more easily influenced, in the hypnotic than in the waking state.

One of the main difficulties in accepting the dissociation theory of hypnosis lies in its dependence on the occurrence of amnesia. The recall of memories depends upon the association of ideas, and the failure to remember events is caused by a break in the chain of ideas which would restore them to consciousness. Whenever this happens, dissociation has occurred and the result is a state of amnesia (loss of recall). Amnesia consequently becomes a necessary element in the theory.

Since the unconscious mind is capable of assuming most of the functions of the conscious mind, Janet concluded that such phenomena as 'fugues' and even ' multiple personalities ' were due to a splitting of consciousness which resulted in the unconscious mind becoming the dominant part for the time being. It is thus often maintained that hypnosis results from a similar splitting of consciousness during which the unconscious part of the mind becomes the dominant one. It should be remembered, however, that in a fugue state the individual has no recollection whatever of his ordinary life and when restored to normality he has a complete amnesia for the events of the fugue. Obviously the dissociation theory depends largely upon the development of amnesia following the trance and is greatly weakened by the fact that deep trances can occur without any appreciable degree of amnesia. Even when present this amnesia is rarely spontaneous and is more often produced by direct suggestion. Moreover, post-hypnotic amnesia can be removed quite easily and the memory restored by suggestion.

6. The Suggestion Theory

Since I have discussed this at considerable length when dealing with the induction of hypnosis (Chapter 2), there is little need to enlarge upon it here except for one or two further points to which attention should be drawn. All the available evidence points to the conclusion that ' suggestibility ' and the ' hypnotic state ' are closely connected, and that the more suggestible the subject is the more easily can hypnosis be induced and deepened.

Bernheim originally maintained that all hypnotism was suggestion, but this is far too sweeping a statement in view of the fact that many phenomena characteristic of the trance can be reproduced in minor form in the waking state.

Much of the practice of medicine cannot be divorced from suggestion. The drugs prescribed by a specialist of renown, who charges the patient a high fee, may sometimes have far more rapid and far-reaching results than the identical preparations ordered by the family doctor. This emphasizes the important part played by ' prestige ', ' authority ', and ' respect ', all of which are factors that are equally significant in facilitating the induction of hypnosis. In hypnosis, suggestion is employed deliberately and dispassionately, and exercises a much greater effect than in the waking state. Even in everyday life most people tend to defer to persons in authority, and this tendency is greatly exaggerated in the hypnotic state. That is one of the reasons why suggestions exercise such a profound effect during hypnosis.

7. The Role-playing Theory

R. W. White formed the conclusion that hypnosis should be regarded as meaningful, goal-directed striving, its most general goal being to behave like a hypnotized person as this is continually defined by the operator and understood by the subject. We suggest, and make it quite clear, to the subject what we expect him to do, and because of the existing rapport he seems to strive to fulfil the role we have outlined. His dominant motive seems to be submission to the operator's demands.

This theory, however, disregards the occurrence of phenomena that are outside voluntary control. Estabrooks tested hypnotic anaesthesia by electric shocks and found that hypnotized subjects could stand without discomfort currents nearly ten times as strong as those that could be tolerated in the waking state. This directly refutes the ' role-playing ' theory for no one trying to behave as a hypnotized person could voluntarily produce such a degree of anaesthesia.

8. The Psycho-analytic Theories

Freud regarded the susceptibility of the hypnotic subject as being due to an unconscious desire for libidinal gratification on his part, and pointed out the similarity of hypnosis to the state of being in love. According to this theory there is an erotic relationship between the hypnotist and his subject which is not usually allowed to progress very far. This seems to be accompanied by the desire for unconditional subjection. Ferenczi agreed with this view and expanded it further by postulating a ' parent-child ' relationship which develops between the hypnotist and his subject.

Both these attitudes, however, tend to exist to some extent between any doctor and patient in ordinary medical practice. The doctor who likes his patient will often be able to get him well more easily than a doctor who dislikes him. And the patient who likes his doctor will put so much trust and confidence in him that he will do much better than when he is treated by a doctor for whom he does not care. Moreover, patients are frequently over-awed by their doctor in exactly the same way as a child by his parent, so that these relationships are certainly not confined to hypnosis.

As with the conditioned-reflex theory, the psycho-analytic theories fail to explain instances of hypnotization by mirrors, rotating discs or metronomes, or the fact that hypnotic states can sometimes be produced by inanimate objects. Since under such conditions no inter-personal relationships are involved, it is difficult to see how any libidinal gratification can ensue.

9. Meares' Theory of ' Atavistic Regression '

This involves the concept that suggestion is an archaic mental function that can be used to explain the nature of hypnosis. In clinical psychiatry, the term ' regression ' is usually applied to the return to a former type of behaviour. When Ferenczi considered hypnosis to be a parent-child relationship developing between the hypnotist and his subject, he was postulating regression as a return to childhood or infantile patterns of behaviour. The atavistic theory requires that regression be applied, not in the field of behaviour, but in the field of mental function. In other words, a regression from normal adult mental function at an intellectual, logical level, to an archaic level of mental function in which the process of suggestion determines the acceptance of ideas. This type of regression is considered to be the basic mechanism in the production of hypnosis.

As Ainslie Meares himself points out, this hypothesis does not in any way suggest that primitive man lived in a state of hypnosis. It assumes that primitive man, before he developed the ability of logically evaluating ideas, accepted them by the more primitive process of suggestion. In fact, the essence of the atavistic theory is that hypnosis is a return to a more primitive form of mental functioning in which suggestion plays a major role. This is a concept which can be of practical value to the clinician, for anything, word or act, which tends to aid this regression will assist the induction of hypnosis. In clinical practice, greater depth of hypnosis is the result of more profound atavistic regression; in lighter hypnosis the regression is less complete.

It would appear then that no single theory of hypnosis is complete enough to explain all the phenomena of the trance. White maintains that no scientific hypothesis can be formulated until it can adequately explain the following facts:

1. That a hypnotized person transcends the normal limits of voluntary control.

2. That he behaves without the experience of will or intention or self-consciousness, and without subsequent memory.

3. That these changes occur because the hypnotist says they will.

None of the theories so far advanced is capable of fulfilling these requirements. It would seem that our present knowledge of human behaviour is not yet sufficiently developed to produce a complete and satisfactory theory of hypnosis. In trying to define it accurately we are only describing an end-result which is often due to a combination of several of the factors already mentioned. I feel that in most trance states suggestion, dissociation and conditioning all play a part to a greater or lesser extent. At least it can be said that an understanding of these mechanisms does much to render trance behaviour intelligible, despite the gaps which still remain to be filled before our knowledge is complete.

The Phenomena of Hypnosis

Curious and unusual as many of the hypnotic phenomena may seem, most of them have their counterpart in everyday life and can be reproduced at least to a minor extent in the waking state. Moreover, they can often be seen and induced in perfectly normal individuals as a result of post-hypnotic suggestion, following which they subsequently appear after the subject has been awakened. Many of them can also be self-induced by those who have mastered the technique of self-hypnosis.

The phenomena of hypnosis have often been separated into two distinct categories—the physiological and the psychological—but it is difficult to draw any hard and fast division between them. As Moll points out, alterations in bodily functions often occur solely as a result of changes in the psychical state. For instance, when a man becomes paralysed by fright his complete inability to move is due to the mental shock he has received, and is certainly not the result of any injury or damage to his muscles. Similarly during the hypnotic state the muscles and sense organs often display abnormalities in function simply because the mental state of the subject has been altered. The alterations usually encountered in the course of hypnosis affect both voluntary and involuntary muscles, the sense organs, the memory, mental activity and the emotions.

Alterations in the Voluntary Muscles

Suggestion exercises an extraordinary influence over the functions of the voluntary muscles, the activity of which can nearly always be influenced to a high degree. During hypnosis, the movements of these muscles can either be inhibited or excited.

1. *Relaxation.* Suggestions of muscular relaxation seem to induce a feeling of laziness in the subject and a pronounced disinclination to move his limbs; he may even feel unable to make up his mind whether

to do so or not. He never actually loses the power to move them, but as hypnosis deepens so muscular tonus diminishes, sometimes to a point beyond voluntary control.

2. *Paralysis of Muscle Groups.* This may effect only small groups of muscles such as those of the eyelids or may be extended to larger groups such as the muscles of the limbs and body. The actual distribution of the paralysis never corresponds exactly to that of the motor nerves but follows the subject's own idea of how a paralysed person would behave. If the subject is told that he has entirely lost the use of all the muscles of his limbs and body he will be quite powerless to get up out of his chair. This occurs simply because the suggestion has aroused in the subject's mind a firm conviction that his muscles are completely useless. Such paralyses are indistinguishable from true hysterical paralyses that arise spontaneously in the absence of hypnosis.

Sometimes the subject is unable to move a paralysed limb because he can no longer voluntarily contact his muscles. In other cases every attempt at voluntary movement is actively opposed and rendered futile by contracture of the antagonistic muscles. The subject may be robbed completely of the power of speech, or told that he will only be able to pronounce his own name and will otherwise be quite dumb. It can be made impossible for him to write whilst still retaining his ability to shuffle a pack of cards or play the piano. The prohibited actions will only become possible again when the necessary permission is given.

These effects will vary greatly from subject to subject. In some people it will be easier to influence one particular set of muscles than any others. For instance, it may be possible to prevent one person from opening his eyes, yet be quite impossible to affect his speech. Another may be rendered quite dumb, yet all attempts to prohibit him from writing will fail completely.

3. *Rigid catalepsies.* Catalepsy is said to occur when a limb remains in any position in which it has been placed by the hypnotist. Such postures can often be maintained for long periods of time far exceeding those possible by voluntary effort, without being followed by the pain and fatigue that one would normally expect after such excessive muscular exertion.

The essential requirement for the production of catalepsy is that the subject should accept the idea of the particular attitude involved. Sometimes you can raise the arm of a hypnotized subject, hold it in the air and then release it, and the limb will remain exactly where it was left although not a word has been spoken. Despite this, the subject firmly believes that his arm must remain so. In another subject the arm will probably fall, yet if you raise it again and tell him that it will now remain in the air, this will undoubtedly happen. Indeed there is no need for you to speak to him at all, for one or two upward jerks of the wrist alone will cause him to understand what is intended to take place. Erickson believes that catalepsy occurs because the subject becomes so intensely absorbed that he is unresponsive to ordinary stimuli.

Cataleptic rigidity can be induced in any limb or even in the entire body by direct suggestion, for example an arm can be stiffened so that it is impossible for a second person to bend it. Moll pointed out that the rigidity could be increased by gently stroking the limb, since touch seems to concentrate the subject's attention upon it. Cataleptic rigidity can be terminated immediately by the appropriate counter-suggestion.

One of the favourite tricks of the stage hypnotist is the production of a cataleptic rigidity of the whole body. The hypnotized subject is then supported by one chair placed under his head and another under his heels. Not only will his body fail to sag, but it will be capable of supporting the weight of a 14-stone man. To heighten the effect, a slimly built girl is usually selected as the subject. Dramatic as this may be, it is unwise to use this particular phenomenon for demonstration purposes. It is bound to involve unwarranted strain upon muscles, joints and ligaments, all of which can be just as easily injured in the hypnotic as in the waking state, for suggested catalepsy is not accompanied by physical changes in the tissues. Consequently bones can be just as easily broken and joints just as easily strained as in the normal state.

4. *Increased muscular performance.* This is largely due to an inability to feel fatigue. Thus in hypnosis we find that the subject can maintain uncomfortable attitudes and perform tasks with much less discomfort and fatigue than when wide awake.

In everyday life, we generally work well below our true capacity and have considerable reserves of power to call upon in times of stress. In the hypnotic state these can be utilized even although they lie outside voluntary effort. Under normal circumstances few of us would be capable of climbing a rope to reach a trap-door in the roof, yet if every exit were blocked by fire and this represented our only means of escape, most of us would be able to manage it. The fact that such reserves can be tapped under hypnosis has been used advantageously in the field of sport. Many athletes have been enabled to attain their maximum effort instead of putting up merely an average performance. It should be remembered, however, that nobody can be caused to exceed their own individual capacity although this is often much greater than would appear from their normal achievements.

5. *Automatic movements.* Not only can muscular action be inhibited by suggestion but it can also be excited and made automatic. If a subject is told that his left arm will gradually rise into the air, it will do so even although he makes no voluntary effort whatever. It will seldom occur to him to resist.

Voluntary movements are not difficult to distinguish from involuntary ones since they are usually smooth and executed with steady ease. On the other hand, even when the subject is passive, involuntary movements are characterized by a certain amount of slowness and jerkiness. This is sometimes greatly exaggerated, and involuntary movements that are executed without the subject's will are often accompanied by strong muscular contractions and trembling. This shows the presence of two antagonistic forces—the suggestion of the hypnotist, and the will of the subject. The latter is fighting against the suggestion that his arm will rise, and this displays itself in the trembling.

A useful test of automatic movement is to rotate the subject's hands around each other in a circular fashion, in front of the body. When his hands are released, the tendency to continue the movement will persist, particularly if he believes that he has to go on turning. If he is then told that he cannot stop, no matter how hard he tries, he will find that although his hands may bump into each other, he will be quite unable to do so. When this phenomenon is elicited, it usually signifies that a medium if not deeper stage of hypnosis has been reached.

Before considering the phenomena affecting the involuntary muscles, there are two specific muscular reactions occurring during the induction of hypnosis which are worthy of attention.

1. *Passive hypnosis.* Occasionally the subject becomes so passive that even the strongest suggestions are insufficient to overcome the muscular relaxation that has occurred. In such cases the arms will drop after having been raised despite all suggestions to the contrary. It may even be difficult to persuade the subject to answer questions.

In most inductions hypnosis will be passive in the early stages. Very often, once the eyes have closed, the head will drop forwards, backwards, or even sideways because the supporting muscles have become so relaxed. Indeed, there are many transitional stages between active and passive hypnosis, and the one can easily pass into the other.

2. *Oculomotor disturbances.* Although in the majority of cases hypnosis is characterized by closure of the eyes, this is by no means essential; but in most cases the eyes do close and, except in somnambulism, cannot be opened again without terminating the hypnosis. Even when the subject remains in a deep trance with his eyes open, he usually feels heaviness in his eyelids and a desire to close them.

The initial closing of the eyes is sometimes gentle, sometimes spasmodic, and is not always complete, but this does not interfere with hypnosis. Once the eyes are closed, the lids frequently quiver, but this is not important and in some instances is a sign of increasing rather than decreasing depth. The eyeballs often roll upwards as the eyes are closing and may remain in this position; in other cases they return to their natural position as soon as the eyes are closed. If they do not only the white sclerotics will be visible if the eyelids are gently raised.

Alterations in the Involuntary Muscles, Organs and Glands

Many functions and activities of the body are quite outside voluntary control. They are controlled and regulated by the unconscious mind acting through the thalamus on the autonomic nervous system. The circulatory, respiratory, alimentary and excretory systems and the endocrine glands are all largely controlled in this manner.

The effects that hypnosis can produce that transcend all voluntary control are important to our understanding of the use of this method in the treatment of psychosomatic conditions, for the activity of both organs and glands can often be influenced by the emotions. Fear, for instance, causes an increase in the secretion of adrenaline and a more rapid heart beat.

Suggestion, particularly in the hypnotic state, can exercise the same effect, which will be greatly heightened if the appropriate emotion is simultaneously evoked. The control by suggestion of the mind and body thus becomes more understandable. The unconscious mind has the power to inhibit or excite the autonomic nervous system, and since in the hypnotic state the unconscious mind becomes more accessible to suggestion, much of the influence exerted under hypnosis becomes explicable. Unfortunately, however, we do not yet know exactly how this comes about.

1. *The Heart.* It has been reported from many sources that the heart rate can be both accelerated and retarded by suggestion during hypnosis.

But the question as to whether or not this can be achieved by direct suggestion alone is still controversial and the available evidence is conflicting. It seems likely that such alterations are usually caused by stimulation of the emotions, but it should be borne in mind that they can be conditioned to verbal cues, once they have resulted from emotional stimulation in the first place.

2. *The Blood-vessels.* Lloyd Tuckey found that the smaller arteries and capillaries were almost invariably contracted in deep hypnosis, so that even deep wounds tended to produce little or no haemorrhage. This is confirmed by many dental surgeons who report a definite decrease in bleeding following the extraction of teeth under deep hypnosis. Subsequent investigations have confirmed the fact that suggestion can exercise a certain amount of influence on the blood-vessels. Forel confirmed the fact that local flushing could be induced by suggestion, and this is not surprising when one considers how easily the vasomotor system is influenced by mental processes. Embarrassment will cause blushing, fear will cause pallor. In the treatment of certain skin conditions I have frequently succeeded in producing a distinct hyperaemia of the skin by direct verbal suggestion accompanied by the lightest stroking of the part to delineate the area. Experiments have also been reported in which local increases and decreases in temperature of one or two degrees centigrade have been achieved by suggestion.

The blood-pressure can also be influenced. Suggestions of relaxation and calmness will lower the blood-pressure and pulse rate, whereas suggestions of excitement and agitation will certainly raise them. Indeed, it is the fact that disturbed emotional states play such an important part in essential hypertension that enables hypnosis to be of value in the treatment of this condition.

3. *The respiratory system.* Vogt found that when the eyes close in response to suggestion during the induction of hypnosis, the respiration rate becomes diminished as the subject experiences a feeling of restful calm. As hypnosis proceeds the breathing becomes slower and more superficial, although it deepens both at the commencement and the termination of the hypnotic state.

Suggestion can also produce considerable variations of both respiration rate and respiratory excursion. Increases in pulmonary ventilation up to 50 per cent have been obtained in a resting hypnotized subject to whom it had been suggested that heavy work was being performed. But though these facts are of some significance in contributing to the success of hypnosis in the treatment of bronchial asthma and bronchospasm, they are not as important as its ability to control the emotional factors underlying the attacks.

4. *The alimentary system.* It has been shown that when a deeply hypnotized subject was told that he was eating an imaginary meal of beef and protein, this suggestion produced an increased secretion of gastric juice. Similarly, when imaginary fats were substituted for the protein, contraction of the gall-bladder followed, accompanied by an increased flow of lipase and bile. These facts are hardly surprising since the mere suggestion of an appetizing meal can cause our mouths to water. It has also been reported that increased and decreased gastric acidity could be produced by suggestions of enjoyment or disgust. Bergman believed that in a case of hyperchlorhydria he succeeded in greatly reducing the acidity and secretion of the gastric juice through therapeutic suggestion.

Peristalsis can frequently be influenced very strongly and efficiently by suggestion, and because of this the bowel actions can often be regulated under hypnosis. If a very deeply hypnotized subject is told that his bowels will act at a specified time, the suggestion is quite likely to succeed. Indeed, when the hypnosis is accompanied by an amnesia, it will seldom fail. It is even possible to arrest the action of aperient drugs by suggestion, although this is less frequent. For instance, a patient has been successfully told that a large dose of castor oil would not take effect for 48 hours. Water has also been given to the hypnotic subject and represented either as a strong purgative or emetic. In each case, the appropriate reaction usually followed.

5. *The secretions.* Secretion of both saliva and perspiration have been reported to have been induced by suggestion. Under hypnosis the eyes can be caused to water if it is suggested to the patient that he is smelling an onion. Similarly, the secretion of tears can be induced by the suggestion of a strong emotion.

Lactation can also be facilitated by hypnotic suggestion and the secretion of milk increased to a considerable extent. However it seems to be doubtful whether the secretion of urine can be affected by suggestion, since in many of the cases reported it is the act of micturition and not that of secretion that has been modified.

6. *Changes in metabolism.* When it is suggested to a deeply hypnotized subject that he has not eaten anything for several days, a fall in blood-sugar results. If it is then suggested that he is enjoying an imaginary

meal of pastry, cream cakes and sugar, a rise in blood-sugar will occur, although he has actually eaten nothing. The blood-sugar level is always increased by adrenaline, so whenever strong emotions such as terror or anger are aroused, more adrenaline is released into the blood-stream and the blood-sugar rises to mobilize the body for action and provide a sufficient fuel supply for anticipated increased muscular demands. Since emotional states such as these can easily be produced by hypnotic suggestion with the consequent release of adrenaline, its effect upon the blood-sugar becomes quite understandable.

7. *Anatomical and biochemical changes.* It would be foolish to deny the possibility of effecting physical change by means of hypnosis, but gullibility should be avoided since the hypnotic subject, knowing that certain things are expected of him, may try to comply with the hypnotist's demands and later develop an amnesia for his actions. There is no doubt, however, that organic changes can be brought about by mental processes.

Menstruation can often be induced or arrested by hypnotic suggestion. This is hardly surprising when one realizes how often psychical influences in everyday life can change the pattern. For instance periods not infrequently become irregular in women who are anxious and apprehensive, as when awaiting a surgical operation.

Bleeding of the nose and skin resulting from suggestion, even when the most elaborate precautions have been taken to prevent the subject from causing a wound, have been reported by many of the older hypnotists. Such phenomena bear a strong resemblance to the stigmata recognized by the Roman Catholic Church when bleeding of the skin is said to occur in sites corresponding to the wounds of Christ. Such reports as these should always be accepted with caution in view of the ever-existing possibility of unconscious deception.

Burns, or marks resembling them, have been reported by many observers. In a typical experiment, a pencil was pressed upon the skin in the morning and the subject was told that it was red-hot and that his skin was being burned. He was then awakened, and after the interval of several hours a blister appeared on the skin in the exact shape of the pencil.

Weals have also been produced by hypnotic suggestion, but it should not be forgotten that some people have been known to develop them under conditions of mental excitement without any hypnosis. It has also been reported in recent years that they have occurred spontaneously in the course of profound emotional drug-induced abreactions. Obviously, reports of these kinds of hypnotic experiment should be received with a certain amount of reserve. Moll states that whilst it is not denied that anatomical changes can be produced by suggestion, *the evidence of such changes having taken place must be unimpeachable before it can be accepted.* Such results, if and when they occur, can only be interpreted as an autonomic response to an emotional stimulus.

Modification of allergic skin responses. It has been known for many years that the symptoms of both asthma and hay-fever could be relieved by direct suggestion under hypnosis. In 1958 A. A. Mason and S. Black described how allergic skin responses were abolished during the treatment of a case of asthma and hay-fever by hypnosis. In addition to the relief of the patient's symptoms, the skin reactions to injected pollens also disappeared. A Prausnitz-Kustner reaction was performed and when the patient's serum was injected into the arm of a non-sensitive volunteer, his skin produced allergic reactions to the allergens to which the patient was now apparently insensitive, proving that although the patient's allergic symptoms had been abolished by hypnotic suggestion, her blood remained unchanged.

In 1963 Black, Humphrey and Niven reported four cases in which the Mantoux reaction was inhibited by direct suggestion under hypnosis. Although histologically there was no observable change in the degree of cellular infiltration, there was evidence that the exudation of fluid had been inhibited. They thus concluded that the Mantoux-positive reaction could be inhibited by direct suggestion under hypnosis to give a Mantoux-negative result, and that a vascular constituent of the reaction is probably involved in the mechanism of inhibition.

CHAPTER 12

Alterations in the Sense Organs: Hypnotic Analgesia

Alterations in the Sense Organs

In deep hypnosis the five special senses, sight, hearing, smell, taste and touch, can all be influenced by suggestion, and the subject's perception through any one of them may be either increased or diminished.

1. *Sight.* The power of vision can often be increased far beyond the subject's normal voluntary effort. In a typical experiment, it is first established that a very short-sighted person, without his glasses, cannot read a printed page at a greater distance than 12 inches. With his glasses he can read the same size of print at the distance of 1 to 2 yards. Under deep hypnosis, he is then told that his sight without glasses will become much keener than normal and that he will be able to read at a much greater distance, but when the hypnotist raps upon the table his sight will immediately revert to normal again. He then opens his eyes whilst still remaining in the trance state, and it will be found that he is able to read a different page of the same print at a distance of over 2 yards *without glasses.* As he continues to read the hypnotist unexpectedly raps upon the table and the subject will immediately break off in the middle of a sentence and will be quite unable to continue until the page is brought to within a distance of 12 inches, which represents his normal performance.

Similarly, the power of vision can be decreased and even abolished if suggestions of partial or total blindness are made. Electro-encephalograph tracings reveal the fact that whenever it was suggested that the subject could not see brain-waves appeared which were identical with those found in the case of a totally blind person, or in one whose eyes were shut. Erickson has also succeeded in inducing colour-blindness through the use of hypnotic suggestion.

2. *Hearing.* This can be rendered much more acute in the hypnotic state. A deeply hypnotized subject can sometimes hear a clock ticking

in an adjoining room which is quite inaudible to him in the waking state, and which nobody else can hear. In fact, it can be stopped and started and the subject will be able to tell exactly when this occurs. Such a case has been described by A. A. Mason, who considers that it is probably due to the fact that, in the hypnotized subject, all external sensory stimuli are minimized so that he is able to bring the whole of his concentration to bear upon whatever task he is called upon to perform. In other words, he hears better because he has nothing to distract him.

Partial or even total deafness can also be induced by hypnotic suggestion. In the case of total deafness, a gun can be fired unexpectedly behind the subject, and not only will he show no sign of having heard anything but he will display no rise of blood-pressure whatever. It should be remembered, however, that in such a case he will also be unable to hear the hypnotist's voice and will lose contact completely unless suitable precautions have been taken. Consequently, before any such experiments are made, the subject should always be given the suggestion that his hearing will become normal again upon a given signal, such as a tap upon his shoulder, in which case he will awaken with his function fully restored.

Both blindness and deafness induced by suggestion are purely mental phenomena. A simple command will suffice to restore the functions of both sight and hearing. The corresponding organ of sense still performs its usual functions, but the impressions and stimuli fail to reach consciousness.

3. *Smell.* The older hypnotists claimed that the sense of smell could be greatly increased by hypnotic suggestion. An acute sense of smell is known to be normal in many animals for a dog will easily recognize his master by the scent. It was held that under certain circumstances this keenness of scent could be attained by human beings as the result of strong suggestion.

Experiments have been described in which gloves and handkerchiefs have been restored to their rightful owners who were guided only by a sense of smell. Braid successfully conducted such experiments but found that when the subject's nose was stopped up all attempts failed. Conversely, the sense of smell can also be diminished or even abolished by suggestion in the deep-trance state, so that irritating vapours can be inhaled without the slightest discomfort.

4. *Taste.* This can be both increased and diminished in hypnosis. A

complete absence of taste can be suggested, or specific taste-sensations only can be obliterated. With hypnotic suggestion, it has been shown to be possible to equalize the taste of sweetness and bitterness to an appreciable extent, and that a tasteless fluid like water can be made to acquire sweetness or bitterness sufficiently to effect measurable changes in salivation.

5. *Touch.* Both Bramwell and Moll claim that the tactile sense can be intensified in hypnosis, and that an improvement in two-point discrimination can be observed (the two points of a compass are used for measuring the least distance between them at which they may be felt as two separate points). Moll states that they can usually be distinguished at a less distance in hypnosis than in the waking state, but Hull does not consider this claim to be valid. Tactual sensibility can also be diminished, or even abolished completely by hypnotic suggestion.

Hypnotic Analgesia and Anaesthesia

There is no doubt that one of the most convincing phenomena that can be produced to demonstrate the validity of hypnosis to a sceptical observer is the ability to abolish all sense of pain. Strictly speaking, the correct term for the loss of feeling of pain is analgesia, for the word anaesthesia really implies a total loss of sensory perception, including touch. Although in common usage the two terms are often employed as if they were interchangeable. I shall refer to loss of the sensation of pain as analgesia, confining anaesthesia to its correct definition.

Unfortunately complete analgesia can only be obtained in rather less than 20 per cent of subjects, and its achievement is usually taken to be a sign that a deep or even somnambulistic trance has occurred. There are, however, a number of subjects who will display partial analgesia of varying degrees when medium depth only has been attained. But in light hypnosis the appreciation of pain generally remains unaltered by suggestion.

Deep-trance Analgesia

In deep hypnosis, since the analgesia is often total and complete, major surgery can sometimes be carried out with no other form of anaesthetic. Amputation of limbs and the removal of breasts have been performed quite painlessly, and in the dental field impacted wisdom teeth have been easily and effectively dealt with. Hypnosis has an advantage over chemical anaesthetic agents that it produces no toxic effects whatever. It is consequently most useful in dealing with patients who are shocked and severely ill. Moreover, the patient's protective reflexes remain unaltered throughout, and should he vomit, the cough reflex is not abolished. He will be in no danger of being burned, for if fluids or hot-water bottles are too hot when he is back in the ward, he will be able to complain about them. He can either swallow blood or spit it out, and if he wants a drink he can safely be given one. In addition to this, post-operative pain or discomfort can readily be relieved and the patient will become ambulant more quickly, thus avoiding chest or other post-operative complications.

When limbs or joints have been operated upon, the patient can be enabled to move them more readily without pain and function is likely to be restored more rapidly. Conversely, in plastic surgery when skin-grafting has been performed, a limb can be totally immobilized in a fixed position by post-hypnotic suggestion. Indeed, such a position can be maintained with a minimum of discomfort for many days or weeks whilst the graft is taking effect.

In view of all these advantages, it is obvious that hypnosis would be the ideal anaesthetic agent were it not for the fact that less than one in every five people are capable of this degree of analgesia. Consequently the use of hypnosis in major surgery remains at present little more than a medical curiosity, and if its value were confined to this field only it might quite easily be discarded.

Medium-trance Analgesia

The degree of analgesia that can be obtained in medium-depth hypnosis may vary from slight to considerable. It is consequently in the medium-trance patient that the greatest use of hypnotic analgesia can be appreciated. Whilst no major surgery can be performed, many minor surgical procedures can be undertaken quite painlessly, probably in some 30 to 40 per cent of medium-depth patients. Pain can either be removed or greatly diminished in such procedures as the dressing of burns, lumbar or abdominal punctures, and certain painful manipulations of injured parts. Hypnotic analgesia can also be of value in conservative dental work such as painful fillings, particularly when the patient dreads the injection of a local anaesthetic, for even should the analgesia obtained be minimal it will often suffice to get him to tolerate the dreaded injection. Sometimes the pain from chronic incurable disease such as cancer can be controlled and diminished in the early stages, thus deferring the need for potent analgesic drugs. But the greatest value of hypnosis by far lies in its ability to produce both mental and physical relaxation and to rid the patient of fear and anxiety prior to an operation. Indeed the reduction of the fear-tension-expectancy syndrome renders it most useful to the general practitioner, the dental surgeon, the midwife and the nurse. Instead of becoming frightened, over-anxious and demoralized, the patient can be rendered calm, co-operative, and much less apprehensive of what lies ahead. The use of hypnosis in obstetrics and for anaesthesia is more fully discussed in Chapter 21.

Sensitivity to Pain

The pain threshold varies tremendously from individual to individual. Some people dread and anticipate pain to such an extent that the moment they are touched they translate this into a feeling of pain. This type of patient is particularly likely to be seen in the dental surgery, and is the kind of person in whom the combination of hypnosis and local analgesia is often most effective.

Most of us have seen a line of patients at a clinic waiting with their arms bared to receive an inoculation. The first feels just a normal prick, the second doesn't feel anything at all, but the third faints either immediately before or after receiving the injection. The actual injection, the method of administration, and even the size of needle are identical in each case. The difference is to be found in the individual patient, for the one who faints is usually tensed up with fear, anxiety and anticipation. This kind of patient is extremely difficult to deal with, and is probably more frequently seen by the dental surgeon than by the doctor. This is the patient who is so terrified by the thought of the dental chair that he will postpone his visit as long as he possibly can, and only turn up once in two years instead of every six months. Even then, he is quite likely to close his mouth as soon as he is approached with the dental drill. Hypnosis can be invaluable in dealing with this type of patient, for with its aid he can be taught to relax physically, and this in itself greatly reduces and relieves mental tension. Used in this way hypnosis can produce relaxed, physically comfortable, co-operative patients who are rendered much more at ease; even should no analgesia be obtained the patient will still be much easier to work upon with the use of orthodox procedures. If an anaesthetic is required, the patient will remain calm and take it without difficulty, so that much less of the anaesthetic agent is likely to be needed. On the other hand, the emotionally disturbed patient will not only require more, but even then the anaesthetic will seldom run smoothly.

The Nature of Hypnotic Analgesia

Suppose an operation has been apparently performed painlessly under deep hypnosis, and when the patient is asked about it afterwards, he says he felt no pain at all. Two very significant questions are bound to arise. Firstly, did he actually feel no pain, or is he merely obliging the hypnotist by saying that he didn't? Secondly, has there been a complete loss of memory for the pain rather than an actual loss of pain itself? In the first case the analgesia would be a simulated one, and in the second case an amnesia for pain rather than a true absence of sensation. In neither instance would the analgesia be a true one. A relatively simple test will establish whether the patient is actually experiencing pain and simply simulating analgesia. If he is really feeling pain under hypnosis his pulse rate will rise and his blood-pressure rise as the needle unexpectedly pierces his skin.

Most hypnotized subjects in whom analgesia is induced have neither an increase in pulse rate nor a rise in blood-pressure, showing that the analgesia is a true one; the few that do have probably felt pain and have developed an amnesia for it afterwards. Even this is not likely to produce any harmful effect, since under chemical anaesthesia it is believed that pain is felt but is immediately forgotten. Laboratory investigations into hypnotic analgesia have demonstrated that no pain is felt, and electro-encephalograms show that the pain threshold is raised during hypnosis. Estabrooks' experiments with a faradic-brush have already been referred to (p. 120).

The 'Distraction' Theory of Hypnotic Analgesia

This is by far the simplest and most credible of the many theories put forward to explain how hypnotic analgesia is produced.

When a patient has music played to him through head-phones whilst he is being operated upon, it has been found that a mixture of gas and oxygen in equal parts will suffice to permit the operation to be effected in comfort. There is certainly not enough gas in this mixture to produce any marked degree of analgesia, yet many minor but painful surgical operations can be carried out comfortably under these conditions. Moreover, it has been noticed that when the music was temporarily stopped in the middle of the operation, the patient immediately showed signs of restlessness and obviously disliked what was taking place, so that the music was definitely having a contributory effect.

Many examples can be quoted from everyday life where, in the heat of the moment, a serious injury will pass unnoticed until the excitement has died down. Soldiers have been seriously wounded in battle but have failed to realize the extent of their injuries until the crisis was past. Another use of the ' distraction ' principle is seen in hospitals, where a nurse will slap a patient on the buttock whilst another nurse simultaneously plunges in the hypodermic needle. And in the old days, the fair-ground dentist would regularly extract teeth without anaesthesia to the banging of a big drum. It used to be thought that this simply drowned the cries of the patient, but it now seems likely that it served to distract his attention and thus diminished his sensitivity to pain.

The Distribution of Hypnotic Analgesia

Hypnotic analgesias *never* correspond to any anatomical distribution. They always coincide with the subject's notion of function, and follow his own idea as to where the loss of pain should occur. Most individuals interpret the word ' arm ' as signifying the whole of the upper limb, so if they are told they will lose all sensation in an arm, they will develop analgesia extending from the shoulder to the wrist. Under similar circumstances, however, a medical student, a nurse or even a person trained in first-aid would only lose sensation from the shoulder to the elbow, since they regard the lower part of the limb as the ' fore-arm '. Consequently, whenever hypnotic analgesia is to be induced, the exact area that is to be rendered anaesthetic must be clearly indicated to the subject. Wherever possible it should be stroked, or even swabbed with spirit or ether to make it feel cold, so that the subject is in no doubt at all as to where the analgesia is to be produced. If this is omitted he will usually produce a ' glove and stocking ' anaesthesia which corresponds exactly to the type that is seen in the hysterical patient. When dental analgesia is required the operator should run his finger along the gum to indicate quite clearly the exact area that is to be made analgesic.

It should never be forgotten that unless some prolongation of hypnotically induced analgesia is needed to relieve post-operative pain, in which case a time limit can be imposed, the analgesia should always be removed before the patient is awakened.

The Induction of Hypnotic Analgesia

This is accomplished by repeated suggestions of progressive loss of sensation in the desired area:

You are now in so deep a sleep . . . that presently, all the feeling is going to disappear from your left hand.

You will not be able to feel anything in your left hand . . . just think of your left hand becoming quite numb . . . as if it had gone to sleep.
Gradually . . . it is becoming more and more numb . . . and all the feeling is going out of it.
And as I go on talking to you . . . your left hand is beginning to feel colder and colder . . . as if it were surrounded with ice.
Just picture your hand being packed round with ice . . . and as you do so . . . it is feeling colder and colder . . . more and more numb and insensitive.
As soon as you feel your hand becoming cold and numb . . . please lift up your other hand.

(After a brief interval during which these suggestions are repeated, the subject's hand rises.)

Your hand has now become so cold and numb . . . that you are losing all feeling in it.
Soon, you will not be able to feel any pain in it at all . . . you will feel no pain at all.
In a moment or two . . . I am going to count slowly up to *three*.
And when I reach the count of *three* . . . *your hand will be completely insensitive to pain . . . and you will be able to feel no pain at all in your hand.*
One . . . Colder and colder . . . more and more numb and insensitive . . . losing all sensation of pain.
Two . . . Your hand is now quite numb and dead . . . there is no feeling in it at all . . . just as if it had gone to sleep.
Three . . . Your hand is completely numb . . . cold . . . and insensitive . . . *you cannot feel any pain in it at all.*

The right hand, upon which the subject has *not* been told to concentrate, is then pricked with a hypodermic needle. The subject usually flinches. The left hand is then pricked, and if the subject neither moves nor flinches some degree of analgesia has been obtained. Further firmer pricking without eliciting any response will establish the extent of the analgesia. If it is complete, the needle may be firmly driven through a fold of the skin without the slightest evidence of pain being felt. Once this demonstration is completed, unless the analgesia is required for therapeutic purposes, it must be removed before the subject is awakened.

In a few moments . . . your left hand will become quite normal again.
It is becoming warmer and warmer . . . and all the feeling of numbness is leaving it . . . and it is now quite normal again . . . just the same as your other hand.
All the sensation has returned . . . and you can now feel everything . . . just the same as with your other hand.

Wolberg finds it advantageous to produce a cutaneous hyperaesthesia before attempting to induce analgesia. This enables the subject to make a comparison between the hypersensitive part and the one that is being anaesthetized. This facilitates the latter process by emphasizing the difference between them.

> Imagine you are walking down a corridor . . . at the end of which you can see a bucket of hot water.
> You know it's hot . . . because you can see the steam rising from the water.
> As soon as you can picture that bucket . . . as soon as you can see it quite clearly in your mind . . . please lift up your left hand.

(The subject's hand slowly rises.)

> Put your hand down again.
> Now, you wonder how hot the water is . . . so you walk over to the bucket . . . and plunge your right hand in the hot water.
> Picture this vividly in your mind . . . so that you will feel the heat.
> Your hand is beginning to smart . . . it feels tender and painful.
> Your hand is tingling . . . and feels warm and tender.
> As soon as you feel these sensations . . . please lift up your left hand again.

(Once again, the subject's hand rises.)

> Right. Put your hand down again.
> Now, I'm going to touch your right hand with a needle.
> Your right hand is so tender and sensitive . . . that it feels just like a stab from a knife.
> So tender and sensitive . . . it feels terribly painful.
> See . . . how tender and painful it feels.
> You'll notice the difference when I touch this hand . . . and when I touch the other hand with the needle.
> I'm now going to touch the other hand . . . now this one, again.
> See the difference!

Good subjects will actually flinch with pain when the hand is touched with the needle. It is important to get the subject to acknowledge that he felt at least some difference in the sensation between the two hands. If he feels no difference, he is told that this requires practice and that he will be able to detect it at his next session.

Occasionally, however, this technique does not succeed and no hyper-sensitivity is produced. In this case, the subject should always be questioned about his difficulties, sometimes with surprising results. A colleague of mine discovered that his patient had no difficulty at all in picturing the bucket of hot water, but was then told ' Surely you didn't think I'd be stupid enough to plunge my hand into water that hot, without cooling it down?'

If successful, an attempt may then be made to induce analgesia. Since this is very rarely complete at the first session, it is necessary to get the subject to admit to some degree of relative insensitivity.

> You'll notice that whilst your right hand is sensitive . . . your left hand is becoming more and more insensitive.
>
> Now, I want you to imagine that you are consulting your doctor because you have a boil on the forefinger of your left hand.
>
> He is going to inject a local anaesthetic around your wrist . . . to cause a wrist-block and remove the pain . . . like this.

(The wrist is then circled with slight needle-pricks.)

> Gradually your left hand is becoming number and number . . . and soon it will become so numb and insensitive . . . you will be able to feel no pain . . . compared with your right hand.
>
> All the feeling will leave your hand . . . and it will become more and more numb.
>
> As you concentrate on your left hand . . . try to imagine that you are wearing a thick, heavy leather glove on your left hand.
>
> As soon as you can picture yourself wearing that glove . . . and feel as if the glove is on your hand . . . please lift up your hand.

(After some delay, during which the suggestions are repeated, the subject's hand eventually rises.)

> Put your hand down, again.
>
> Your hand now feels as if you are wearing a thick, heavy, leather glove . . . so that when I touch it with a needle . . . it will feel just as if I am touching leather.
>
> You will feel no pain at all . . . just a dull feeling.
>
> Now, I'm going to show you the difference, by first touching your right hand . . . the sensitive one . . . and then the left one.
>
> Do you see the difference ?
>
> And now, your hand is becoming more and more numb . . . more and more insensitive . . . and all sensations of pain are disappearing completely.
>
> This dull feeling is spreading over your whole hand . . . over the back of your hand . . . your fingers and thumb . . . over the front of your hand.
>
> This feeling is becoming duller and duller . . . your hand is beginning to feel as if it were made of wood.
>
> I can stick a needle in it . . . and you will feel no real pain.
>
> It has become so numb and insensitive . . . that you can feel no real pain at all.

(The hand is now pricked, and the subject questioned.)

See how numb it feels!

(Should the subject say that he feels pain, he must be reassured.)

Although you still feel slight pain . . . it is less than in the other hand, isn't it ?

(He will usually admit to feeling a difference.)

That's good . . . it shows that the suggestions are beginning to work.
Let yourself relax completely . . . and you will fall into an even deeper sleep.
And next time you come . . . you will not only fall into a deeper, deeper sleep . . . but the feeling in your hand will disappear completely.

Demonstrations of Hypnotic Analgesia

Experiment 1. A subject is induced into deep hypnosis, his sleeve rolled up, and a circle of about two to three inches diameter drawn on his fore-arm. He remains lying back in the chair, *with his eyes closed*. He is then told: ' When I count up to five, inside that circle your arm will become cold and numb. You will be able to feel no pain at all . . . *inside the circle*. The rest of your arm will remain normal . . . and you will be able to feel pain everywhere else. But, inside the circle . . . you will not be able to feel pain.'

First, the arm is pricked *well inside the circle*, and the subject takes no notice. Then it is firmly pricked again, *well outside the circle*, and the subject flinches. Finally, it is firmly pricked again, *inside the circle but close to the perimeter*, and the subject flinches again. This experiment shows that because he cannot see the circle, the subject is not quite sure where it is, and is thus unable to produce an accurately defined area of analgesia.

Experiment 2. The same subject is then told to open his eyes without waking up from his trance, that he will be able to see quite clearly but will not wake up. He is then told to look at the circle and that once again he will not be able to feel any pain inside the circle.

His arm is then firmly pricked again, *inside the circle*, but this time it will not matter where his arm is pricked, even up to the periphery of the circle. He will show no response whatever. When the arm is pricked, *outside the circle* the subject will flinch, but when it is pricked *inside the circle, no matter how close to the perimeter*, he will fail to display any reaction at all. This demonstrates the fact that, with his eyes open, the subject is now able to define accurately the precise area that is to become analgesic. It thus emphasizes the fact that if the subject is to produce the desired analgesia he must be left in no doubt as to exactly where it is to take effect. Methods of ensuring this have already been mentioned on page 143.

Experiment 3. The same deeply hypnotized subject is told that his arm has become normal again and that the feeling has returned. He is then told: ' When you, yourself, count up to three . . . your arm inside the circle will become quite numb and insensitive to pain.

' You will be able to prick yourself . . . but you will be able to feel no pain at all . . . *inside the circle.*

' But when you count backwards . . . from three to one . . . your arm will return to normal . . . and you will feel pain everywhere in your arm.'

This demonstrates the fact that the subject can be enabled to produce and abolish analgesia for himself upon a given signal. He can also be taught how to do this, to a strictly limited extent, in the waking state as the result of post-hypnotic suggestion.

Experiment 4. Before he is finally awakened, the subject is given the following instructions: ' You will be able to produce this same numbness for yourself . . . after you wake up. *For the next five minutes only* . . . you will be able to make any part of your body that you wish, become completely numb and insensitive to pain.

' When you wish to produce numbness . . . you will be able to do so by counting . . . one . . . two . . . three.

' When you wish to remove the numbness and restore the part to normal . . . you will be able to do so by counting backwards . . . three . . . two . . . one.'

The ability on the part of a good subject to produce self-induced analgesias must always be severely restricted, either to a limited period of time, or to a specific situation or occasion. Hence the five-minute spell imposed above. The subject must never be allowed to leave with the ability to relieve pain in himself for an indefinite period. He might otherwise mask some serious condition such as acute appendicitis, with the grave danger of subsequent perforation.

On the other hand, such a subject can be safely told that he will always be able to produce analgesia for himself *whenever he sits in his dentist's chair*, but under no other circumstances. In this case a very useful procedure is for him to produce complete analgesia of his forefinger. He will then rub the desired area of his gum with this finger, and as he does so the finger will return to normal and the gum will become completely insensitive and analgesic. In other words, the analgesia will become transferred from his finger to his gum. It has been claimed that when this transference occurs, a more profound analgesia is likely to result.

The use of self-induced analgesia in child-birth is discussed on page 307.

Paraesthesias

Numbness, tingling, itching, sensations of coldness, and increased sensitivity to pain, pressure, temperature and touch may be relatively easy to induce under hypnosis. Paraesthesias of vision, taste and smell can also be suggested. A somnambulist can be told that when he smokes a cigarette, he will get a horrible taste in his mouth, just like dead leaves. When he tries to smoke after he wakes up, he will only be able to take one or two puffs before he throws the cigarette away in disgust (*see also* p. 275).

CHAPTER 13

Somnambulism and the Psychological Phenomena of Hypnosis

All kinds of sense-delusions can be produced in deep hypnotic states, many of which are so remarkable that anyone seeing them for the first time may well be excused for doubting the reality of the phenomena. In everyday life, we all depend so completely upon our sense organs that it seems incredible that a few words or phrases can succeed in placing the hypnotic subject in entirely different surroundings. But before many phenomena such as these can be elicited, a very deep or even somnambulistic trance is usually essential.

Somnambulism

This is generally considered to be one of the deepest stages of hypnosis, and one of the most reliable tests of this condition is to cause the subject to open his eyes without awakening from his trance. He will be able to see quite clearly, to talk, and to walk about whilst still remaining deeply hypnotized, and will continue to carry out all the suggestions made to him by the hypnotist. Occasionally, but not very often, the subject may appear drowsy in the somnambulistic state; this can easily be remedied if suggestions of alertness are given to him when he will become just as wide awake as in his normal state. Indeed, it can sometimes be very difficult to tell whether a good somnambule is actually in a hypnotic state or not, as Estabrooks has pointed out. Possibly the only criterion by which this may be judged is the extent to which the subject will respond to suggestion. Other tests of somnambulism are found in the subject's ability to produce hallucinations, to carry out bizarre and complicated post-hypnotic suggestions, to establish major anaesthesia to pain, and to produce complete amnesia for the events of the trance state. Some of these phenomena have already been discussed, but others, such as illusions and hallucinations, must now be considered in some detail.

Unfortunately, under ordinary circumstances only some 15 to 20 per cent of the population are capable of achieving somnambulistic trances, and in medical work the average will probably prove to be no more than one person in ten. Generally speaking, it can be said that children are more readily induced into somnambulism than adults, and people who are natural sleep-walkers or automatic writers will often prove to be potential somnambules. With careful training, however, these figures can be considerably improved upon. Erickson has succeeded in inducing somnambulism in difficult subjects only after several hours of continuous sleep suggestions, but very few hypnotists possess either his patience or the necessary skill to induce these deep states in average individuals.

Illusions and Hallucinations

Delusions of the senses are usually classified as ' *illusions* ' or ' *hallucinations* ', and before considering them, it is as well to define exactly what is meant by these terms: *a delusion* is a false belief, *an illusion* is a false interpretation of an existing object, and *a hallucination* is the perception of an object or person where nothing really exists.

For instance, if a cushion is taken for a cat, we speak of an illusion. But if a cat is perceived when there is actually nothing there, we call it a hallucination. On the whole, it is easier to induce an illusion than a hallucination, for in the absence of an external object the suggestion will frequently fail. Both illusions and hallucinations can be produced in connection with any of the five senses, and may be either positive or negative. If a subject is told that he can see something that is not really there, the resulting hallucination is a positive one, but when he is told that he cannot see something that is actually present, a negative hallucination is produced. However, it should be noted that in order not to see something that is really there, the object must first be perceived before it can be abolished, although this is an unconscious perception of which the subject is unaware.

Moll describes a convincing experiment which tends to prove that the subject recognizes the object of a negative hallucination, even though there is no conscious perception of it. He took a match and marked it with a spot of ink, and suggested to a somnambulistic subject that this match would become invisible. He then took twenty-nine other matches and put the whole thirty on the table in such a manner that the subject could still see the ink spot.

When asked how many matches were on the table, the subject replied, ' Twenty-nine '. Whilst his back was turned, the marked match was ' moved in such a way that the ink spot could no longer be seen.

The subject once again counted the matches and said there were now thirty of them on the table. This shows clearly that the marked match could only remain invisible as long as the subject could distinguish it from the others. It seems certain that in negative hallucinations the subject always retains a dim consciousness of the true situation.

It is generally considered that the negative hallucination is probably the deepest of all hypnotic phenomena, and as such is the most difficult to obtain.

1. *Positive hallucinations.* Hallucinations of sight are usually more readily induced when the subject's eyes remain closed. He will then see objects or persons with his eyes shut exactly as he does in dreams. It will even seem to him that his eyes are open since we are all unaware in our dreams that our eyes are shut. It should be noted, however, that hallucinations of sight and hearing are only likely to succeed when very deep trance states have been achieved. Generally speaking, it is found that the senses of taste and touch are more easily influenced than others. All the organs of sense can be deceived in this way. A sudden blow upon a desk may be interpreted as a gun shot. A subject can be induced to hear music in the absence of any external stimulus. Water may be represented as neat whisky, and its consumption will be followed by the usual manifestations of insobriety. Told that a raw potato is an apple, the subject will eat it with every appearance of enjoyment, and strong ammonia will be smelt with pleasure if it has been presented as Eau-de-Cologne. If given a rubber ball for an onion, when the subject smells it his eyes will fill with tears.

The expression on the subject's face as he complies with such suggestions corresponds exactly with what one would expect had the real article been employed and the thoroughness of the deception is clearly reflected in his reactions. No epicure could show more delight than does the hypnotic who sits down to a hallucinated meal of his favourite dishes.

The stage hypnotist depends upon the production of hallucinations such as these for the entertainment value of his performance, but it cannot be too strongly emphasized that hallucinations of this kind which violate the dignity of the subject should never be indulged in by the medical profession. Even when demonstrating hallucinations for scientific purposes the approval of the subject should be sought before any experiments are made and he should always be treated with the same consideration and respect that he would receive if he were awake. Although mild hallucinations are sometimes possible in medium-depth hypnosis, one can be sure that the more bizarre and complex they become, the deeper the trance that has been achieved.

When the deeper somnambulistic stages have been reached, the subject is able to open his eyes without awakening from his trance. In order to test this, I usually instruct him in the following manner:

> In a few moments . . . when I count up to *five* . . . you will open your eyes . . . but you will *not* wake up from this deep sleep.
> You will be able to see quite clearly . . . but you will still remain very, very deeply asleep.
> It may be that things will seem a little hazy or blurred at first . . . but in a few moments . . . everything will become quite clear . . . although you will still remain in this very, very deep sleep.
> You will be able to see clearly . . . everything that I point out to you!

In this state positive visual hallucinations can be produced which will evoke exactly the same emotional reactions and behaviour that would be expected were the stimulus a real one. The subject will shrink with terror when told that he is confronted with a tiger, or will pick up and fondle a cat.

Hallucinations can also be produced as a result of post-hypnotic suggestion. A subject can be told during hypnosis that at 12 o'clock tomorrow morning his forehead will begin to itch and will continue to do so until he relieves it by rubbing. This will actually occur at the stated time.

2. *Negative hallucinations.* These are possible only in the deepest somnambulistic states, and even then the instructions given to the subject have to be very carefully and precisely worded. When successful, he will be unable to recognize the presence of either an object or a person with which he is confronted. The importance of framing suggestions explicitly with the utmost care is shown in the two following examples, which produce widely different results.

1. If the subject is told: ' From now on you will only be able to see me. You will not be able to see Mr Blank although he is still here ', he will be able to talk to Mr Blank, to answer his questions, and even be able to feel him. But he will *not* be able to see him.

2. If, on the other hand, the subject is told: ' After you wake up Mr Blank will have disappeared completely. You will not be able to see Mr Blank, to hear Mr Blank or to feel Mr Blank ', he will stare straight at the chair in which Mr Blank is sitting and ask where he has gone. If spoken to by Mr Blank he will be unable to hear him, and if he is asked

to examine the chair still occupied by Mr Blank he will feel something there but will be unable to interpret it correctly and will probably suggest that Mr Blank has left his overcoat on the chair.

When a fountain-pen is held in front of the subject's eyes, he will recognize it, but if it is then relinquished to Mr Blank, one of two things will happen according to the interpretation he puts upon it. If he then considers that when Mr Blank is holding it, it has become his property and consequently a part of him, the pen will vanish completely. But if he still interprets the pen as belonging to someone else, it will appear to him to be floating unsupported in the air. In this particular experiment the senses of vision, hearing, and touch are all simultaneously affected.

Interesting although they may be, hallucinations are not solely of academic interest and sometimes have therapeutic applications. Crystal and mirror-gazing under hypnosis are both forms of visual hallucination. When instructed to gaze into the crystal or mirror, the subject will both see and describe scenes that arise from his own unconscious conflicts and emotional disturbances. This technique is frequently used in hypno-analysis.

As in the case of hypnotic analgesia, hallucinations that have been induced must always be removed before the subject is awakened and allowed to leave.

Methods of producing hallucinations. Although in somnambulism it is not difficult to enable the subject to remain in his trance with his eyes open, it is not always easy to get him to hallucinate objects or persons under these conditions. Wolberg has described two excellent techniques for achieving these results.

1. The hypnotist tells the subject that he is going to pick up a small bottle, and to picture him doing so. He will feel curious as to what is in the bottle and will notice a flower on the label. He will realize that the bottle contains perfume and he will picture a flower. As he does so, he will smell the perfume. The hypnotist then places the bottle under the subject's nose whilst simultaneously removing a cork from an actual bottle to convey the necessary sound. The subject is then told that as soon as he smells the perfume, he is to raise his hand. This experiment is carried out with the subject's eyes closed, and when successful produces a positive hallucination of smell.

2. The hypnotist then teaches the subject how to open his eyes without awakening, by giving him the following suggestions.

I want you to imagine that I am holding a bottle of water in front of your eyes.
You will notice that it is colourless . . . but as you watch it . . . it is gradually becoming pinker and pinker . . . and changing to a reddish colour.
As soon as you see the colour changing . . . please raise your hand.

(As soon as the subject's hand rises, the suggestions are continued.)

Although you are still deeply asleep . . . you are going to be able to open your eyes without waking up.
Your eyes will open slowly . . . but you will *not* wake up from this deep, deep sleep.
Things may seem a little hazy at first . . . but they will gradually become quite clear . . . and you will remain very, very deeply asleep . . . even though your eyes are wide open.
You will stay asleep with your eyes open . . . until I tell you to close them again.
You will be able to stand up . . . or walk about . . . just as a person walks in his sleep.
You will see everything that I point out to you.
When you open your eyes . . . you will notice that I am holding a bottle of clear fluid in front of your eyes.
As you watch it . . . you will see the colour of the fluid slowly becoming pinker and pinker . . . until it becomes quite red . . . just as it did when your eyes were shut.
As soon as you see the colour changing . . . please lift up your hand.
Now open your eyes, slowly . . . very slowly . . . open your eyes.
Never mind if things look a little blurred at first . . . as you look at the bottle . . . they will gradually become clear . . . and you will see the colour changing . . . first to pink . . . then to red.
Open your eyes slowly . . . wider and wider.

As the subject does so, a bottle of water is held in front of his eyes, which he gazes at until he notices the colour change, and raises his hand. Once this has occurred, he can be told that as he looks at the table, he will see a candlestick with a burning candle. He is told to go over to the table and blow out the candle. This suggestion is repeated several times.

When subjects are able to hallucinate well with their eyes closed, but have difficulty in doing so with their eyes open, Weitzenhoffer suggests that they will picture a simple object such as a red index card. When they signify that they can see this clearly, he tells them that when they open their eyes they will remain deeply hypnotized, but will still be able to see the red card once their eyes are open.

Four Effective Demonstrations

For each of the following demonstrations a deeply hypnotized somnambulistic subject, capable of opening his or her eyes without awakening from the trance, is required.

1. The hypnotized subject reclines in a chair with eyes closed. A volunteer sits close by, and is instructed to close his eyes and to try to simulate the hypnotic state. The hypnotist then produces a small bottle containing fluid which he represents to be a very delightful perfume. He tells them that they will each smell it in turn and derive the greatest pleasure and enjoyment from doing so. The bottle is then placed under the nose of the hypnotized subject, who smells it repeatedly with enthusiasm. When asked what it smells like, the subject invariably names a favourite scent. The bottle is then presented to the non-hypnotized volunteer, who takes one deep sniff only and turns his head away in disgust. It actually contains strong ammonia.

2. The deeply hypnotized subject is told that presently he will open his eyes and will be able to see quite clearly, without awakening from his trance. One minute after his eyes open, he will hear a noise like a cat mewing, and will look around to see where it is coming from. He will then see a kitten walk round the side of his chair, and will bend down, pick it up, and stroke it. He is then told to open his eyes without waking up, and within the prescribed time-limit he will comply with these suggestions in a most convincing manner.

This experiment demonstrates hallucinations of hearing, sight and touch. Before embarking upon it, however, it is always advisable to make sure that the subject neither dislikes, nor is allergic to cats. If fond of dogs, the suggestion of a puppy barking can be substituted.

3. Once again, the hypnotic subject is told that he will presently be able to open his eyes without awakening. He is also told that, when his eyes are open, a tall ashtray standing on the table will have completely disappeared and that he will not be able to see it. After he has opened his eyes, he is asked to pass the ashtray which is on the table, in full view. He will carefully scrutinize the table and fail to discover any ashtray there. A packet of cigarettes can then be placed on top of the ashtray and, to the utter astonishment of the subject, will appear to be floating unsupported in the air just above the table.

This experiment demonstrates a negative hallucination of sight. With a good somnambule, both this demonstration and the last one can be even more effectively performed in the waking state, as the result of post-hypnotic suggestion.

4. A new pack of playing-cards is required, in which to all outward appearances the back of one cannot be distinguished from the others. A card is chosen, the face of which is noted, and its reverse side only is shown to the deeply hypnotized subject, whose eyes are open. He is told that he will see a black cross appear on the back of the selected card, and that he will raise his hand as soon as he sees it. He is told to study it carefully so that he will recognize it easily. The card is then shuffled amongst twenty others from the rest of the pack, and these are presented to him with their backs uppermost. He is then asked to pick out the one with the black cross upon it. It is helpful to add that since it is the only one bearing this design, he will have no difficulty in distinguishing it from the others. He will usually be able to do this quite successfully. Even if the whole pack is used, the experiment rarely fails. The limitation to fewer cards only avoids prolonging it unduly.

This experiment is supposed to demonstrate some hyperaesthesia of vision, for if the backs of playing-cards (even new ones) are closely scrutinized with a lens, minute differences and defects in the pattern can be detected that are almost invisible to the naked eye. The hypnotic subject can see these quite easily as he studies the selected card, and when he identifies them again, these points of difference are so closely associated with the suggested image that they invariably call it up again. I have often performed this experiment successfully by suggesting that the card would be identified by a familiar smell such as ammonia or paint, in place of a visual image. The fact that the same method of identification is employed in this case is proved by the fact that when the subject is blindfolded, the task becomes impossible.

The Psychological Phenomena of Hypnosis

The psychological phenomena characteristic of the hypnotic state can be most conveniently discussed under the headings of memory, mental activity and emotions.

Memory

This determines every other psychical activity for all the higher mental functions are dependent upon memory, which consists essentially of four important factors:

1. The power of assimilating ideas.
2. The power of retaining ideas.

3. The power of recalling ideas.
4. The power of recognizing ideas and locating them accurately in the past.

The part these play is clearly shown in the following example. Let us take some event we can remember from the past, such as a severe reprimanding from a teacher. In such a case, the memory acts in four ways:

1. What was said at the time was assimilated by it.
2. What was said at the time was retained in it.
3. The memory can recall and reproduce exactly what was said.
4. It can be placed in its exact position in time by recalling its relation to other events, such as being at the school.

There are also three other factors upon which the powers of retention and recall ultimately depend: firstly, the more forcibly or dramatically an event or idea strikes us at the time, the more likely it is to be remembered; secondly, the more frequently an experience is repeated, the more easily it will be remembered; thirdly, the more distant such an experience is in time, the more difficult it will be to remember.

It was originally thought that the subject always forgot upon awakening everything that had happened during the trance, but this is certainly not correct. In the lighter hypnotic stages, the memory is usually unaffected. During the trance, the subject will remember everything of which he was conscious in everyday life, and when it is terminated he will recollect accurately everything that has occurred during his hypnosis. In the deeper hypnotic states, however, it is a very different matter. There is frequently a complete amnesia upon awakening, and the subject is astonished to hear what he has actually been doing during the trance. But it must not be assumed that this is necessarily the case, since certain individuals who readily achieve deep trances can still recall spontaneously everything that has occurred during the trance. And in other cases, the mere association of ideas will be sufficient to restore the missing memory. Moll quotes the following example.

'I suggest to a hypnotic that he is at a concert. He hears various pieces of music amongst which is the overture to *Martha*. He goes into the bar, drinks his beer, and talks to imaginary people. On awakening, he can remember nothing of all this. I then ask him if he knows the opera *Martha*. This one word will suffice to recall nearly all the events of the hypnosis.'

Bernheim went so far as to state that the memory could be recovered in all cases by means of strong, persistent suggestion in the subsequent waking state. Indeed, it was one of his experiments to illustrate this that caused Freud to develop the technique of psycho-analysis (Chapter 22). Amnesia is more fully discussed on page 166.

It is a well-known fact that memories which have been entirely forgotten, and consequently inaccessible in the waking state, can be recalled during hypnosis. This remarkable phenomenon is termed hyperamnesia, and is the opposite to amnesia. None of life's experiences are ever completely lost. All are perceived in consciousness and recorded in the mind. Most of them, however, are trivial. Since it would be impossible to retain everything, they are discarded and become no longer subject to recall. On the other hand, more significant events that are charged with emotion, pleasant or unpleasant, can usually be recalled at will, or through an association of ideas. Even so, if these memories are associated with such humiliating and painful experiences that their restoration to consciousness would arouse considerable anxiety, it will be impossible to revive them. Nevertheless, hypnosis is still capable of removing the inhibitions and repressions that keep them from awareness. This object is often achieved in a deep trance state by employing the technique known as age-regression, in itself a most fascinating phenomenon.

Age-regression

In deep hypnosis, an adult can be told that he is going back in time, perhaps even to childhood, and that he will be able to relive experiences that he underwent at that particular age. If he is regressed to the age of 5 years, he will begin to talk and act exactly as if he were a small boy again, and will be able to recount experiences and events of that period which he could not possibly remember in the waking state. Indeed, if he is taken back successively through several different ages and is asked to write his name at each age, his handwriting will change progressively until it becomes quite childish both in character and performance.

Some authorities consider that hypnotic regression is an artefact and that the subject is merely playing a role, but the general view nowadays is that the regressed subject frequently does reproduce early patterns of behaviour far too accurately to permit the possibility of simulation alone. Erickson and Kubie recognize two distinct types of age-regression:

1. In the first type, the subject does actually return to an earlier stage of development, with a total amnesia for all events subsequent to that

period. When regressed to 5 years of age he will readily remember things that happened to him at this period of his life but will have completely forgotten everything that followed. He may even fail to recognize the hypnotist himself, whom naturally enough he has not yet met, and who may consequently have to identify himself with someone with whom the subject was familiar at this particular age.

2. In the second type the subject never succeeds in actually returning to an earlier stage of development but behaves exactly as he imagines a child of that age would behave. Despite this, the hypnotic subject will always be able to simulate earlier patterns of behaviour far more accurately than a subject in the waking state, and he will still be able to remember at the regressed level things that are beyond conscious recall in his adult life. All this can happen without any subsequent amnesia for the trance.

In true regression of the first type (which is sometimes referred to as *revivification*) the changed immature handwriting will often be found to correspond closely to that in old school-books of that particular period. Moreover, the way in which it is performed will sometimes carry further conviction.

I can recall the case of a man, aged 42 years, whom I regressed quite easily to the age of 5. When asked to write his name, he started to do so immediately in the painstaking, laborious manner of a child. At the ages of 10 and 15 years, he put pencil to paper as soon as he was told to write, but at the age of 20, he paused and carefully dipped the pencil in an ashtray before starting to write. From 25 years onwards, he once again started to write immediately with no preliminaries whatsoever. Being curious about this, I questioned him and discovered that, up to the age of 18, he had always been accustomed to writing with a pencil or fountain-pen. Between the ages of 18 and 23, he had been employed as a clerk and compelled to use an ordinary pen and ink, the use of fountain-pens being forbidden. But after he changed his job at the age of 23, he had once again reverted to his former habits.

Sometimes the revived memories of the regressed subject can be checked. It has been reported that when an adult subject, regressed to her seventh birthday, was asked what day of the week it was, she replied ' Friday ' without the slightest hesitation, and subsequent investigation proved this to be true. This is a feat of memory that I think few of us could accomplish in the waking state.

Platonov reported in 1933 that he had regressed a number of subjects to the ages of 4 years, 6 years and 10 years. He then subjected them to intelligence tests and found that each of the subjects, at the suggested age, was unable to pass tests which went beyond those for the corresponding age according to the Binet-Simon scale. He also observed that their behaviour corresponded exactly to that one would expect at each particular age. On the other hand, Young regressed fourteen subjects to their third birthday, yet found intelligence tests to reveal an average mental age of six. He also claimed that seven unhypnotized subjects were able to simulate the performance of a three-year-old child more closely than the hypnotized subjects did. He considers that a role is being played and that hypnotic regression is an artefact.

Be that as it may, it is an undisputed fact that hypnotic regression will often succeed in uncovering unconscious mental and emotional conflicts that underlie neurotic illness, and it thus plays an important part as a technique in analytical psychotherapy. Even in this field, however, it will sometimes prove impractical. I have had a patient, an excellent somnambule with complete amnesia, who I had reason to believe had undergone an extremely distressing emotional experience of a sexual nature at the age of 7 years. She would readily regress to the age of 8 years, and to the age of 6 years, but nothing would induce her to go back to the age of 7. I might add that these painful memories were subsequently recovered under an intravenous amylobarbitone sodium abreaction.

Methods of producing age-regression. There are several different methods of producing age-regression. The simplest of these is just to tell the deeply hypnotized subject that, upon a given signal, he will once again feel that he is at a particular age—say 10 years old. It is always wise to specify some special day such as a birthday or Christmas day. The subject is told that he will feel exactly as if he were 10 years old again, and will experience everything that he formerly did upon that occasion. A little time should be allowed for these suggestions to take effect, and then the signal should be given. It is helpful to ask the subject to raise one hand as soon as he feels that he is 10 years old. He can then be questioned as to who he is, where he is, how old he is, what he is doing and what presents he has received.

No matter what technique is used, it is necessary that the hypnotist should be fitted into the regressive pattern. It is obvious that if the subject is taken back to a period of his life prior to meeting the hypnotist, as far as he is concerned the latter does not even exist. It is true that such a situation seems to arise but rarely, for in most cases the subject either continues to accept the hypnotist as such, or spontaneously fits him into the regressive situation. There would, however, be a real danger of losing contact if he failed to do so. It is consequently wise for the hypnotist to include in his instructions to the subject the suggestion that he will become identified with someone the subject knew well at that particular time of his life.

Once any specific phase of regression is ended, the subject should be told to sleep deeply again before any further regression is attempted, or before he is returned to his normal age. Weitzenhoffer advises that the subject should be previously conditioned to two non-verbal signals, one to produce instantaneous hypnosis, and the other to cause the subject to return to the present. Should verbal contact then be lost, these signals would enable the hypnotist to retain control over the situation. In attempting regression for the first time, I usually employ a relatively simple and uncomplicated technique:

> Whilst you are in this deep sleep . . . time no longer matters . . . you will presently be able to go back quite easily to any earlier period of your life. You are gradually going back to the time when you were 6 years old . . . you will feel that you are gradually getting smaller . . . smaller and smaller . . . that your arms and legs are getting smaller . . . that your body is getting smaller . . . and that I am someone that you know and like.
> In a few moments now . . . you will feel that you are 6 years old again . . . and that it is your birthday.
> You are exactly 6 years old.
> As soon as you feel that you are exactly 6 years old . . . please lift up your hand.

Wolberg precedes this by first taking the subject back to yesterday, and questioning him about what he did and what meals he ate. He then takes him back to the very first consultation. He is asked to describe it, how he was feeling, and what clothes he wore. He is told that he will actually see himself talking to the doctor once again. This is a modification of the most powerful of all methods which was originally described by Erickson. It consists of a combination of disorientation and reorientation. The subject is slowly but completely disorientated both for time and place. A general state of confusion is first produced by suggesting to the subject that he finds it more and more difficult to remember what day of the week it is, what the date is, what the month is and what year it is. It is suggested to him that he is gradually becoming more and more mixed up, and when this occurs he is slowly reorientated to the particular age required.

Although it is necessary that age-regression should be both fully described and demonstrated when teaching hypnosis, it should never be used for idle experimentation. There is always the risk of unwittingly regressing a subject to an age at which some traumatic emotional experience had occurred, in which case the reactions might be both severe and difficult to deal with. For this reason alone, I believe that the technique of age-regression is ordinarily best restricted to those with psychiatric or clinical psychological experience, and that even for treatment purposes it is best avoided by general medical and dental practitioners.

Mental Activity

Just as in the normal state, the mental activity in hypnosis depends upon the attention paid by the subject. In deep hypnosis, the subject's attention is primarily directed towards the hypnotist, so that other objects or persons hardly seem to exist so far as he is concerned.

Rapport. This can best be defined as a state of affinity existing between subject and hypnotist and is present at the very onset of hypnosis. It is of such a nature that it tends to prevent the subject from responding to any stimuli other than those arising from the hypnotist himself unless he instructs the subject otherwise. Even when it is not as strong as this, it will still cause the subject to respond more effectively to suggestions from the hypnotist, himself, than those from other people. Moll distinguishes two kinds of rapport. When the subject responds only to the hypnotist, he speaks of isolated rapport, but when the subject responds most strongly to the hypnotist and more weakly to other persons, he refers to it as plain rapport.

In the early days of hypnosis, it was believed that a subject would only respond to the suggestions of his original hypnotist, and would ignore those from anyone else unless instructed otherwise. This rapport could easily be transferred to another person, in which case the hypnotist himself would lose contact with the subject. It was also thought that the subject could only be awakened by the individual with whom he was in rapport.

Although such complete rapport does sometimes occur, it is more frequently present to a lesser degree. It is, however, mistaken to consider rapport as being merely the product of suggestion. It is very much more than that. Erickson remarks that one can never be sure what it actually includes, and feels that it expresses the attitude of the subject towards his surroundings and is very definitely a phenomenon of hypnosis. Essentially, rapport seems to be a kind of mental sympathy which gradually develops through repetition into a state of exaggerated belief and trust on the part of the subject which often leads to a form of emotional attachment between subject and hypnotist.

We have already seen that these conditions begin to exist before trance induction is even attempted. Indeed, induction will only be likely to succeed when the hypnotist has first convinced the subject that he is to be trusted implicitly and that whatever he says is to be believed and relied upon. Only in this way can anxieties relating to the trance be reduced to a bare minimum. But one must not think that rapport consists of nothing more than this initial approach, strengthened by various deepening techniques which result in increasing the subject's trust and belief. The work of Freud and the psycho-analytical school has demonstrated that something much more fundamental exists. They consider rapport between subject and hypnotist to resemble a child-parent relationship. This is a phenomenon that regularly occurs in psycho-analysis, and is a state in which the subject unconsciously regresses and adopts the attitude of a child towards his parent, with all its exaggerated trust, belief, affection and acceptance of authority. In this respect, it can be said to resemble the transference situation that exists in most doctor-patient relationships, the difference being merely one of degree. In hypnosis this regression is much more complete and results in a diminution of the subject's ability to evaluate critically the situation that has developed.

The fact that rapport can either be transferred to, or shared with another person should the hypnotist so desire, can often be important in the therapeutic field. This applies particularly to obstetrics, for should the hypnotist be unable to attend the confinement, the patient can be placed in rapport with the obstetrician or midwife, and will then follow their instructions just as faithfully as if they had been given by the hypnotist.

The sense and judgement of time. The evidence as to whether in the hypnotic state a subject is able to judge the passage of time more accurately than in the waking state is conflicting in nature.

It is certainly true that if the hypnotized subject is asked to perform a task after a specified number of minutes, he will usually do so with a fair degree of accuracy. Similarly, he will perform an act as the result of a post-hypnotic suggestion, after a prescribed interval of time. The most comprehensive account of this phenomenon was given by Bramwell, whose hypnotic subjects were unbelievably accurate in their judgement of time. Unfortunately, however, no subsequent investigator has succeeded in duplicating his results. Indeed, controlled experiments tend to show that the ability to estimate time is no greater in the hypnotic than in the waking state, provided that sufficient concentration is devoted to the task.

Calculations carried out in the unconscious mind are not invariably exact. Sometimes suggestions are not executed punctually when an abstract period of time has been given. Even so, they will usually approximate fairly closely to the specified moment. This unconscious estimation of time is not unknown in everyday life. Some people can judge time in the waking state with remarkable accuracy, whilst others can do the same during sleep. They are able to waken themselves up at a predetermined hour without hearing a clock strike or an alarm bell ring.

Personality changes. Under deep hypnosis, the subject can be made to believe that he is a totally different personality, and will act the role of the suggested character in a most convincing manner. Moll points out that in such cases not only do many memories connected with the subject's own personality disappear, but he tries to connect the remaining ones with his suggested personality and will sometimes create new ones appropriate to it. For instance, when a subject was told that he was Frederick the Great, he promptly walked with a crutch in the well-known gait, *but he knew nothing of railways.*

If during hypnosis several different personalities are suggested, each successive change is usually accompanied by a loss of memory of that which preceded it. One hypnotized subject was unable to remember as Napoleon what he had done as Frederick the Great. These changes of personality in hypnotic subjects have often been compared with the performances of actors, yet few actors seem to identify themselves so completely with a character as the hypnotic does. This is because the hypnotic subject is not distracted in any way by sense-perceptions, whereas the actor cannot avoid being affected to some extent by them.

The Emotions

The emotional changes that arise spontaneously as feelings towards the hypnotic state and the hypnotist have already been discussed. But quite apart from these, the general feelings of the subject can be readily influenced by hypnotic suggestion. Desire and dislike can easily be suggested, particularly in deep hypnotic states. Sadness or cheerfulness can readily be induced in deep hypnosis and may alternate very quickly. Similarly, emotions such as love, hate, fear, anger and anxiety are easy to evoke by means of suggestion. Indeed, many moods can be artificially induced under hypnosis if a specific situation is suggested which tends to arouse that mood. For instance, if after being told to hallucinate some person he dislikes intensely, he is told that he is being insulted by him, the hypnotic subject will promptly fly into a rage. Under such circumstances, the facial expression, attitude and behaviour of the subject show quite convincingly what he is actually feeling.

Post-hypnotic Amnesia

After somnambulism, the subject usually experiences a loss of memory on awakening, the extent of which varies with the depth of the trance. This may or may not occur following medium or even deep trances, and when it does, the resulting amnesia is only partial. Indeed, it can be said that complete post-hypnotic amnesia is only likely to be found in the deepest of hypnotic states.

Although no amnesia may be observed following the first few hypnotic sessions, it can still appear upon some subsequent occasion. It is sometimes spontaneous and occurs in the absence of any suggestions from the hypnotist. At other times, it can be induced by direct suggestions to this effect. When it appears, it always means that some degree of dissociation has actually occurred. The events of the trance state are forgotten, and the amnesia seems to resemble that for dreams which follows normal sleep. Even a good subject will be unlikely to develop an amnesia if he is instructed to remember what has occurred during his trance.

Amnesia will only arise if the subject has no objection to it, conscious or unconscious. I have often found that whilst the subject is perfectly willing and anxious for me to induce an amnesia, he is still incapable of developing one, no matter what technique is used. Subsequent enquiry usually reveals the fact that his memory is vitally important to him in his job, and despite all reassurances to the contrary, he has an unconscious fear that if he allows his memory to be tampered with in any way, there is a risk that it might also be affected in everyday life. Observations such as these over many years have led me to the conclusion that, except in the deepest forms of somnambulism, the more important the memory is to a subject in his occupation, the more difficulty there is likely to be in successfully inducing an amnesia. I have had several subjects of this type who could not only open their eyes and remain deeply hypnotized, but could also produce negative hallucinations yet were quite incapable of developing an amnesia, even after slow and painstaking attempts at training.

Another unconscious obstacle that is difficult to overcome arises when the personality of the subject is such that he feels that at all costs he must retain some degree of control. Although he may enter the deep trance state, he will either remember everything that has occurred, or at least sufficient to satisfy his needs. This can sometimes be countered by telling him that he will remember one or two of the more trivial incidents, but will forget all the rest. On the whole, I think it is true to say that if the subject does wish to remember something, he will almost certainly do so.

Amnesia is most complete immediately the trance state is terminated, but sometimes begins to break down, hours, days or weeks later. In this case, it is probable that fresh associations enter the subject's mind which tend to restore his memory. When complete amnesia can be induced in a somnambulistic subject, he may often be caused to forget certain aspects of his waking life. He can even be told that he will not remember being hypnotized, and will subsequently deny that anything has happened.

Complete amnesia is an invaluable asset when it can be secured. It convinces the subject in no uncertain manner that he has really been hypnotized, and ensures deep-trance production on future occasions. Amnesia always seems to strengthen the effect of post-hypnotic suggestion and is most useful from the therapeutic point of view, for since the patient will have no recollection of what has been said, he will be unable to criticize the suggestions he has been given during the trance. They will consequently take effect much more rapidly and powerfully. Although the events of the trance are forgotten when complete amnesia occurs, they can usually be remembered in subsequent trance states, unless instructions to the contrary have been given.

Methods of producing post-hypnotic amnesia. At each hypnotic session, before awakening the subject it is wise to suggest that every time he enters a trance, he will remember less and less of what has occurred, until eventually he will be able to remember nothing at all concerning his hypnosis. If this occurs, it will obviously be the result of continued post-hypnotic suggestion.

1. Amnesia can sometimes be produced in the deep trance state by

direct suggestion alone. When applied forcefully, it can be very powerful indeed and, provided that the trance is deep enough, will often prove successful.

> You are now in a very, very deep sleep indeed . . . so deep, in fact . . . that, after you wake up . . . *you will not be able to remember anything that has happened during this deep sleep.*
> After you wake up . . . *if you try to remember what has occurred during your sleep . . . your mind will go completely blank . . . and you will not be able to remember anything that has taken place.*
> After you wake up . . . *you will not be able to remember anything that has been said . . . or done . . . during this deep sleep.*

As a test of amnesia, I often tie a handkerchief around the subject's wrist, before I awaken him. I never refer to this, but leave him to discover it for himself. When he does so, the bewildered look upon his face leaves little doubt as to the success of the suggestions, and a simple question or two as to how it got there, or who put it there, will readily confirm this fact. It occasionally happens that the subject seems to avoid looking at his wrist and makes no comment. In this case, I also ignore it completely and discuss various other matters until he is about to leave. I then say quite quietly to him, ' By the way, you might let me have my handkerchief back before you go,' and this remark usually produces exactly the same effect. It seems to me that this brief interval of time allows the amnesia to consolidate and become firmly established.

The greatest disadvantage of this method lies in the fact that failure seems to render the induction of amnesia by any subsequent procedures much more difficult, and often impossible.

2. Sometimes it is wiser to adopt a much milder, more persuasive approach, which will be much less likely to prejudice further attempts.

> You are now in so deep a sleep . . . that, after you wake up . . . *you will have no desire whatever to remember what has occurred during your sleep.*
> *You won't feel that you want to remember anything that has happened during this deep sleep.*
> *Your sleep is becoming so deep . . . that you will tend to forget everything that has happened since you went to sleep.*

In therapeutic work I generally add the following suggestions to provide increased motivation.

The less you remember of what I say to you, during this sleep . . . the more quickly and powerfully this treatment will act . . . so that you will not want to remember anything . . . after you wake up.

I find that amnesias produced by this method are seldom complete at first, but can sometimes be rendered total by constant repetition over a number of sessions.

We have already noted the fact that both hypnosis itself, and loss of memory seem to offer a threat to the peace of mind of certain subjects. In such cases, Wolberg suggests to the subject that he will remember some trivial event of the trance, but will develop amnesia for the rest of it. This allays the subject's fear of losing control completely. Should this fail, and the subject remembers everything, Wolberg proceeds in the following manner during the next trance session:

3. The subject is told that he is to imagine that he is at home, asleep. He will then have a short dream, after which his eyes will open and he will wake up with a start. He will feel that he has just awakened from a sound sleep. He will remember the dream vividly, but immediately after describing it, he will only have a vague recollection of other events of the trance and may even forget some of them when questioned.

4. If a partial amnesia is secured as a result of these suggestions, they are followed up in the next trance, and the subject is told:

Forgetting is a perfectly normal process . . . it is easy to forget if you divert your attention to other things.
Last time, you forgot certain things that happened whilst you were asleep.
Today you will probably forget many more . . . possibly everything that happens during your trance.

Before awakening the subject, the above dream sequence is repeated. These two techniques can be constantly repeated over a number of sessions to train the subject to gradually achieve amnesia.

Weitzenhoffer finds it effective to use a modified 'fractionation' method. He repeatedly awakens and rehypnotizes his subjects, each time suggesting that they will forget more and more of the happenings in the trance. He points out that since amnesia and depth of hypnosis are intimately related, this is a very convenient way of dealing with the two problems simultaneously.

5. A method which I have sometimes used with success is the so-called blackboard technique.

I want you to imagine that you can see a blackboard . . . and that I am standing in front of it with a piece of chalk in my hand.
Just picture that blackboard . . . and as soon as you can see it quite clearly . . . please raise your hand.

(The subject's hand rises.)

Now, as you watch that blackboard . . . you can see me writing on it with the chalk.
You can see what I am writing . . . I am writing the word MEMORY.
You can see that word quite clearly.
As soon as you can see that word . . . please raise your hand.

(Once again, the subject's hand rises.)

As you go on watching the blackboard . . . you can see that I have taken a wet duster . . . and am cleaning the writing off the board.
And as the word . . . MEMORY . . . disappears from the blackboard . . . so will everything that has happened during your sleep also disappear from your mind . . . just as if your mind were being cleaned like the blackboard.
As soon as you can see that the word has disappeared . . . and the blackboard is clear and blank . . . please raise your hand.

(The subject's hand rises.)

In a few moments . . . when I wake you up . . . you will not be able to remember anything that has happened whilst you were asleep.
If you try to remember what has happened . . . your mind will remain quite blank . . . just like that blackboard, after it had been cleaned.
After you wake up . . . you will not be able to remember anything that has happened during your deep sleep.

Amnesia is a complicated and sometimes unpredictable phenomenon. As we have seen, it can vary from the simple forgetting that is found in hypnosis, to the much more significant and severe loss of memory caused by the repression of traumatic experiences, the recollection of which would arouse acute anxiety. This type of amnesia is considered in Chapter 22.

Paramnesias

These can be readily induced in hypnosis, particularly in the deeper stages. They differ from the amnesias in that the subject is told that he will only forget specific things, such as his name, his birthday or even the meanings of words. Aphasias can thus be produced. The subject may be deprived of the power to speak at all, or simply rendered unable to pronounce a particular word or consonant. Moreover, false memories can also be induced. If the subject is told in deep hypnosis that a number of entirely imaginary events have occurred, when he awakens he will remember them as actual facts.

CHAPTER 14

Post-hypnotic Suggestion: Self-hypnosis

Post-hypnotic Suggestion

This is the phenomenon in which suggestions that are given during the trance state are caused to take effect after the subject has been awakened. But for this, the therapeutic value of hypnosis would be almost negligible. Sometimes these post-hypnotic suggestions will be faithfully executed when only a medium or relatively light depth of trance has been obtained, despite the fact that the subject remembers the instructions that have been given. Such subjects, however, must necessarily be very suggestible, and it is possible that they would respond fairly readily to suggestion in the waking state. Generally speaking, it may be said that most post-hypnotic suggestions (except the very simple ones) are only likely to be effective when a deep trance state, followed by amnesia, has been produced. There is no doubt that amnesia greatly increases the force of post-hypnotic suggestion.

Moll considers that this phenomenon is hardly as curious as it may seem, since it can be compared to a similar kind of behaviour that occurs in everyday life. He quotes the following example:

I give a letter to Mr X who has called on me, and ask him to post it on his way home if he passes a letter-box. He puts the letter in his pocket and subsequently meets a friend and walks home with him, passing a letter-box on the way. Whilst engaged in conversation, Mr X apparently did not notice the box, but threw the letter into it without interrupting the conversation. Later on, it occurred to him that he had a letter to post. He had only a dim recollection of having done so, and only by feeling in his pocket and finding no letter there could he convince himself that he had indeed executed the commission.

The particular feature to be noticed here is that Mr X has performed a specified act *without the intervention of his will,* and one of the most striking features of post-hypnotic suggestion is the fact that it is carried out under precisely the same conditions. Moll also calls attention to the fact that it is not the post-hypnotic command itself—not what was actually said to the subject at the time—*but the idea of carrying out the instruction* that becomes conscious at the appointed time. For instance, if it is suggested to the hypnotic subject that he will ask for an apple, half an hour after he wakes up, he will certainly do so. But it is not the fact that he has been told to ask for an apple that will occur to him at the appropriate moment. It will be the idea that he would like an apple and had better ask for one that will rise into his conscious mind. Even in normal life, ordinary occurrences can sometimes produce similar ideas through suggestion. A healthy patient has frequently become convinced that he is suffering from heart disease as a result of overhearing some casual conversation about a severe cardiac condition.

It is remarkable to what extent post-hypnotic suggestions are carried out at the right moment. This can be appointed in two ways: (1) *By a concrete external signal* such as a sign given by the hypnotist, or the striking of a clock. (2) *By fixing an abstract period*—after so many minutes, hours or days. In the latter case, the accuracy is often less precise than in the former, although a very close approximation will usually occur.

The first of these methods involves no new mental phenomenon at all, for in normal life the striking of a clock often calls to mind something that we wished to do at a particular time, and we promptly proceed to do it. How often have you wanted to write a letter tomorrow, and have tied a knot in your handkerchief to remind you of the fact. The knot and the letter have become so closely associated in your consciousness that, although you may have completely forgotten what you intended to do, when you see the knot the next day the idea of writing the letter arises from your unconscious mind into consciousness again.

The following examples illustrate the various kinds of predetermined signals used in post-hypnotic suggestion:

1. ' When you hear me rap on the table twice . . . you will lie back in your chair and fall into a deep sleep.'

This is an audible external signal.

2. ' When you see me light a cigarette . . . you will get up from your chair and open the window.'

This is a predetermined visual signal, suggested by the hypnotist.

3. ' Ten minutes after you wake up . . . you will bend down and take off your right shoe.'

In this case a period of time—10 minutes—has been fixed. Specifying the time in this way, however, may not always be successful, for some subjects' perception of time may be poorer than others, or they may even become so interested in what is taking place that they tend to lose track of time. But even after the specified interval has elapsed and the subject has shown no sign of complying with the instruction, it does not necessarily mean that the suggestion has failed. Indeed, it is more than likely that if in general conversation some casual remark is made about the subject's shoes, he will probably become restless, look down at his feet, and eventually take off his shoe.

Although one of the most characteristic features of the post-hypnotic act is its compulsive nature, this certainly does not mean that it cannot sometimes be resisted. But even when there is no amnesia and the subject remembers the instruction he has been given, he will still need to make a tremendous effort to resist, and will usually end up by complying with the suggestion after a greater or lesser interval of time.

Supposing the subject has been told during hypnosis that, five minutes after he wakes up, he will fetch a book from the shelf and place it on the desk. He will remember this when he awakens and may decide that he is not going to do it. Consequently, when the five minutes have expired, nothing will happen. But as time goes on the subject will gradually become more and more restless and uneasy. A mental conflict has been aroused. On the one hand, he feels that he *must* fetch the book as instructed, and on the other hand, he feels that he *needn't* do so because he doesn't want to. Now any conflict of this nature invariably arouses anxiety, and after prolonging his resistance successfully for some considerable time, the odds are that the subject will eventually comply with the suggestion if only to gain peace of mind.

This important fact should always be borne in mind when demonstrating or attempting post-hypnotic suggestion, for *no subjects should ever be allowed to leave without having complied with any such suggestion that they have been given.* Alternatively, if they fail to do so, they must be rehypnotized and the appropriate suggestion cancelled before they are allowed to go home.

Post-hypnotic suggestions of a reasonable kind, that are not out of keeping with the subject's personality, will generally be acted upon quite readily. But inconsiderate, ridiculous or improper suggestions which are repugnant to the subject will often fail to be acted upon, despite the fact that he is a somnambule. There are several ways in which he can avoid complying with such suggestions. He may wake up spontaneously, his hypnotic sleep may change into ordinary sleep, he may become hysterical and throw a fit, or he may develop such severe signs of increasing anxiety and nervous agitation that the hypnotist will have no choice but to awaken him, after cancelling the offending instruction. Under these circumstances, however, the hypnotist is present and able to take prompt steps to counter the suggestion, or replace it with one that is more acceptable. *It is not always the actual suggestion that is made, but the way the subject interprets it that determines the way he responds, and whether he finds it acceptable or not.*

This question of interpretation is of the greatest possible importance. Suggestions to be acted upon post-hypnotically must always be most carefully and precisely worded, not only to ensure that their meaning is fully understood by the subject, but also to avoid the slightest risk of ambiguity or possibility of misinterpretation. It is not always easy to foresee the latter occurrence, for our intentions often seem so clear to us that we are only too prone to assume that they are equally clear to the subject. This is not invariably the case, as the following example will show:

During the last war, I had a patient who was a member of a British Red Cross Detachment. He was a man in his late thirties, strictly brought up, very religious, and who never in his life had been known to use bad language. He was sadly lacking in self-confidence and dreaded one of his tests for promotion, in which he had to command a squad in stretcher drill. He was an excellent somnambule with complete amnesia, and I gave him the post-hypnotic suggestions that the moment he stood up in front of his squad, all traces of nervousness would disappear and he would be able to give his commands and drill the men *just like an army sergeant-major*. During the actual tests, much to my discomfiture he proceeded to address his squad in the following terms: ' Squad 'shun! As you were! Jump to it, you blankety-blank, pot-bellied lot of so-and-so's! '

It is obvious that his own literal interpretation of my instruction varied widely from my own innocent intention that he should drill his squad ' with the confidence of an army sergeant-major '. Careless wording was entirely responsible for this unfortunate and embarrassing incident which took place in the presence of a large number of onlookers. This need for formulating one's instructions clearly and unambiguously is equally important at every stage of hypnosis, for it should never be forgotten that the hypnotic subject tends to take everything literally, sometimes with unexpected and surprising results.

Sometimes a post-hypnotic suggestion will only be carried out if the subject has been provided with a logical reason for the suggested act.

If I tell a subject to take a glass of water and throw it over my desk, he may well refrain from doing so, but if I first suggest to him that the desk is on fire, he will comply without the slightest hesitation. Similarly, if I tell him to steal Dr Blank's fountain-pen when his back is turned, he will certainly not do so. But if I represent to him that it is really my fountain-pen, which Dr Blank has pocketed, and that my only chance of regaining my property is for him to steal it back for me, he will probably oblige.

In certain cases, seemingly harmless suggestions can arouse sufficient anxiety to prevent their fulfilment because of an association with the subject's own unconscious mental conflicts. For this reason, you should always watch your subject's reactions carefully, so that any such suggestion can either be rephrased or withdrawn if it appears to arouse uneasiness or anxiety. This can be important, for if such suggestions are post-hypnotic and the subject fails to realize their full implications at the time, severe psychological disturbances could quite easily result.

The phrasing of post-hypnotic suggestions may also determine whether they are executed or not. If either the wording or manner of delivery of such suggestions betrays the slightest lack of confidence on the part of the hypnotist that they will be carried out, the subject will detect this immediately and will be better able to resist. When, however, the suggestion conveys to him the belief and conviction that he is expected to comply, he will be much more likely to do so.

The effect and duration of post-hypnotic suggestions can be very prolonged. Many authentic instances have been reported in which they have been carried out months or even years after they have been given. The passage of time does not seem to diminish the intensity of the compulsion.

I taught a woman who was expecting her first baby to go to sleep whenever I suggested she should do so. She was a complete somnambule and had a painless confinement, after which I did not see her again for 7 years. She then returned for her second confinement, and in the course of an ordinary conversation, without altering the tone of my voice, I quite unexpectedly said, ' Go to sleep, Mrs Blank,' upon which she immediately sank back in the chair in a deep somnambulistic sleep.

Since writing the above, I have encountered another similar example of the same phenomenon.

A young married woman aged 26 years, sought hypnotic treatment for her psoriasis. In the course of her interview she asked me if I remembered her. When I apologized she reminded me that I had treated her previously for insomnia when she was only 11 years old. Once again I just told her to go to sleep and she lapsed into complete somnambulism after an interval of 15 years.

Estabrooks described a case in which a post-hypnotic suggestion was realized after 20 years, and believes that if it is occasionally reinforced, it can be made to last indefinitely.

There is no doubt that the effects of post-hypnotic suggestion can be greatly enhanced if the suggestion is repeated frequently. Indeed, if repeated often enough, such suggestions tend to become permanent since it is probable that a conditioned reflex becomes established. This may partly explain why patients who have improved under hypnotherapy do not generally tend to relapse.

Another method of increasing the strength of a post-hypnotic suggestion is to couple it with some normal experience, so that a reasonable explanation becomes possible in the subject's mind. Under hypnosis, a subject can be told:

After you wake up . . . you will drink a glass of water.

Better still, a much clearer indication can be given by saying:

Five minutes after you wake up . . . you will drink a glass of water.

The best way of putting it, however, would be to say:

As soon as you wake up . . . you will begin to feel thirsty.
Your mouth will become dry and parched . . . and in a few minutes . . . you will drink a glass of water.

Each of these suggestions would need to be repeated, but the last would require less frequent repetition than either of the others. It would none the less influence the subject far more powerfully for, once again, he has been given a logical reason for the suggested act.

Rationalization

When post-hypnotic amnesia is present, and the subject upon awakening is unable to remember the particular instruction that has been given, once the action has been performed and he is asked why he had done it, he will usually produce the most ingenious rationalizations for his conduct. Suppose he has been told that, two minutes after he wakes up, he will take off his right shoe. Provided that he has developed a deep trance followed by amnesia, he will faithfully carry out this instructtion. Since he is quite unable to remember having been told to do this, when he is asked why he has removed his shoe, he will generally give some plausible yet entirely false explanation of his action which completely satisfies himself. He will probably say, ' My foot was itching,' or ' My sock had become creased and uncomfortable.' Indeed, the more bizarre or incongruous the post-hypnotic suggestion is, the more astonishing such rationalizations are likely to be. Several instances have been recorded in which post-hypnotic suggestions have been chosen for which it would be difficult to find logical explanations:

1. A subject was told that five minutes after he woke up, he would leave the lecture room and return with an umbrella from the hall. He would then unfurl the umbrella and walk round the room with it open. When asked why he had done this, he calmly remarked, ' I thought I would like to find out if anybody present was superstitious.'

Moll gives an account of some really incongruous post-hypnotic suggestions which were none the less explained by the subject to his own complete satisfaction.

2. A subject was told that when he woke up, he would take a flower-pot from the window-sill, wrap it in a cloth, put it on the couch and bow to it three times. When asked for his reasons for performing this remarkable series of actions, he replied, ' When I woke up and saw the flower-pot there, I thought that since it happens to be a cold day, the flower-pot ought to be warmed a little or else the plant might die. So I wrapped it in a cloth, and as the couch is nearer to the fire I thought I had better put the flower-pot on it. I then bowed because I was so pleased with myself for having such a bright idea.'

Although most amnesic subjects do rationalize, this is not always the case. Sometimes a subject will say, ' The idea just occurred to me to do so,' or ' Something made me feel that I should do it.' Generally speaking, however, no matter how silly or absurd the suggested action may be, it has to be performed, and thus the subject feels it necessary to provide himself with a logical reason for doing it. Such explanations are needed because, being wide awake, the subject is fully aware of what he has just done.

To the stage hypnotist, the post-hypnotic suggestion is the mainstay of his performance, and the more amusing he can make such suggestions, the better the audience is pleased. One well-known performer used to return several subjects to their places in the audience with the post-hypnotic suggestion that whenever he snapped his fingers, they would stand upon their seats and cry ' pea-nuts '. Such exhibitions may be undesirable and degrading and there is always the risk that when a number of subjects are being used in this way, the hypnotist may lose track of some of the suggestions he has given and the subject return home without the instruction having been removed.

An instance is reported in which a secretary had been told by a stage hypnotist that, whenever she heard the tune *I'm so tired*, she would immediately fall into a deep hypnotic sleep. During his performance, he secretly signalled to the orchestra from time to time, and on each occasion the tune was played, the subject promptly fell asleep. Unfortunately, the performer omitted to cancel this instruction with the result that two days later when she heard an office-boy whistling this tune she promptly fell asleep at her work.

A great deal of discussion has taken place as to whether the post-hypnotic performance of a suggested act occurs in the normal waking state, or whether at the moment of its execution the subject re-enters a spontaneous self-limiting trance. Quite often a good subject will seem rather dazed and develop a rather glassy far-away look in his eyes as he carries out the suggested action, as if he were behaving quite automatically. It has also been noticed that, the more incongruous or ridiculous the post-hypnotic suggestion may be, the more likely the subject is to develop a complete amnesia, possibly in order to avoid embarrassment or anxiety.

Erickson and his wife conducted a systematic investigation of post-hypnotic behaviour and concluded that when the hypnotized subject is instructed to execute some act post-hypnotically, he invariably develops spontaneously a hypnotic trance. This trance is of brief duration, occurs in direct relation to the performance of the post-hypnotic act, and apparently constitutes an essential part of the process of response to, and execution of the post-hypnotic command. They further pointed out that the development of this trance state as part of the post-hypnotic performance requires for its appearance neither suggestion nor instruction. It develops at the moment of initiation of the post-hypnotic act, and usually persists for only a moment or two, so that it is easily overlooked. If there is no amnesia for the original trance and the post-hypnotic suggestion that has been given, or if the amnesia is weakened so that the subject remembers it before he carries it out, this spontaneous trance may not develop. In this case, the suggestion is complied with either voluntarily or through a feeling of compulsion.

Post-hypnotic Conditioning in Hypnosis

Post-hypnotic suggestion is not only invaluable in the therapeutic application of hypnosis, but is also extremely useful in facilitating future trance induction and protecting the subject against accidental hypnosis. In the latter case, an easily hypnotized person may even be prevented from being hypnotized by some unqualified individual.

The induction of a hypnotic trance for the first time can occasionally be a laborious and time-consuming process. Indeed, it may take anything from 15 minutes up to many hours to secure satisfactory depth, and if it were necessary to repeat this procedure in full on every subsequent occasion, the practical uses of hypnosis would be limited indeed. So much time and energy would have to be spent upon induction alone that there would be little left for therapeutic purposes. As already described, conditioning the subject by post-hypnotic suggestion to enter the trance state upon a given signal, verbal or otherwise, is easily accomplished. This can always be done for deep-trance subjects, and for many who achieve medium-depth hypnosis only.

The somnambulistic subject is so highly suggestible, even in the waking state, that it is wise to protect him against unexpected hypnosis. This can easily be effected by telling him, in the deep hypnotic state, that under normal circumstances nobody except yourself will be able to hypnotize him in future. Should, however, the necessity for this ever arise, he will then be able to respond to any other doctor or dental surgeon who possesses special knowledge and experience of hypnosis. Various authorities have doubted whether this does afford complete protection. Moll considers that the chief danger does not arise from susceptibility to hypnosis as such, but from susceptibility to accidental hypnosis, or hypnosis against the subject's will. As an example of the efficiency of such protective suggestions, I can quote one case of mine in which, entirely without my knowledge or intention, it was actually put to the test.

I had been treating a schoolgirl, aged 14 years, who was so excellent a somnambule that I judged it wise to protect her in this manner. About 12 months later, I met her father socially and he told me that whilst they were on holiday they went to see a stage exhibition of hypnosis. In the course of this, the performer rashly claimed that he would guarantee to hypnotize anyone in the theatre. This so annoyed the father that, knowing the protection I had given, he promptly challenged the hypnotist to hypnotize his daughter. Despite his efforts, the performer was quite unable to induce even the lightest hypnotic state, and excused himself to the audience on the grounds that this was one of the very rare cases in which a person was completely unhypnotizable. The father then announced that this was very curious, since the child was accustomed to enter the deep hypnotic state whenever her doctor simply told her to go to sleep.

Auto-hypnosis or Self-hypnosis

This involves the production of a self-induced hypnotic trance without the intervention of another person. The subject either learns or is taught how to enter the hypnotic state on his own, whenever he needs to make use of it. Although the technique is more easily learned by subjects who have previously entered medium or deep trance states, it is not difficult to acquire without any former subjective experience of hypnosis. Most persons who practise hypnosis have generally taught themselves self-hypnosis at some time or other.

Whilst eye-closure and light or even medium-depth hypnosis are relatively easy to obtain, deep hypnosis is a much more difficult matter. Part of this difficulty lies in the fact that since the subject has to be his own hypnotist, he is faced with the problem of having to play both an active and a passive role at one and the same time. Because of this, although the state of mind that is self-induced is very similar to that produced by a hypnotist, it is usually on a lighter plane. The subject has to retain a certain degree of conscious control and activity in order to direct operations, and thus cannot allow himself to go too deeply. On the other hand, when he enters a trance state induced by a hypnotist, he can let himself go completely and doesn't need to worry about anything that is likely to happen or anything that is being done. He can consequently allow himself to go so deeply that his conscious mind becomes inactive and needs to play no part in what is taking place. In self-hypnosis, a part of the conscious mind must necessarily remain active in order to control the hypnosis and direct what is to happen in the self-induced trance. Roughly speaking, it is as though the conscious mind assumes the role of the hypnotist in making the suggestions which enter the unconscious part of the mind, where they are first accepted and then acted upon.

One of the easiest ways of teaching a subject to induce self-hypnosis is through the use of post-hypnotic suggestion. It seems to me to be doubtful, however, as to whether this procedure is really entitled to be called self-hypnosis since it has certainly not been initiated by the subject's unaided efforts. It is a power that has been delegated to him by the hypnotist which is indistinguishable in its mode of operation from any other form of post-hypnotic suggestion. As might be expected, the subject who is taught in this way will be able to enter the trance state much more rapidly, often in response to a self-administered signal, and will probably be able to achieve greater depth. This can be very useful therapeutically when it is necessary for the patient to induce the trance state rapidly, in order to avert a threatened attack of asthma or migraine. Unless needed for such purposes, however, I prefer not to use this method since I believe that the patient who has been taught to achieve self-hypnosis on his own, without the active intervention of the hypnotist, will always feel that he has much more control over the proceedings. Moreover, the increased confidence that he develops in his own unaided capacity for producing hypnosis when required does a great deal to add force to his own auto-suggestions, and thus tends to offset the dis-advantage of a rather lighter trance.

No matter what particular method I propose to use, before teaching a subject self-hypnosis I always discuss the matter with him in the waking state:

> I am going to teach you how to put yourself into the hypnotic state when-ever you need to make use of it. You will not run the slightest risk because you will always be able to waken yourself up whenever you wish to do so. If you go to sleep whenever I tell you to, you are equally bound to wake up when I tell you to do so. This is because I am in control of what is taking place.
>
> Similarly, if you go to sleep on your own when you tell yourself that this will happen, then you are equally bound to wake up when you tell yourself to do so. This time, you see, *you* are in complete control of what is happening. So there is no risk whatever of putting yourself to sleep and being unable to wake yourself up whenever you wish to do so.
>
> During your hypnotic sleep, you will be able to relax completely . . . you will be able to think clearly . . . and you will be able to give yourself what-ever suggestions you wish . . . and they will act just as if I had given them to you, myself.
>
> Whenever you hypnotize yourself . . . you will be able to remember the kind of suggestions I have been giving you . . . and you will be able to administer them·to yourself.

I also tell the patient that if he uses and practises self-hypnosis in this way, it will help him to improve even more quickly. I usually explain it to him in this way:

> It's just as if each time you came to me, you brought with you a block of wood and a 6-inch nail.
>
> Whilst you are with me, I produce a heavy hammer and strike the nail a powerful blow which drives it an appreciable distance into the wood.
>
> You then take it home with you, and every day you do the same.

But you don't possess a heavy hammer. You've only got a light one. Nevertheless, if you use that regularly and give the nail a larger number of lighter blows, you will still succeed in driving it home although it will necessarily take more time.

Auto-hypnosis Through Post-hypnotic Suggestion

When teaching auto-hypnosis through post-hypnotic suggestion, I put the subject into as deep a trance as possible and proceed to give him the following instructions:

> You are now in so deep a sleep . . . *that everything that I tell you that is going to happen . . . will happen . . . exactly as I tell you.*
> *And every feeling . . . that I tell you that you will experience . . . you will experience . . . exactly as I tell you.*
> *And these same things will continue to happen to you . . . and you will continue to experience these same feelings . . . just as strongly . . . just as surely . . . just as powerfully . . . when you are back home . . . as when you are with me, in this room.*
> I am now going to teach you how to go into this deep sleep, whenever you wish to do so . . . even though you are no longer with me.
> All you will have to do is to lie back in a chair . . . fix your eyes upon a spot on the ceiling . . . and count slowly up to *five.*
> As you do so . . . your eyes will rapidly become more and more tired . . . your eyelids heavier and heavier . . . *and the moment you have reached the count of five . . . your eyes will close immediately . . . and you will fall immediately into a sleep . . . just as deep as this one.*
> Whilst you are in this deep sleep . . . stage by stage, you will be able to suggest complete relaxation of all the muscles of your body . . . exactly as I do . . . and all other suggestions that you give yourself for your own good . . . will act . . . just as effectively as if I had given them to you, myself. Should any unexpected emergency arise during your deep sleep . . . you will automatically wake up immediately . . . fully prepared to take any necessary action.
> After you have given yourself treatment . . . as soon as you are ready to wake yourself up . . . you will count slowly up to *seven . . . and the moment you reach the count of seven . . . your eyes will open . . . and you will be wide awake again . . . feeling much better than when you went to sleep.*

I then awaken the subject and talk to him for a few minutes, after which I tell him to lie back in the chair and put himself straight off to sleep again. Whilst asleep, he is to relax all his muscles, and once he feels this relaxation he is to waken himself up. I usually rehearse him in this procedure several times until it occurs quite automatically. I conclude by putting him back into a deep trance again, and adding these further instructions:

> Whenever you are with me . . . and you put yourself into this deep sleep . . . you will always be able to hear everything that I say to you . . . and you will always carry out any instructions that I give you.
> *Even when you are no longer with me . . . you will always be able to put yourself into this deep sleep . . . whenever you wish to do so . . . by lying back in a chair . . . staring at a spot on the ceiling . . . and counting slowly up to five.*
> Whilst you are in this deep sleep . . . you will neither listen to . . . nor accept suggestions from anyone other than myself.
> But your own suggestions will always take effect . . . more and more powerfully as you become more proficient.
> You will only use this self-hypnosis for your own benefit . . . *you will never use it for the purpose of demonstration or entertainment.*

There are many other ways, of course, in which the subject can be taught to produce the trance post-hypnotically. He can be instructed to induce it for himself by more orthodox methods of trance induction, or in cases where speed is essential to produce it upon a given signal such as a predetermined word. In the latter case, however, it is wise to condition him to enter the trance only when he repeats the selected word three times in rapid succession. This will prevent anything happening should he inadvertently use the key word in an ordinary conversation.

Self-hypnosis Without Post-hypnotic Suggestion

When teaching self-hypnosis in the waking state without the use of post-hypnotic suggestion, after having given the preliminary explanations and assurances, I usually proceed in the following manner:

> Now, I want you to listen carefully to the instructions I am going to give you . . . and after I have finished . . . I shall ask you to lie back in the chair and put yourself right off to sleep . . . by doing exactly what I've told you.
> When I tell you to put yourself to sleep . . . you will lie back in the chair . . . and fix your eyes upon a spot on the ceiling.
> Don't let your eyes wander from this spot . . . and while you are staring at it . . . you will repeat to yourself . . . over and over again . . . that your eyes are becoming very, very tired . . . that your eyelids are feeling heavier and heavier . . . that they will want to blink . . . and that as they blink . . . they will feel that they want to close . . . that they are wanting to close . . . that you want them to close . . . and that you will let them close as soon as they want to.
> You'll find that if you keep on saying these things over and over again to

yourself . . . your eyes will very soon close of their own accord . . . and you will have no desire to open them . . . until you tell yourself to do so. Once your eyes have closed . . . and you have fallen into a light hypnotic sleep . . . I want you to tell yourself . . . that all the muscles of your legs and thighs are becoming completely relaxed . . . all the muscles of your chest, body, and stomach are becoming limp and slack . . . and that all the muscles of your neck, your shoulders and your arms are becoming completely and utterly relaxed.

Keep on repeating these suggestions . . . over and over again . . . until you do feel relaxed . . . then, tell yourself that you will open your eyes and be wide awake again, the moment you count *seven* . . . feeling very much better than when you went to sleep.

I usually repeat these instructions once, to make sure that the subject knows exactly what he has to do. Then I tell him to put himself to sleep, and that I shall not utter another word until he has done so and awakened himself again. This procedure rarely fails. Indeed, it often succeeds in people who have never previously been hypnotized, provided that the preliminary talk and explanations have carried conviction. As one would expect, the previous subjective experience of hetero-hypnosis facilitates it greatly, even though no post-hypnotic suggestion is used.

The subject is told to practise this daily until he sees me again. On the next occasion, I tell him that after he has put himself to sleep and produced relaxation, before he wakens himself up he is to hold his arm out stiff and straight, level with his shoulder and with the palm upwards facing the ceiling. He is then to tell himself, over and over again, that his arm is becoming stiff and straight from the shoulder to the wrist, just like a steel poker, and that it will feel so stiff and straight that he will be quite unable to bend it until he counts up to three. In fact, the harder he tries to bend it, the stiffer and straighter it will become. As soon as he feels this stiffness, he is to try to bend it and when he finds that he cannot, he is to relax it again by counting up to three. Then he is to waken himself up.

This often succeeds at the first attempt. If it doesn't, it is important to get him to admit that he did feel some stiffness, and to tell him that as he practises and becomes more proficient, he will eventually succeed. If, on the other hand, he does succeed in producing arm-rigidity, I follow it up by teaching him how to induce automatic movement, by resting his elbow on the arm of the chair and imagining the cord tied round his wrist as already described in the orthodox deepening techniques.

Finally, I try to prove to him that other suggestions that he gives himself will also work. I tell him that I am going out of the room and that whilst I am absent, he will put himself to sleep. Once his eyes have closed, before he continues with his relaxation and deepening techniques he is to tell himself that should anyone touch the handle of the door to enter the room before he counts up to seven, his eyes will open immediately and he will be wide awake again. I then leave him for 2 or 3 minutes, after which the moment he hears me turn the handle of the door, he awakens immediately. I point out to him that just as this suggestion worked, so other suggestions that he gives himself, for his own good, will also work, but that treatment suggestions are bound to take longer and require frequent repetition before they take full effect. I also tell him that it is quite useful to give himself this particular suggestion each time he induces hypnosis, since it will ensure that he will never be taken unawares by someone entering the room unexpectedly. Once he has mastered the technique and whilst he is still in a self-induced trance, I am in the habit of imposing the same safeguards that have already been described in connection with the post-hypnotic method of induction.

No matter what method of instruction has been adopted, once the subject has mastered the technique of the self-induced trance, he will be able to apply suggestion to himself exactly as the hypnotist does. He will normally remember the therapeutic suggestions he has been given and will make use of these, rewording and rephrasing them to suit himself. Normally, he will not go beyond this, but since in deep-trance subjects it is sometimes possible to enlarge the field of auto-hypnotic phenomena to include self-induced analgesias, it is necessary for the hypnotist to take the protective measure of imposing strict limitations upon such capabilities. It could be extremely dangerous if the subject were left with the ability to remove pain or other symptoms at will, in the absence of medical supervision. In the case of such complaints as dysmenorrhoea or migraine, the ability to remove pain auto-hypnotically can be restricted by the hypnotist to this particular pain alone, as and when it occurs. Similarly, a subject can be told that he will only be able to produce dental analgesia for himself when he is actually sitting in his dentist's chair.

The Use of Gramophone Records or Tape-recordings

Subjects can easily be conditioned by post-hypnotic suggestion to enter the trance state in response to a gramophone record or tape-recording, either through listening to a full induction routine, or the simple instruction 'go to sleep'. There are certain disadvantages in using a full induction technique, since the suggestions cannot be accurately timed to the actual rate of trance induction, and cannot be worded in the most appropriate way to suit the individual at each step.

The method offers far more scope when it is used for the recording of therapeutic suggestions, the patient having already been conditioned to enter the trance state immediately upon being instructed to do so. Here the use of tape affords the great advantage that recordings can be altered or adjusted from time to time to suit changing conditions. Used in this way, the tape-recorder has become a very valuable therapeutic tool. It enables the patient to receive treatment more frequently, daily if required, and in such conditions as asthma and migraine, it can be put to good use in inhibiting the development of a threatened attack. And in obstetrics, it can play an invaluable part in the collective training of expectant mothers in hypnotic relaxation. As might be expected, the depth of hypnosis achieved by a recording is usually greater than that obtained in self-hypnosis, since it frees the subject from the need to exercise conscious control over the proceedings. The depth does, however, seem to be rather less than that produced in the actual presence of the hypnotist.

The preparation of a therapeutic tape-recording is quite a simple matter. My usual practice is to record an ordinary treatment session as it progresses. This obviates any difficulty in the timing of certain suggestions, which will consequently conform to the requirements of the individual patient. Before starting, I switch on the recorder and tell the patient to lie back in the chair and allow himself to relax. I then say, ' Go to sleep, Mr Blank! ' and proceed with his customary relaxation and treatment routine. When this is concluded, before awakening him, I give the following instructions:

From now on . . . whenever you wish to give yourself treatment at home . . . all you have to do is to lie back comfortably in a chair . . . and switch on this recording.

The moment you hear my voice, on the tape, say, ' Go to sleep, Mr Blank ' . . . your eyes will close immediately . . . and you will fall immediately into a sleep, just as deep as this one.

During this deep sleep . . . as you listen to my instructions and suggestions . . . they will take effect just as powerfully as if I, myself, were giving them to you in this room.

And the moment you hear my voice, on the tape, count up to ' seven ' . . . your eyes will open immediately . . . and you will be wide awake again . . . feeling wonderfully better for your deep sleep.

If, at any time during your treatment . . . before you hear me count up to ' seven '

. . . the machine should stop unexpectedly . . . or the tape break . . . you will immediately realize that something is wrong . . . and that your treatment has been interrupted.

You will consequently count up to ' seven ', yourself . . . and your eyes will open immediately . . . and you will be wide awake again.

Similarly . . . should any other emergency arise during your treatment . . . you will be fully conscious of it . . . and will wake up immediately . . . fully prepared to take any necessary action.

In a few moments . . . I am going to count up to ' seven ' . . . and you will open your eyes and be wide awake again.

You will wake up feeling wonderfully better for this long sleep . . . feeling really fit and well . . . completely relaxed, mentally and physically . . . feeling quite calm and composed . . . and with much more confidence, both in yourself and in the future.

One . . . two . . . three . . . four . . . five . . . six . . . seven !

Once the subject is awake, I re-wind and switch on the recording again, and watch him go off to sleep. I let it play for 2 or 3 minutes and then stop the machine, unexpectedly. The subject always awakens spontaneously with little delay. This is a useful check to ensure that everything is going to plan, and also gives the subject complete confidence in the recording.

PART THREE

THE CLINICAL APPLICATIONS
OF HYPNOSIS

CHAPTER 15

General Considerations of Hypnosis in Medical Treatment

The Therapeutic Applications of Hypnosis

Every illness with which the general practitioner has to deal is primarily organic, functional or psychosomatic in origin. In the last two instances, the importance of mental and emotional attitudes is fully recognized, but in the case of physical complaints too little notice is apt to be taken of the extent to which they can be aggravated and prolonged by psychological factors. Mind and body can never be separated. Each reacts on the other, and consequently needs to be taken into account in every case.

Physical disease is always accompanied by pain, discomfort, or impairment of function, sometimes all three. But these will almost invariably be accompanied by some disturbance of emotional balance and harmony. The patient who is suffering pain cannot help worrying about the significance of his symptom. He constantly asks himself, ' Is it a sign of cancer? ' or ' How long am I likely to be ill and unable to earn my living?' In the first case, his fear may be so great that he cannot summon up the courage to seek advice. And when he eventually does so, he may be quite unable to convince himself that the doctor, being human, may not be mistaken in his opinion. In the second instance, he may be afraid to resume his work for fear of breaking down again, and destroying all hope of being able to earn his living in the future. This is particularly prone to occur when he has a wife and family to support. Furthermore, such fears and anxieties are far from being the only emotions that can be aroused by illness. The patient may feel bitter resentment at his ill-luck or even depressed as to his prospects, all the more if he has previously enjoyed good health. And then, there is another aspect of the picture which strikes us even more forcibly, namely, the individual who seems to enjoy bad health. Such people often receive so much more consideration, kindness and attention than when they are well that it is hardly surprising that they are so reluctant to give up these advantages. They consequently make very little effort to recover. Now this is extremely important, for without the co-operation of the patient, there are few illnesses from which recovery can be made either quickly or completely.

Every single case, medical, surgical, or psychiatric, needs to be approached from three angles—the physical, the psychological, and the environmental. Indeed, the importance of viewing every illness against the background of the various stresses and strains to which the patient has been subjected cannot be over-emphasized. This is particularly essential when hypnotic treatment is considered, for lack of success can often be traced to an insufficient knowledge of the patient's personality and life-history. Both the choice of the best method of induction and the approach to treatment may well depend upon these factors.

Nevertheless, it should not be thought that case-taking on these lines need necessarily be a prolonged or arduous task. Provided that the right questions are asked systematically, it is surprising how much relevant information can be elicited with ease. The following scheme should be of assistance in this respect since it incorporates the important points to which attention should be directed.

1. *History of present illness.* Time and mode of onset. Description of symptoms. Details of previous medical or other treatment.

2. *Family history.* Description of father, mother, sisters and brothers. Family relationships, past and present. Attitudes and feelings towards each other.

3. *Childhood history.* Childish illnesses, particularly bed-wetting and sleep-walking. Educational history. Reactions to various schools and other children.

4. *Occupational history.* Ambitions as a child. History of various occupations after leaving school. Reasons for changes. Present employment, and reactions to work-mates and environment.

5. *Psycho-sexual history.* Childish knowledge of sexual matters, and how acquired. Bad habits (masturbation, etc.). Past and present emotional affairs. Marriages (if any). Marital relationships or difficulties. Financial status.

6. *Past medical history.* Previous illnesses, operations, accidents and treatment. In the case of a woman, menstrual history, pregnancies, confinements or miscarriages.

7. *Present state of mind.* Depression. Anxiety. Phobias. Insomnia. Lack of concentration or interest. Memory. Suicidal thoughts (where depression is present). Fear of insanity.

8. *Mental or nervous disturbances.* Insanity, neurosis or epilepsy in parents, close relations or members of the family.

I have intentionally made the above scheme of case-taking comprehensive enough to enable the general practitioner to undertake the hypnotic treatment of the milder forms of psychosomatic or functional nervous conditions, should he wish to do so. It should, moreover, help him to be able to discriminate between the cases which are likely to fall within his province, and those which would be best referred to a psychiatrist. But in the course of his everyday work he will encounter a large number of medical conditions in which the taking of such a comprehensive history will seem neither necessary nor desirable. Yet, even in these cases it will be possible to select certain important questions from the above list, the answers to which will throw a flood of light upon the patient's underlying attitudes towards his illness.

When dealing with the anxious or apprehensive patient never ask bluntly whether any of his relatives have ever been in a mental hospital. This will simply frighten him and you will probably make very little further headway. Similarly, never ask him directly whether he is afraid of insanity, as very many anxious patients nurse a secret fear of ultimately becoming insane. Since the patient will obviously never mention this fear himself it is necessary to enquire about it so that he may be given the reassurance for which he secretly craves. I find that putting the question in the following way usually produces a frank admission, without causing undue alarm: ' If this condition of yours were to get worse, have you ever been afraid that you might have to go away for treatment ? '

Under these circumstances, since the term ' going away for treatment ' is almost invariably interpreted by the patient as applying to a mental hospital, he will usually unburden himself quite freely. Then, in the course of the ensuing discussion, discreet questions can be interpolated regarding any possible mental disturbances in his close relatives. In many cases the question of sexual attitudes must also be approached with caution. It may be most unwise to ask intimate and embarrassing questions during the first interview. These are frequently best deferred until closer contact with the patient has been established when the more general and harmless aspects of the situation have first been explored. Although much of such detailed case-taking appears to belong more to psychological than general medicine, the importance of psychological, emotional and environmental factors in such general conditions as asthma, insomnia, migraine and certain dermatological disorders can not be ignored.

Hypnosis in General Medicine

The reassurance and encouragement that can be given under hypnosis to patients with any complaint, functional or organic, should not be underestimated. Although hypnosis can be extremely useful in many organic illnesses, it will always prove most effective in those conditions accompanied by strong emotional components. In cardiac disturbance, which is physically determined by the presence of organic disease, hypnosis can help considerably in the alleviation of the patient's symptoms. It will do this by modifying his reactions to such symptoms, by lowering emotional tension and by reducing his fears, particularly the fear of death; cardiac disturbances that originate from emotional disturbances or psychological stress and not from organic disease will yield much more easily and completely to hypnotic treatment. It is necessary to inculcate in the patient a strong faith in his ability to recover, and to try to teach him to readjust to himself to reality and to his environment; in talks such as these, hypnotic suggestion can be of the greatest possible assistance.

Hypnosis can sometimes be used to afford symptomatic relief in certain chronic physical diseases. It does this partly by reducing tension, anxiety and apprehension, and partly by exercising a direct influence over the threshold of pain itself. In the latter case, however, considerable depth will almost certainly be necessary, so that the degree of success achieved in difficult cases such as cancer will be bound to depend largely upon the susceptibility of the individual patient. Even so, hypnosis has been found to assist greatly in controlling pain in the earlier stages, thus postponing the need for powerful drugs, and even when these are employed, a much lower dosage will be effective. Since, under these circumstances, the motivation for hypnosis is exceedingly strong, the attempt is often well worth while.

There are three main methods of employing hypnosis therapeutically:

1. Hypnosis in symptom removal.
2. Hypnosis in simple psychotherapy.
3. Hypnosis in analytical psychotherapy.

Normally only the first two of these will fall within the province of the general practitioner, and there is no doubt that symptom removal will be the one that he will find most useful in his practice. This is in fact the oldest of the hypnotic techniques, but has often been criticized as being the least successful. The objections are usually made that the indiscriminate removal of symptoms is dangerous; that sufficient depth of hypnosis can rarely be obtained; and that the results will seldom be sufficiently permanent.

Such criticism is no longer justified. Nevertheless, it must be admitted that since symptom removal deals with effects rather than causes, it must necessarily possess certain limitations. Its best results will always be obtained where the symptom has a minimal defensive value. That is why it can frequently be used with success in the treatment of many conditions that are seen in the average surgery, the defensive functions of which are almost negligible. In cases such as these, little danger is likely to result from the simple removal of the offending symptom by direct hypnotic suggestion. The analytically orientated psychiatrist is tireless in emphasizing the fact that symptom-removal is dangerous since it will often be followed by the release of anxiety or even the formation of substitute symptoms. There is no doubt that in certain of the severer neuroses such as the hysterias, and others arising from deep-seated fundamental conflicts, such difficulties may well be encountered, and under these circumstances the argument that direct symptom-removal under hypnosis is both undesirable and dangerous is fully justified unless the therapist has undergone the necessary psychiatric training to enable him to deal with the situation. Sometimes the analytically trained psychiatrist can use direct hypnotic suggestion himself to avoid these difficulties and afford much needed relief in cases in which the symptom possesses a strong defensive value by deliberately leaving the patient with some residual symptom which is less disabling than the original one. For instance a paralysis may be removed from an arm and induced in the little finger instead. It is then suggested to the patient that the finger paralysis will have exactly the same meaning for him as the arm paralysis, and will remain until he fully understands the reason for his original paralysis and no longer needs it. In this way, he may be enabled to resume work whilst still continuing treatment. Nevertheless, in recent years the dangers of ' direct symptom-removal ' have been so grossly exaggerated that one wonders whether the adherents to this school of thought would be equally vociferous in demanding that no physician should prescribe aspirin for a headache without first seeing an angiogram. Such generalizations drawn from practice largely confined to dealing with deep-seated problems are not only suspect but also dangerous in the limitations they seek to impose. After thirty years experience in the field of hypnotherapy both in general and psychiatric practice, I believe that the general practitioner using hypnosis is most unlikely to attempt to treat cases which properly fall within the realm of the psychiatrist, and even if he were to do so by direct suggestion under hypnosis, little or no damage would result. In fact, unless he possessed talent much above the average in the art of hypnosis, and happened to be dealing with a subject who was unusually susceptible, I doubt whether his efforts would attain the slightest success, since most patients of this type would be unwilling to surrender their symptoms until they felt strong enough to do without them. In other words, *the greater the need of the patient for the symptom as a defence mechanism, the more intractable it will prove to be to any method of psychotherapy.* In so far as the second objection is concerned, the practitioner should experience little difficulty in securing sufficient depth for ordinary treatment purposes in the majority of his cases.

The third objection, that the results of symptom-removal will seldom be permanent, is largely invalid provided that measures are taken during the treatment to strengthen the patient's ability to cope with his difficulties and to encourage him to begin to stand upon his own feet. This task is not nearly as formidable or time-consuming as it sounds, but I consider it to be of vital importance. Many years ago in a paper dealing with these so called dangers of direct symptom-removal (the subsequent production of acute anxiety, the appearance of substitute symptoms, and the inevitability of relapse) I called attention to the following principle:

In all cases, direct symptom-removal will be most successful and such dangers entirely avoided if, at each and every session, it is preceded by a sequence of simple psychotherapeutic suggestions designed to remove tension, anxiety and apprehension, and to gradually restore the patient's confidence in himself and his ability to cope with his problems.

This was the principle upon which was based the subsequent development of the *ego-strengthening technique*, a procedure which I have been employing successfully for many years, during which I have hardly ever seen either the release of undue anxiety or the occurrence of substitute symptoms. Moreover, once treatment has been successfully completed, only rarely have I been confronted with any relapse, which could always be attributed to some entirely new and unanticipated emotional disturbances, equally easy to deal with. The significance of this lies in the fact that when symptom-removal is preceded by simple psychotherapy, it is not only greatly facilitated but becomes much more effective and produces more permanent results. Indeed, the patient's ability to adjust himself to his difficulties is strengthened to such an extent that relapses are much less likely to occur.

The Ego-strengthening Technique

Psychotherapy of this kind need be neither difficult nor complicated, provided that certain fundamental requirements of the patient are borne in mind. For this purpose his psychological reactions to his illness can be conveniently divided into two groups:

1. Those arising as a consequence of the illness itself, such as anxiety, fear, tension and agitation.
2. Those arising from defects in his own personality, such as nervousness, lack of confidence, dependence and maladjustment.

In planning your general psychotherapeutic suggestions to combat these, many can be adopted as standard ones which remain unchanged from case to case. Others will naturally have to be added or varied to suit each individual and his particular complaint. If once you develop the habit of using such a technique in every case that you treat under hypnosis before you proceed either with direct symptom-removal or hypno-analysis as the main object of your therapy, you will find it will pay handsome dividends. Not only will the patient obtain more rapid relief from his symptoms, but he will display obvious improvement in other ways. You will notice him becoming more self-reliant, more confident and more able to adjust to his environment, and thus much less prone to relapse. In fact, my own experience has led me to believe, and this has been confirmed by innumerable reports from professional colleagues, medical and dental both in this country and overseas, that *this combination of what I call ' ego-strengthening ' suggestions and symptom-removal will enable the general practitioner to deal successfully with the majority of his cases without having to resort to hypno-analytical procedures.* Naturally, he will still encounter some cases in which a relatively simple investigation and superficial analysis of the patient's current environmental difficulties and his reactions to them will render his treatment both speedier and more effective. Even under these circumstances, I still adopt the same basic scheme in framing my therapeutic suggestions, incorporating any additions that may seem desirable as a result of analytical investigation. It has been especially interesting to hear how many dental surgeons are successfully using a specially constructed and shortened version of the standard technique in their everyday work.

In the construction of an ego-strengthening technique, quite apart from the actual suggestions themselves, it is essential that particular attention should be paid to such significant factors as ' *rhythm* ', ' *repetition* ', the *interpolation of appropriate* ' *pauses* ', and the ' *stressing of certain important words and phrases* '. The verbalization that I devised for my own use, even in psychiatric work, has been carefully constructed in accordance with these principles. In this connection, I consider certain points to be worthy of your attention. You will notice that repetition is often achieved by expressing the same fundamental idea in two or three different ways. This tends to avoid excessive monotony. Some words and phrases are stressed because of their importance and significance to the patient himself. Other words are stressed and suitable pauses included with the sole purpose of emphasizing the rhythm of the whole delivery which, in my opinion contributes considerably to its success. The manipulation of these factors should become self-evident as I describe the whole routine.

First, I must refer briefly to the question of trance depth. One of the advantages of this technique is the fact that deep trances are certainly not essential. Nevertheless, as in most hypnotherapeutic methods, the deeper the trance, the more rapidly improvement will occur and the shorter the duration of a course of treatment will be. The patient who has been conditioned to enter the hypnotic state upon a given signal, verbal or otherwise, can usually be regarded as having attained sufficient depth for treatment to be effective. Yet even this is not absolutely necessary since a satisfactory response can often be obtained in light trance states only. Under these circumstances, however, one would naturally expect treatment to be continued over a longer period and the results to manifest themselves more slowly. Methods of trance induction and deepening are of little significance and can be safely left to individual preference, although I do consider it important that the patient should be rendered as fully relaxed, mentally and physically, as possible and it is well worth while spending a little extra time to attain this objective.

In the following detailed account and analysis, I am describing in full the routine I use successfully in dealing with such cases as anxiety states, tension states, phobias, etc. Most of it is equally applicable as a prelude to the treatment of asthmas, migraines and various psychosomatic conditions. It lends itself admirably to shortening, adaptation and the addition of specialized suggestions in accordance with individual needs, both of the patient and of the therapist.

A Typical Ego-strengthening Routine

Once the patient is in a trance state and is as fully relaxed as possible, I proceed as follows:

> You have now become *so* deeply relaxed . . . *so* deeply asleep . . . that your mind has become *so* sensitive . . . *so* receptive to what I say . . . that *everything* that I put into your mind . . . will sink *so* deeply into the unconscious part of your mind . . . and will cause so deep and lasting an impression there . . . that *nothing* will eradicate it.

This tends to prepare the patient's mind to receive the suggestions that follow. Notice the stressing and repetition of the word ' *so* ' which not only adds force to the ideas presented, but also strongly emphasizes the rhythmic quality of the delivery.

> Consequently . . . these things that I put into your unconscious mind . . . will begin to exercise a greater and greater influence over the way you think . . . over the way you feel . . over the way you behave.

This is the first indication to the patient that he will begin to feel a gradual change in his thoughts, feelings and actions, as a result of the suggestions he is about to receive.

> And . . . because these things *will* remain . . . firmly imbedded in the unconscious part of your mind . . . after you have left here . . . when you are no longer with me . . . they will continue to exercise that same great influence . . . over your *thoughts* . . . your *feelings* . . . and your *actions* . . . *just* as strongly . . . *just* as surely . . . *just* as powerfully . . . when you are back home . . . or at work . . . as when you are with me in this room.

Here you will notice the introduction of the first unobtrusive post-hypnotic suggestion to the effect that the patient can expect the same changes to continue in his everyday life, after the trance state has been terminated. Note also that so far, all the suggestions have been directed towards the modification of the three fundamental psychological processes —' *thinking* ', ' *feeling* ', and ' *acting* '. These words have been stressed because of their importance to the patient, and the word ' *just* ', in order to add to the rhythmic quality of the delivery. Repetition has been ensured by the use of three different words—' *strongly* ', ' *surely* ', ' *powerfully* '—all of which convey the same essential idea. Those familiar with my original descriptions of this technique will realize that these groups of suggestions are entirely new. Judging by clinical results, I am convinced that their addition has given increased force to the effectiveness of the basic routine.

You are now so *very deeply asleep* . . . that *everything* that I tell you that is going to happen to you . . . *for your own good* . . . *will* happen . . . *exactly* as I tell you.

And *every feeling* . . . that I tell you that you will experience . . . you *will* experience . . . *exactly* as I tell you.

And these same things *will continue to happen* to you . . . *every day* . . . and you *will continue to experience* these same feelings . . . *every day* . . . just as strongly *just* as surely . . . *just* as powerfully . . . when you are back home . . . or at work . . . as when you are with me in this room.

Here we have repetition, not only of single words or phrases, but of the same group of expectations and ideas already expressed—' driving them home '—as it were. The patient begins to expect that he will not only experience something in the course of the trance, but that he will continue to benefit from this even when he is no longer receiving active treatment! I attach the greatest importance to this ' post-hypnotic ' effect, for surely the whole success of treatment under hypnosis depends upon the simple fact that the suggestions last longer than the trance itself. The words ' *will* ' and ' *exactly* ', together with other phrases of significance to the patient, are pronounced with increased emphasis to add force and authority to the suggestions, and although you will have noticed the continued interpolation of ' *pauses* ', I have not drawn particular attention to them. Let me repeat one phrase in a slightly different manner:

Just as strongly . . . (pause) . . . *just* as surely . . . (pause) . . . *just* as powerfully . . . (pause).

and observe how the stressing of the word ' *just* ' helps to drive the idea home, almost like the blows of a hammer, and this, taken in conjunction with the pauses, establishes a rhythmical quality to the delivery similar to the beat of a metronome. In this connection, I think most of us tend to pay far too little attention to the importance of pauses in our work with hypnosis. Although this may be partly due to the limitations on our time, I am sure that this is not invariably the case. After all, when we give the patient a drug we are quite content to allow sufficient time for it to take effect, and if only we adopted the same attitude of mind when working with a patient in a hypnotic trance I am convinced that our results would become greatly enhanced.

As a result of this brief analysis of the mode of construction and delivery of these suggestive routines, you should now be able to detect these devices whenever they are used. You will find that, throughout the rest of this technique, I have strictly observed the same cardinal principles of 'repetition', 'stressing', and the use of 'synonymous words and phrases' intermingled with 'pauses' to secure a smooth, rhythmic delivery.

During this deep sleep . . . *you* are going to feel physically *stronger* and *fitter* in every way.

You will feel *more* alert . . . *more* wide-awake . . . *more* energetic.

You will become *much* less easily tired . . . *much* less easily fatigued . . . *much* less easily discouraged . . . *much* less easily depressed.

Every day . . . you will become *so deeply interested* in whatever you are doing . . . in whatever is going on around you . . . that your mind will become *completely distracted away from yourself.*

You will no longer *think nearly so much about yourself* . . . you will no longer *dwell nearly so much upon yourself and your difficulties* . . . and you will become *much less conscious of yourself* . . . *much less pre-occupied with yourself* . . . *and with your own feelings.*

Every day . . . your nerves will become *stronger and steadier* . . . your mind *calmer and clearer* . . . *more composed* . . . *more placid* . . . *more tranquil.* You will become *much less easily worried* . . . *much less easily agitated* . . . *much less easily fearful and apprehensive* . . . *much less easily upset.*

Here are the first group of actual 'ego-strengthening' suggestions, intended to improve the patient's general condition, to strengthen his weaknesses, to increase his confidence and to allay his anxieties. You will notice as we proceed how they have been designed, not only to alleviate most of the complaints made by the average neurotic, but also to improve and mitigate those defects which have contributed largely to his illness.

You will be able to *think more clearly* . . . you will be able to *concentrate more easily.*

You will be able to *give up your whole undivided attention to whatever you are doing* . . . *to the complete exclusion of everything else.*

Consequently . . . *your memory will rapidly improve* . . . and you will be able to *see things in their true perspective* . . . *without magnifying your difficulties* . . . *without ever allowing them to get out of proportion.*

Every day . . . you will become *emotionally much calmer* . . . *much more settled* . . . *much less easily disturbed.*

Every day . . . *you* will become . . . and *you* will remain . . . *more and more completely relaxed* . . . and *less tense* each day . . . *both mentally and physically* . . . even when you are no longer with me.

And *as you become* . . . and *as you remain* . . . *more relaxed* . . . *and less tense* each day . . . *so* . . . you will develop *much more confidence in yourself* . . . more confidence in your ability to *do* . . . not only what you *have* . . . to do each day . . . but more confidence in your ability to do whatever you *ought* to be able to do . . . *without fear of failure* . . . *without fear of consequences* . . . *without unnecessary anxiety* . . . *without uneasiness.*

Because of this . . . *every day* . . . you will feel *more and more independent* . . . *more able to ' stick up for yourself '* . . . *to stand upon your own feet* . . . *to hold your own* . . . no matter how difficult or trying things may be.

You have probably noticed how much more positive and definitive the suggestions have become as the treatment proceeded.

Every day . . . you will feel a *greater feeling of personal well-being* . . . *A greater feeling of personal safety* . . . *and security* . . . than you have felt for a long, long time.

And because all these things *will* begin to happen . . . *exactly* as I tell you they will happen . . . *more and more rapidly* . . . *powerfully* . . . *and completely* . . . with every treatment I give you . . . you will feel *much happier* . . . *much more contented* . . . *much more optimistic* in every way.

You will consequently become much more able to *rely upon* . . . *to depend upon* . . . *yourself* . . . *your own efforts* . . . *your own judgement* . . . *your own opinions.* You will feel *much less need* . . . to have to *rely upon* . . . or to *depend upon* . . . *other people.*

I have found this routine, the full and unabbreviated version of which I have just described, to be equally valuable in preceding direct symptom-removal or the more involved hypno-analytical techniques. Constant repetition at the beginning of each treatment session strengthens the ' ego-defences ' to such an extent that it not only renders the symptoms more vulnerable to direct suggestion and lessens the likelihood of relapse, but will often enable a patient to co-operate eventually in an analytical investigation he was formerly ill-equipped to face.

No matter what particular branch of therapeutic activity in which you are engaged, I have always found that patients will respond much more rapidly and effectively to treatment if you will only deal with them as intelligent individuals, and explain in advance exactly what you propose to do, why you are doing it, and what they can reasonably expect to happen. Consequently, I invariably find it helpful to explain to the patient, in the waking state, why and how he can expect this method to work.

When you first went to school, I'm sure you can remember sometimes being given a short piece of poetry to learn off by heart so that you could recite it next morning without the book.

And how did you set about this task ?

I expect that you read the poem over and over again at home, possibly aloud, and each time you did so, a little bit more of it became stuck in your mind until eventually you could recite the whole of it from memory, without referring to the book.

Now this treatment acts in exactly the same way because it is also a ' *learning process* ', only instead of having to do it all yourself, every time I repeat these suggestions to you, more and more of them will stick in your unconscious mind so that you will gradually notice yourself improving in your everyday life, even when you are no longer with me.

This will happen more quickly and easily than when you are wide-awake because, whenever you enter a trance state, your memory becomes greatly improved, and your powers of concentration greatly increased.

I always begin every treatment session with this particular sequence of suggestions as soon as the induction and deepening of hypnosis have been completed. The suggestions are given slowly and deliberately, and I prefer to leave those specifically directed towards symptom-removal to the end, since this seems to render them more effective. Indeed, in certain psychosomatic cases in which symptom-removal is the principal objective, a somewhat abbreviated version may be used before proceeding with the main suggestions to that effect. In neurotic, anxiety, tension and phobic states, however, I always employ it in full, coupled at times with a relatively superficial analysis of the patient's current problems and difficulties. Used regularly in this way, its efficacy can be surprising. In my own psychiatric practice, some 70 per cent of my patients recover as a result of this technique alone, usually within Wolberg's suggested limit of twenty sessions of short-term psychotherapy.

It is certainly not intended that this verbatim account should be adopted in the precise form I have described. It is the principle that I consider worthy of attention, and the sequence I have outlined should be regarded simply as a guide to the individual therapist in framing his own suggestions to conform with his own personality, method of approach, and style of delivery. It is impossible to suggest here the varying inflections of the voice, but the same cardinal rules of construction, stresses and pauses etc. should be used in order to maintain a rhythmical quality from start to finish.

The following case history, with a somewhat unexpected result, seems to illustrate the effectiveness of this technique:

The patient was a young man, a salesman aged 28, and happily married. He had been suffering from ' *claustrophobia* ' for about 7 years and was quite incapable of remaining in confined spaces without developing acute attacks of panic and anxiety. Curiously enough, he had never sought treatment for this before I saw him. Recently, he had been moved to the top floor of an eight-storey block of flats. Since he found it impossible to use the lift (or elevator) he was compelled to climb the stairs several times a day, and this was making his life intolerable. Obviously motivation was strong. He was a highly-strung, anxious individual, lacking in confidence, but otherwise fairly well-integrated, with no gross personality defects. No significant factors emerged from routine investigation of his childhood, his family history, or his prevailing environmental circumstances.

I concluded that only an analytical approach would be likely to solve this problem. Unfortunately, however, whilst he was easily taught to enter the hypnotic state upon a given signal, the simpler methods of analytical investigation failed to produce any clues whatsoever, and it proved impossible to deepen his hypnosis sufficiently to use the more involved hypno-analytical techniques.

He attended for treatment once a week, and since mentioning his incapacity seemed to distress him greatly, I ceased to refer either to ' claustrophobia' or to the difficulty he was experiencing with the lift, I consequently continued with the ' ego-strengthening ' technique alone. and made no attempt whatever at direct symptom-removal. I hoped that he would eventually improve sufficiently to permit this, or that it would become possible to obtain the greater depth necessary for further analysis. Certainly after a few weeks he became much calmer and less tense, and seemed to be gaining more confidence in himself. Nevertheless, I was both surprised and gratified when he attended for his eleventh session, looking extremely pleased with himself. Apparently, several days before, he was carrying home a load of timber with which he intended to make book-cases, and whilst passing the lift and faced with eight flights of stairs to climb, he suddenly felt that he might be able to overcome his fears sufficiently to try to use it. This he did, on the spur of the moment, and subsequently experienced no further difficulty whatever. In view of many past experiences in dealing with this kind of symptom, I can only say that such a quick and satisfactory result was entirely unexpected.

Suggestion in Symptom-removal

When using hypnotic suggestion in a direct attack upon symptoms, certain basic principles must be observed in order to succeed. One of the first and most important things to do is to try to increase the patient's motivation before starting treatment. You should always discuss his symptoms in some detail, emphasizing how inconvenient and distressing they are, and pointing out how different and more enjoyable life will become once they have disappeared. You should then explain to him how hypnosis can help to get rid of them by producing complete mental and physical relaxation. Naturally, you must speak with the utmost conviction, for the patient will always accept suggestions much more readily when he feels that you have a firm belief in what you are saying.

The suggestions made should always be positive, direct, logical and accompanied by sound reasons for their acceptance. You should certainly give them with authority, whilst also taking care that the patient does not feel that he is being dominated. It is not a difficult matter to phrase suggestions in such a way as to avoid this, and yet convey your confidence that they will be accepted. The application of these principles can best be illustrated by considering the use of the hypnosis in the alleviation of pain.

Hypnosis in the Relief of Pain

The ability to control pain and sometimes to abolish it completely in the hypnotic state is one of the most remarkable and impressive phenomena we can observe. Unfortunately it has one main drawback in that it is unpredictable and even unreliable in any individual case. I have seen cases in which pain could be completely abolished when the patient was only in medium-depth hypnosis and others in which little or no analgesia could be produced in deep or even somnambulistic trances. Much may therefore depend upon the normal threshold of pain in the individual patient. Since the production of satisfactory analgesia seems to be extremely capricious, it would appear to offer only limited scope in the hypnotic treatment of painful conditions; this, however, is far from being the case.

Some years ago I was undertaking the hypnotic training of a young married woman in preparation for her confinement. She was a good subject, and I had already taught her self-hypnosis as a result of which she was able to produce a state of complete relaxation whenever she wished to do so. She had previously achieved so deep a state of hypnosis that I had no doubt that I should easily succeed in inducing a complete analgesia to pin-prick. Unfortunately I was mistaken and this did not occur, and the most I was able to achieve was a slight blunting of sensation to painful stimuli—all attempts to secure a complete analgesia failed completely. Despite this, I continued to impress upon her mind the fact that during her confinement she would be able to relax and free herself from tension so completely that she would still be able to abolish pain and merely experience the discomfort of her uterine contractions. Several weeks later she appeared with her right arm in a sling. It seemed that she and her husband had been involved in a car accident, as a result of which she had developed acute pain in her right arm and shoulder. Worried at her distress, he left her sitting by the road-side and hurried to the nearest farmhouse to seek assistance. When he returned, he was amazed to find that during his absence she had put herself into the hypnotic state and had completely abolished all pain and discomfort.

It must, therefore, sometimes be possible for hypnosis to secure complete relief from pain arising from pathological or physiological processes in cases in which it was impossible to produce any marked degree of insensitivity to pain caused by an artificial, external stimulus. Certain carefully controlled experiments carried out in the research laboratories of Harvard University led to the conclusion that pain of the pathological variety is much more susceptible to suggestion than artificially induced pain.

The importance of this can hardly be over-estimated. It means that even if you fail to produce any significant degree of analgesia to pin-prick, you may still succeed in relieving pain that is organically or psychologically determined. Of these two, it is probable that the latter will prove the easier to deal with.

Several years ago, Goldie discovered that many patients arriving in a Casualty Department with severe pain due to injury were not only capable of being induced into deep hypnosis on the spot, but could also have fractures set and injuries dressed quite painlessly under no other form of anaesthesia or sedation. This is particularly likely to occur if the patient happens to be terrified of having a general anaesthetic. Once again, we can trace the all-important question of motivation. It can truly be said that the greater the patient feels the need for hypnotic treatment, the more readily and deeply he will respond.

The technique of pain-removal. Whenever you attempt to remove symptoms by attacking them directly, it is always wise to give logical reasons for the disappearance of the symptom which support the actual suggestions you are using. It is quite useless to say to a patient, ' Your pain has gone. It has disappeared completely.' Being acutely aware of discomfort, he knows that it hasn't, and can see no reason why it should just because you say so. He will consequently reject the suggestion completely. On the other hand, if you adopt the following approach, not only are your suggestions more likely to be accepted, but treatment will be much more effective:

> Pain is often caused . . . and is always aggravated by tension.
> Consequently . . . as you become more relaxed and less tense . . . so you are beginning to feel more comfortable.
> As this relaxation increases . . . so your pain is gradually becoming easier and easier . . . and presently you will feel so completely and utterly relaxed that the pain will disappear completely.

Here you will notice that the phrasing of the suggestions explains to the patient why he can expect to experience relief. There is no doubt that as his hypnosis became deeper, he did in fact feel more and more relaxed. This will certainly have produced a greater feeling of comfort. Consequently, by relating the suggested disappearance of the pain to these two established facts, the patient is much more ready to believe that this also will presently occur. Moreover, ample time has been afforded for the desired suggestion to take effect.

Another useful technique in the relief of pain is the production of a suggested feeling of warmth in the affected part. Even in the lighter stages of hypnosis this is fairly easy to secure. It used to be considered quite important by the earlier medical hypnotists, many of whom held its appearance to be an accurate test of the genuineness of the hypnotic state. It can be greatly facilitated by gently stroking the appropriate area, and in evoking this phenomenon it should be remembered that two important principles of suggestion are involved: the giving of a positive rather than a negative suggestion, and the coupling of a desired effect with one that is already taking place. The following example shows its application in the removal of headache:

> As I stroke your forehead . . . you can feel a feeling of warmth . . . spreading all over your head, face, and neck.
> That feeling of warmth is increasing . . . with every stroke of my hands.
> As soon as you can feel this warmth . . . please lift up your hand.

(The patient's hand slowly rises.)

> Good. Put your hand down again.
> And as this feeling of warmth increases . . . with every stroke of my hands . . . so your head is beginning to feel more and more comfortable.
> As the warmth increases . . . so your pain is becoming less and less . . . and in a few moments . . . your head will feel so warm and comfortable . . . that all the pain will have disappeared completely . . . and your head will feel quite free from all pain . . . aching . . . and discomfort.

As soon as your head feels quite warm and comfortable . . . and all the pain and aching has disappeared completely . . . please lift up your hand.

(The patient's hand slowly rises again.)

Good. Put it down again.
And in a few moments . . . when I count up to *seven* . . . you will wake up again . . . feeling perfectly fit and well . . . with your head completely clear and comfortable . . . without the slightest trace of pain . . . aching . . . or discomfort.

Suggested alterations in the sensation of the affected part can be advantageously used in conditions other than pain. I always use this technique in conjunction with the suggested shrinkage and disappearance of warts. In this connection, either suggested warmth or coldness can be equally effective. But in certain skin conditions where it is necessary to allay irritation, to prevent itching or to produce analgesia, the suggested cooling of the desired area is likely to prove more successful.

Initial Preparation for Simple Hypnotherapy
Whilst the deepest trance state possible is always advantageous but rarely essential, I have found that the patient who has been conditioned to enter the hypnotic state immediately upon receiving the instruction to do so, has usually attained sufficient depth to be effective for all ordinary treatment purposes. Even this depth is not absolutely necessary, for a satisfactory response may often be obtained in the lighter stages of hypnosis. Under such circumstances, however, treatment will naturally have to be extended over a longer period. In the case of the patient who readily enters the trance state when instructed to do so, I usually adopt the following routine at each treatment session:

1. I tell the patient to lie back comfortably in the chair, to let himself relax as much as possible, and to breathe quietly, in and out. I then tell him to go to sleep, upon which his eyes close immediately.
2. I take him through the complete relaxation sequence, used in his initial induction, starting with his feet and ankles and finishing with his neck, shoulders and arms, coupling each stage with suggestions of increasing depth.
3. I follow this with the counting and breathing technique for further deepening, as already described on page 76.

Although the last two steps are certainly not essential and may be omitted, they exercise a valuable deepening effect and allow time for the hypnosis to become firmly established. Since they can be completed in some 5 or 6 minutes the extra time is well spent for it seems to render the patient much more receptive to the therapeutic suggestions which follow.

4. I start treatment with the ego-strengthening routine, which occupies a further 7 to 8 minutes, and only when this has been completed do I proceed with the suggestions directed towards symptom removal.

CHAPTER 16

Nocturnal Enuresis and Asthma

Hypnosis in Nocturnal Enuresis

This troublesome and distressing condition is often met in general practice, usually in children. Whilst in most cases it proves to be psychogenic in origin, a physical and urological examination is always necessary to exclude any organic factor. Even such simple conditions as over-acidity of the urine and an irritable bladder should be treated by the administration of alkalis and hyoscyamus, in addition to whatever psychotherapeutic methods may be employed.

The power of retention of urine is a habit which can be cultivated in childhood. In many cases of bed-wetting, it will be found that the child passes water too frequently during the day as well as at night, with the result that the bladder capacity becomes smaller than normal. It is possible to increase this by training if the child is encouraged to hold his water as long as possible during the day, and only to pass it when the urge to do so can no longer be resisted. Moreover, a greater degree of control can gradually be established if the child is taught to make a habit of interrupting the stream two or three times whenever he passes water in the daytime.

The psychogenic factors underlying this habit are now generally accepted. It may arise from defective toilet-training, or as a result of certain childish illnesses. In many cases it follows the birth of another child when it is the outward expression of unconscious anxiety. The mother's attention has to be shared with the newcomer, and the child not only resents this, but also develops an unconscious feeling of insecurity. It is prolonged into later childhood because it provides the means of attracting the mother's interest and anxiety, and is sometimes employed as a defence against an over-fussy or nagging parent. Prognosis will thus depend largely upon the successful modification of unfavourable environmental influences.

The attitude of the parents, particularly that of the mother may well determine the difference between success and failure. The extra work imposed by the daily washing of soiled bed-linen, together with the worry caused by an increasing sense of hopelessness and defeatism, only too often lead to a complete lack of sympathy and understanding. The wretched child is not only scolded, sometimes even punished, but also has to endure the humiliation of ridicule at the hands of brothers, sisters and other children, so it is hardly surprising that it so frequently remains sodden, unhappy and miserable.

Before treating the child, the parent, usually the mother, should be interviewed. Explain to her how the condition probably arose, and lay particular emphasis on the fact that the child is to be pitied rather than blamed, since it is unable to help itself. Sympathize with her own difficulties and concern, but point out that in showing her anxiety to the child, she is creating the very conditions that tend to prolong the habit. Tell her that if treatment is to succeed, she must try to ignore the wet beds and treat them with indifference, never even referring to them in the child's presence. She must never give the child anything to drink last thing at night, and should always see that he passes water immediately before getting into bed. If, as so often happens, the child is put to bed early in the evening, then before going to bed herself she should pick him up and see that he empties his bladder once more. These points may seem very obvious and trivial, but they are all-important and should never be omitted.

You should then talk to the child, and try to gain his confidence and co-operation. Tell him that he can be cured if he wishes, that whilst he is getting better he is bound to have a certain number of accidents, but that gradually he will begin to be dry more and more often. Tell the child and his parents that they must stop thinking and talking about wet beds. After all, a bed that is half-wet can be equally accurately described as half-dry. They should begin to think solely in terms of dry beds, and the parents should try to encourage a sense of pride and achievement whenever the child has one. I always insist upon a weekly record being kept of what happens each night. For this purpose I adopt a simple sub-division into *dry*, *partly dry* and *no change*. The record provides a valuable indication as to the progress of treatment. It is kept by the mother if the child is very young, but otherwise I ask the child to do this himself in his own writing as this provides a great incentive to progress.

In most cases of enuresis the child will invariably wet the bed when it is afraid that it will do so. Consequently, it is necessary to deal with this fear during treatment, and to encourage an expectation of dry beds.

Sporadic relapses can often be directly traced to emotional disturbances, so when these occur it is always wise to question the child as to what has happened the previous day, either at school or at home. Suitable suggestions can then be included in the treatment. Although many enuretics sleep too deeply, it is usually unnecessary to correct this by means of drugs since it is relatively easy to adjust it by hypnotic suggestion.

Routine Hypnotic Treatment

I prefer to have the child sitting comfortably in a chair. I then induce as deep a trance state as possible. If somnambulism can be achieved (and this is not difficult in many cases) so much the better, and whilst certainly not essential, amnesia will always lead to more rapid results.

> As a result of this deep sleep, you are going to feel stronger and better every day. You will become *much* calmer . . . *much* quieter . . . *much* less easily excited . . . *much* less nervous . . . *much* less easily upset.
> Every day, you will feel *much more confidence* in yourself . . . you will feel more able to *stick up for yourself* . . . to *hold your own* . . . *without becoming worried* . . . *without becoming frightened* . . . *without becoming anxious.*

This is a brief, modified version of my routine ego-strengthening suggestions, which I have found to be extremely useful in dealing with the nervous, highly strung child.

Following this, I then sit down beside the child, and gently massage his stomach.

> As I stroke your tummy like this . . . you will feel a feeling of warmth in your tummy . . . your tummy is getting warmer and warmer, with every stroke of my hand.
> As soon as you feel your tummy getting warmer . . . please lift up your hand.

Both the stroking and the suggestions of increasing warmth are continued until the hand rises:

> Good. Now, put your hand down again.
> And as I continue to stroke your tummy, that warmth is spreading deep down into the lower part of your tummy . . . into the bladder, that holds your water. And, as your bladder becomes warmer . . . so, it is becoming stronger . . . so that it will be able to hold your water, all night long, and in the morning your bed will be dry.
> With every treatment I give you, it will become stronger and stronger . . .

the nerves that control your bladder will become stronger, and less irritable
. . . so that you will begin to get more and more dry beds . . . until, eventually, you will have a dry bed *every morning*.

Here, direct suggestions are being made with regard to improvement
in bladder capacity and control, and the expectation of improved performance is being emphasized.

You will *never* have anything to drink just before your bed-time.
You will *always* remember to pass water, *immediately* before you get into bed.
You *won't worry* about whether you will have a dry bed or not, because,
presently, there will be no need for you to do so . . . and the less you worry
about it . . . the quicker the beds will become dry.
You will sleep well . . . but you will *not* sleep so deeply . . . so that if there
is any need for you to pass water during the night, your tummy will begin
to feel *so uncomfortable* that it will wake you up in plenty of time for you to
get out of bed, and pass water in the proper place. When you get back
into bed again, you will fall asleep right away . . . and when you wake up
in the morning, *your bed will be dry*.

Post-hypnotic suggestion is now being used, and is often most useful
in establishing some control over the situation.

And, during the daytime, whenever you feel you want to pass water, I
want you to hold it back, as long as you can . . . and only go to the toilet
when you feel you can't possibly last much longer.
If you get into the habit of doing this, you will find that you will gradually
be able to hold your water longer and longer during the day . . . and as
this happens, you will be able to hold it longer and longer during the night
. . . all night long, in fact . . . so that in the morning your bed will be dry.
Whenever you do pass water, during the day, as soon as you have started,
I want you to get into the habit of stopping yourself before you have
finished . . . starting again . . . then stopping again . . . and then finishing
completely. If you do this, it will help you to get complete control over
it, even during the night.

These suggestions relating to bladder exercises will be found most
useful in increasing both the bladder capacity, and control.

And because these things *will happen* . . . *exactly as I tell you they will happen*
. . . you will feel *much* happier . . . *much* more contented . . . *much* less
easily worried . . . *much* less easily upset.
And, in a few moments, when I count up to *seven* . . . you will open your
eyes and be wide awake again . . . feeling very much better for this long
sleep.

I have described the above treatment in terms that are quite applicable to the average schoolchild. Naturally, the child's age and intelligence must be taken into account, and the wording of the suggestions varied accordingly. In some cases, certain omissions may also have to be made.

Whenever very deep hypnosis, or somnambulism has been achieved, I use the following procedure instead which, when successful, greatly increases the force of the post-hypnotic suggestion:

> In a few moments, your tummy is going to feel more and more uncomfortable. You will begin to feel that you want to pass water ... and your tummy will feel so uncomfortable that it will wake you up, out of this sleep, in plenty of time to go to the toilet.
> As soon as your tummy feels uncomfortable . . . your eyes will open, and you will be wide awake again . . . feeling that you want to pass water.

I then stop speaking, and wait. Presently, the child will probably wriggle a little in the chair, but his eyes will open, and he will say that he wants to go to the toilet. If he says nothing, ask him if he feels anything wrong, and this will almost always elicit the response that he wants to pass water. Send him off to the toilet immediately, and as soon as he returns, put him straight off to sleep again.

> If ever there is any need for you to pass water during the night, your tummy will begin to feel more and more uncomfortable . . . and will wake you up, out of your sleep . . . *just as it did, a few minutes ago* . . . feeling that you want to pass water . . . *in plenty of time to get out of bed, and pass it in the proper place* . . . *so that every morning, your bed will be dry.*

The suggestions for bladder training can follow this and the treatment completed as already described.

Nocturnal Enuresis in Adults

It is often mistakenly thought that nocturnal enuresis is only a childish complaint, and that most children grow out of it. Whilst many of them do, there are other unfortunates who retain the habit into adult life and in whom it causes untold misery and mental distress. Difficult though these cases prove to be, hypnosis usually offers a greater chance of improvement than any other form of treatment, depending largely upon the depth of trance that can be achieved. Even so, because of the prolonged duration of the complaint, it is bound to be more time-consuming than in the case of children although the results, when satisfactory, render the extra effort well worth while.

It usually starts, in childhood, as a result of the factors already discussed, and its persistence into adult life is frequently associated with some degree of emotional immaturity. Wolberg considers that it is often maintained by unconscious mental conflicts, sexual or aggressive in nature, and sometimes represents a masturbatory equivalent. Aggression is generally directed either against the parents or circumstances in general. In other cases, he thinks it denotes an appeal for dependence on the part of a childish, passive personality. Cases in which sexual or aggressive conflicts predominate will usually need the deeper hypno-analytical approach, which rarely falls within the scope of the general practitioner. On the other hand, many in whom emotional disturbances and the need for dependence are prominent factors, respond extremely well to symptom removal preceded by the ego-strengthening routine in an adult form. Careful history-taking will greatly assist in the selection of cases suitable for this form of treatment.

The part that emotional stress can play in enuresis is often seen in everyday life. Although ordinarily continent, the candidate waiting for a viva-voce examination will not infrequently need to pay several visits to the toilet. The threat of imminent danger can also produce the same result. The need for dependence is generally a prolongation into adult life of the same unconscious motives that operated in childhood.

I have found that there often exists a much greater conscious desire for cure in adults, than in many children. In several cases, it has been regarded as a barrier to marriage, or to the adoption of a much desired career. Consequently it is possible to make use of this motivation and to strengthen it, thereby rendering both the induction of hypnosis and the deepening process much easier. As deep a trance state as possible is always advisable, the attempt at which I prefer to extend over three consecutive sessions. In most instances, sufficient depth can be obtained for adequate therapy, although where somnambulism can be achieved, the task will be greatly simplified. Instructions and treatment follow the same pattern as that described for childish enuresis, with such re-wording and rephrasing as would seem necessary to suit an adult. Not only do I give the ego-strengthening suggestions in full, but I augment them by explaining to the patient how his trouble arises from a continuation of a childish feeling of helplessness, and a fear of accepting adult responsibilities. Moreover, I give the strongest possible suggestions that, with each treatment, he will find it easier to stop behaving like a child, and will be able to face his difficulties like a man. When somnambulism is achieved, it is just as effective to secure the awakening of the patient from hypnosis, with a feeling of discomfort and desire to pass water, as it is in the case of a child, particularly if care is taken to associate this action in the patient's mind with a feeling of satisfaction and achievement.

It will occasionally be found, both in the case of adults and children, that the depth of sleep is too great for the patient to respond to the need to urinate and that even hypnotic suggestion that the sleep will be lighter fails to have any effect. In such cases the use of a drug will be necessary and amphetamine sulphate is the one of choice. Curiously enough, even when the dosage is large, few patients seem to complain of insomnia although the drug is taken last thing at night. Once the correct dosage has been established, patients seem to enjoy just as refreshing a sleep as they did previously. The effective dosage will vary from patient to patient, and can only be established by experience. Even children may require one or two tablets of dextro-amphetamine to start with, and this dose will often have to be greatly exceeded in the case of adults. Should any initial difficulty in getting off to sleep occur, this can often be successfully dealt with by post-hypnotic suggestion. Dosage should be maintained until the bed-wetting ceases, and should then be reduced very gradually. It may, however, have to be adjusted from time to time during the period of treatment if the patient does complain of wakeful nights. As an alternative, good results have been reported in the case of children from the administration of a single paediatric dose of Syrup of Tryptizol (amitryptyline), last thing at night.

It is also possible to teach the patient to use auto-hypnosis each night before he goes to sleep. With suitable suggestions, this can sometimes enable him to control the level of his sleep much better, thus avoiding the necessity for using the undesirable amphetamine drugs.

Occasionally a post-hypnotic suggestion can be given (to both children and adults) that the patient will awaken at a given time during the night and get out of bed to pass water, or even that he will be able to sleep the whole night through. The best criterion for the latter suggestion lies in the fact that if the patient can hold his water for four hours during the day, he is likely to hold it for eight hours during the night when the kidney secretes only half the amount of urine. Consequently, when there is *no* frequency by day, it can be suggested that the patient will be able to hold his water all night.

Finally, it should be borne in mind that very deep sleep is sometimes a neurotic reaction, in which the individual is so unhappy that instead of merely sleeping, he goes into a comatose-like state in order to escape from his difficulties.

Hypnosis in Asthma

By far the most important truth that has to be accepted concerning the hypnotic treatment of asthma is briefly this: *the more the attacks are precipitated by psychological or emotional disturbances, the better will be the prognosis.*

Nevertheless, even when the asthma is determined by organic factors, such as bronchitis, emphysema, allergies or cardiac disturbances, considerable relief can still be afforded and the frequency and severity of the attacks diminished through the reduction of the fear and anxiety caused by each impending threat of breathlessness. Moreover children who suffer from asthma are generally so responsive to hypnosis that, were its use restricted to the treatment of this complaint alone it would still, I believe, justify itself in general practice.

Only too frequently asthma is regarded as if it were a disease in its own right, but of course it is merely a symptom (paroxysmal dyspnoea) of several different conditions and is due to a variety of causes, some organic and some psychological. Even in those cases arising from organic disease the attacks can be affected by emotional disturbances, so that obviously the family doctor is in far the most favourable position to assess the illness accurately against the psychological background. To do this, it is necessary to seek the answers to the following three questions:

1. Why did this patient become ill, in the first place?
2. What kind of an individual is he?
3. Why did he develop this particular complaint?

The personality of the patient, the attitude of the parents, his reactions to brothers and sisters, to school, or to over-excitement or stress should all be the subject of enquiry. Information should also be sought as to the presence of allergies, and his food-habits. This applies equally in the case of adults, as to children. Indeed, the answers to these three questions are of the utmost importance in all cases of psychosomatic illness, no matter what the particular symptomatology may be.

Asthma in Children

The typical asthmatic child is usually both bright and intelligent. At the same time he will frequently be found to be over-anxious, dependent, and lacking in confidence; in many instances he is an only child. In other cases the onset of asthma will often follow the birth of a second child and represents both an unconscious feeling of insecurity and a repressed aggression towards the new arrival.

The attitude of the parents is of great importance. They will generally prove to be unduly anxious, fussy and concerned, and their well-meaning, over-solicitude for the child's welfare exaggerates its feeling of insecurity and produces the fear and tension that both provoke and prolong its attacks of asthma. Discordant home conditions will have the same effect. Where the parents are unhappy or quarrel in the presence of the child, severe emotional conflicts are bound to ensue, its need for dependence will become increased, and its confidence still further undermined. Such factors will inevitably be reflected in the increased frequency and severity of the asthma. The significance of parental attitudes and home conditions is amply illustrated by the fact that, no matter how bad the child has been, the attacks usually stop very quickly once it has been admitted to hospital, only to return shortly after its discharge.

The investigation of possible allergies usually results in the avoidance of certain foods or conditions, without the anticipated degree of improvement in the asthma. In this connection, it should be remembered that whilst the presence of real allergies may have been proved, once the patient is informed of these, fear alone may still precipitate an attack. The classical example is that of the patient who was found to be allergic to roses, and who developed an attack when he approached a bowl of artificial roses, believing them to be real at the time. Moreover, too many precautions such as the avoidance of eggs, milk, dust, certain smells, feathers and domestic animals frequently increase the misery of the child's existence without having any marked effect upon its asthma.

Once established, asthma may offer the child an unconscious means of escape from situations that it either dreads or dislikes. Attacks are not uncommon on the eve of school examinations, or when homework has been too difficult, and has not been completed. Sometimes it becomes the excuse for not taking part in physical exercises, or organized sport at school. On other occasions, an attack may occur simply as the result of emotional disturbance such as over-excitement following a party or a visit to the circus.

Asthma in children can be both easily and effectively treated by hypnosis in general practice. Only in the case of very young or excessively nervous children is there likely to be any difficulty in securing adequate depth. Below the age of 5 to 6 years it is sometimes impossible to hold the child's attention long enough for the induction to succeed.

Before starting treatment, it is most important to interview the parents. The effect that their attitude of over-concern and anxiety has upon the child must be explained to them, until they fully understand and accept it. They must be told that, no matter how worried they may feel, they must never show it in the child's presence, since if they do, it will not only aggravate its feeling of fear and insecurity, but will completely nullify all attempts at reassurance.

I usually start treatment in the following manner, once I have obtained adequate depth:

> As a result of this deep, deep sleep . . . during this next week, you are going to feel better and better each day.
> Every day, your chest will become stronger and clearer . . . the wheezing will become less and less . . . and your breathing will become easier and easier, each day.
> You will become *much* calmer . . . *much* quieter . . . *much* less easily excited . . . *much* less nervous . . . *much* less easily frightened . . . *much* less easily upset.
> Every day, you will feel *much more confidence* in yourself . . . you will feel *much safer* . . . *much more secure*.
> You will feel much more able to *stick up for yourself* . . . to *hold your own* . . . *both at home* . . . *and at school* . . . *without becoming worried* . . . *without becoming frightened* . . . *without feeling anxious or insecure*.

The precise wording of these modified ego-strengthening suggestions often has to be altered to suit the age and the intelligence of the child. Since, in the course of routine case-taking, certain provoking causes of the attacks will have emerged, specific suggestions may be added that these will no longer be followed by asthma:

> Every day, your chest will become *much stronger* . . . *much less wheezy* . . . Your chest muscles will become . . . and will remain more relaxed . . . your air-passages will remain relaxed . . . you will lose all feelings of tightness in your chest . . . and your breathing will become easier and easier.
> If, at any time, you do begin to feel a little wheezy, or short of breath . . . you will *not become frightened* . . . you will *not become worried or afraid of developing a bad attack* . . . because, with my help, you will learn how to stop it.
> If ever you do become a little wheezy, or short of breath . . . *you will stop whatever you are doing* . . . *you will lie back, in a chair, and let yourself go* . . . *as limp and slack as possible*.
> *Close your eyes* . . . *and try to imagine that you are back in this room, listening to me*.

At the same time . . . *just press one hand, lightly, over the lower part of your chest.*
And, as you do so . . . *you will feel your chest muscles beginning to relax again . . . the air-passages, beginning to relax . . .* and in a very few moments, *you will feel your breathing becoming easier and easier.*
In a few more minutes . . . *the breathlessness will disappear completely . . . your breathing will become perfectly free and easy again . . . without ever developing into a severe attack.*

You will notice here the use of post-hypnotic suggestion (pressing the hand on the chest) as a signal to initiate the relaxation of the chest muscles. This device seems to work very well indeed and many mothers have told how they have observed the child aborting a threatened attack simply by carrying out this procedure. Naturally, it is important to start right away, before the asthma has a chance of establishing itself. To begin with, at least, I do not believe in forbidding the use of inhalers or tablets since this may well lead to an increased feeling of anxiety and insecurity. I find that as the child begins to gather confidence, its reliance upon these gradually diminishes, until they are only rarely used, when the attack develops too quickly for the suggestions to take effect. As improvement takes place such attacks occur much less frequently and, in favourable cases, die away completely. It is also surprising to see how successfully the frequency and severity of the attacks subside once the fear and expectation begin to yield to suggestion. This, of course, explains the effectiveness of hypnotic treatment in affording relief in those cases in which asthma is not psychologically determined, but is more physical in origin. Although it cannot be expected to cure the condition under these circumstances, its use can still prove an invaluable adjunct to more orthodox methods.

Asthma in Adults
In addition to the all too familiar cases that are primarily physical in origin, asthma often develops in adults who have been subjected to periods of excessive mental stress and strain. Jealousy, anger, anxiety and sexual excitement can play an important part. Emotional shocks, such as bereavements, financial worries and marital difficulties are, not infrequently, followed by the development of asthma. In women, attacks that are prone to precede a period may be determined by an unconscious fear of pregnancy. When they occur mostly during menstruation, they may even represent unconscious disappointment at

the failure to become pregnant. Such factors surely underline the importance of treating the patient, rather than the symptom.

As in the case of children, hypnosis and psychotherapy can prove valuable even in the somatic type of case, although the best results will always be obtained in those cases in which strong emotional conflicts or disturbances are involved. Improvement occurs, not only as a result of direct suggestion, but also through the increased insight gained by re-education during hypnotic treatment. Where insufficient evidence of underlying emotional factors emerges from the history, it is often surprising how much important information can be obtained from simple questioning under hypnosis. Conflicts of a predominantly sexual or aggressive nature are, however, likely to prove too deep-seated to yield to anything but an analytical approach. Since most adult asthmatics are of the dependent type, mere reassurance will usually be insufficient. Psychotherapeutic suggestions must also be directed towards strengthening the patient's feelings, self-assurance and independence. Where the individual is known to react to certain emotional stimuli by an asthmatic attack, provided that the hypnosis is deep enough, he will be found to respond in exactly the same way to suggested emotional situations of a similar nature.

Whilst medium-depth hypnosis will often be sufficient to obtain some degree of improvement, the best and most rapid results will always occur when the deeper stages have been achieved. I always begin treatment with the adult form of ego-strengthening suggestions (p. 191) and following the last section I proceed with the general psychotherapeutic suggestions aimed at the alleviation of the asthma itself:

Because of this . . . every day . . . you will feel *more and more independent* . . . *more able to 'stick up' for yourself* . . . *to 'stand upon your own feet'* . . . *to hold your own* . . . no matter how difficult or trying things may be.

You will feel more able to *rely upon yourself* . . . *to depend upon yourself* . . . upon your *own* efforts . . . your *own* judgement . . . your *own* opinions.

You will feel *much less need to rely upon* . . . *or to depend upon other people.* And *as* you become . . . and *as* you remain . . . *more and more relaxed*, each day . . . *even when you are no longer with me* . . . *so* . . . *your chest muscles will become* . . . *and will remain relaxed* . . . *the air-passages will become* . . . *and will remain relaxed* . . . *and your breathing will become* . . . *and will remain* . . . *easier and easier* . . . *each day* . . . *not only first thing in the morning* . . . *and throughout the day* . . . *but throughout the night as well.*

If . . . at any moment . . . for any reason . . . you *do* begin to feel a little

short of breath . . . *you will not panic . . . you will not become alarmed . . . you will remain perfectly calm and composed . . . you will no longer be afraid of developing a severe attack.*
The moment you feel your breathlessness increasing . . . *just stop whatever you are doing . . . lie back in a chair . . . let yourself relax . . . as much as possible . . . close your eyes . . . and try to imagine that you are back in this room . . . listening to me.*
As you do this . . . *just press one hand . . . lightly . . . over the lower part of your chest.*
And . . . within a very few minutes, you will find that *your chest muscles are beginning to relax again . . . that your air-passages are beginning to relax . . . and that your breathing is gradually becoming easier and easier.*
Very soon . . . you will be breathing quite freely and easily again . . . without developing a severe attack.

In proceeding from the initial ego-strengthening suggestions to the treatment of the asthma itself, the suggestions directed to relaxation of the chest muscles and air passages are deliberately linked with those of general relaxation, that have already been given. Later, in stating that relaxation of the chest muscles will follow the pressure of the hand on the chest, advantage is being taken of post-hypnotic suggestion.

The ability of the patient to induce auto-hypnosis can greatly increase his chances of inhibiting threatened attacks. Consequently, whenever he has attained a deep stage, I invariably try to train him in this technique. Since the time factor is important, and it is necessary for him to achieve the hypnotic state without delay, the best method is obviously the one that conditions him to fall immediately into a trance state upon a given signal. This can easily be done as the result of a post-hypnotic suggestion. With the patient in a deep hypnotic state, I usually proceed as follows:

You are now in so deep a sleep . . . that *everything that I tell you that is going to happen . . . will happen . . . exactly as I tell you.*
And every feeling . . . that I tell you that you will experience . . . you will experience . . . exactly, as I tell you.
And these same things will continue to happen to you . . . and you will continue to experience these same feelings . . . just as strongly . . . just as surely . . . just as powerfully . . . when you are back home . . . as when you are with me, in this room.
Now . . . in a few moments . . . I am going to wake you up by counting seven.
After I have wakened you up . . . I shall talk to you . . . and I shall then ask you to put yourself into this deep sleep again.

You will then lie back in the chair . . . fix your eyes upon a spot on the ceiling . . . and count slowly up to *five*.

The moment you have reached the count of five . . . your eyes will close immediately . . . and you will fall, immediately, into a sleep . . . just as deep as this one.

After one minute . . . you will say to yourself . . . ' *my eyes will open . . . and I shall be wide awake again . . . the moment I count seven* '.

Then . . . count up to *seven* . . . and wake yourself up.

And . . . because this *will* happen . . . *exactly* as I tell you it will happen . . . you will open your eyes, and be wide awake again . . . the moment I count *seven* . . . feeling *much happier* . . . *much more contented* . . . *much more cheerful* . . . *much more optimistic.*

I then awaken the patient, and after talking to him for a few minutes, I tell him to lie back in the chair, and put himself off to sleep again. He is usually surprised to find that this happens without the slightest difficulty, so I immediately rehypnotize him, and give him the following instructions:

Just as you put yourself to sleep, a few moments ago, by counting up to *five . . . so . . . you will always be able to do this, immediately . . . whenever* you need to control your breathlessness.

Once your eyes have closed . . . *you will press one hand . . . lightly . . . over the lower part of your chest . . .* and you will say to yourself . . . ' *as I press my hand on my chest . . . my chest muscles are beginning to relax . . . the air passages are beginning to relax . . . my breathing is becoming easier and easier . . . and, in a few minutes, I shall be breathing quite freely and easily, again . . . without developing any severe attack* '.

You will continue to say this, over and over again . . . until you feel your chest muscles relaxing . . . and your breathing becoming easier.

Then . . . as soon as you are ready . . . you will say to yourself . . . ' *my eyes will open . . . and I shall be wide awake, again . . . the moment I count seven . . . feeling much better . . . much more relaxed . . . with no feeling of tightness in my chest . . . and my breathing much easier . . . much more normal* '.

Once I have trained the patient in this technique, I always substitute the above suggestions for those already described in the normal treatment routine:

The moment you feel your breathlessness increasing . . . just stop whatever you are doing . . . lie back in a chair . . . and, put yourself off into a deep sleep . . . by counting up to five.

Once your eyes have closed . . .

One great advantage of this procedure lies in the increased self-confidence the patient seems to acquire as a result. The fact that he has gained, from his own point of view, sufficient control to be able to induce the hypnotic state whenever he requires it, usually enhances his confidence in his ability to ward off a threatened attack of asthma to a remarkable extent.

The true efficiency of hypnosis in the treatment of asthma has too frequently been obscured by the largely objective nature of the experimental approach to the subject. Conclusions have been wrongly drawn from the inconclusive and unconvincing figures obtained from the measurement of vital capacity, forced expiratory volume, and peak flow. These tend to ignore the degree of subjective improvement which, it must be admitted, is much more difficult to assess with accuracy. Fortunately the controlled trials reported by Maher-Loughnan, Macdonald, Mason and Fry have gone a long way towards restoring the matter to its true perspective. Their conclusions confirm the fact that hypnosis can produce more symptomatic improvement than treatment by the antispasmodics.

From the purely clinical point of view it is very easy to assess progress on the basis of subjective observations made by the individual patient. Attacks tend to become less frequent, shorter in duration, and of gradually diminishing intensity. Moreover the patient soon learns to exercise a sufficient degree of confidence and control in the early stages of an attack to be able to inhibit its further development. Improvement of this kind is amply confirmed by relatives, and not infrequently by the family doctor who is only too pleased to find himself relieved of the burden of several visits per week, to say nothing of out-of-hours calls necessitating injections of adrenaline.

Finally, there are two points worthy of attention. When first interviewing the patient, great care should be taken not to promise too much. This can easily be avoided without conveying any lack of confidence in the ability of hypnosis to assist. I begin by explaining that the less the asthma depends upon physical causes, the better the prospect will be but in any case treatment should still be able to produce a considerable amount of relief through the reduction in frequency and severity of the attacks. I also point out that people vary a great deal in their susceptibility to hypnosis, so that much will depend upon the depth that can be achieved. Until this has been ascertained, it is impossible to predict with any accuracy the degree of improvement that can be expected. This method of approach seems to increase rather than diminish the patient's confidence since, on previous occasions, the high hopes they had entertained regarding other treatments had so frequently failed to be realized. I almost invariably aim at securing the greatest possible depth in three consecutive sessions. It is seldom possible to administer treatment more than once a week.

I also find it helpful to impress upon the patient's mind that ' wheezing ' and ' asthma ' are not necessarily the same thing. It is true that most asthmatics suffer from wheezing, but so do many chronic bronchitics who never develop asthma. Obviously wheezing in the chest is not invariably followed by an attack of asthma. Once the patient accepts this fact his fear of developing an attack, should his chest become a little wheezy, will be greatly diminished. This explanation is particularly advisable in cases which are predominantly physical in origin.

Results are particularly gratifying on the whole, especially in the case of children. Much unnecessary running about may be avoided, but it must be realized that treatment will usually have to be continued for a period of at least two to three months. Despite this it will generally prove to be well worth the expenditure of time and effort.

CHAPTER 17

Migraine and Insomnia

Hypnosis in Migraine

This distressing and incapacitating complaint consists of recurrent paroxysms of intense headache, generally preceded by visual or sensory phenomena and accompanied by nausea. Actual vomiting may or may not occur. An impending attack is sometimes heralded by vague feelings of malaise. Visual or sensory auras such as flashes of light, or shimmering spots, tingling in the limbs, lips or tongue, may follow, which within 10 to 20 minutes are usually replaced by the typical headache. It is usually unilateral and temporal at first, but may become bilateral later. It is extremely severe and the patient often has intense pain on moving his eyes, and suffers from photophobia which necessitates his lying down in a darkened room. Nausea is almost invariably present and vomiting may take place. When the warning auras are absent the headache is more of the throbbing type and seems to be prone to occur in the early morning. Individual attacks may last only for an hour or two, or may continue all day. They are generally followed by feelings of prostration and exhaustion, and their frequency may vary from once or twice a week, to every few months.

Although it occurs in both sexes, it is usually more common in women, in whom it is often exacerbated by the menopause. Exciting factors are often found in eye strain, gastric disturbances and dietetic indiscretions, menstruation and emotional stress. These patients are usually well balanced, often artistic, intelligent and industrious members of the community. They tend, however, to be over-anxious and dependent, and may sometimes display introverted and obsessional characteristics. Attacks are often precipitated by mental fatigue, worry or anxiety. Emotional tension such as that caused by fear, frustration, anger, resentment, insecurity, inadequacy or even guilt, can also play an important part. Sometimes an unconscious feeling of inferiority will cause the patient to conceal it from himself by undertaking responsibilities which are frankly too much for him, and with which he finds it increasingly difficult to cope. In such instances the ensuing emotions of anger, hostility and frustration are diverted into physical channels and gain expression in attacks of migraine. Obviously psychotherapy can be extremely useful in certain cases, and hypnosis is always well worth trying, particularly when orthodox medicinal control has proved ineffective.

Before hypnotic treatment is even considered, it is essential that the patient should be thoroughly investigated to exclude any possible organic cause. Such conditions as occipital lobe tumours, or chronic nephritis with uraemia must be eliminated. Migraine has also been associated with allergies, cyclical vomiting and epilepsy. Today, it is generally accepted that it is accompanied by some changes in the calibre of the cerebral blood-vessels.

In diagnosing true migraine, it is necessary to differentiate from other forms of psychogenic headache. This does not usually present much difficulty, since the typical psychoneurotic headaches are rarely true pain. They are commonly described by the patient as being something rather worse, and even less bearable than pain. He will complain of an intolerable feeling of weight or pressure on top of his head, or a feeling of a tight band around his temples. This kind of headache may be occipital, frontal or even generalized, *but it is characteristically bilateral, whereas migraine is almost invariably unilateral* in its onset.

Whilst often successful, treatment is by no means easy, and it is almost impossible to give the prognosis. The severity and duration of individual attacks, and the length of time the patient has suffered from the complaint offer little or no guidance. Neither does the response to medicinal treatment. Fortunately, many of these patients are capable of achieving the deeper stages of hypnosis which greatly facilitates their treatment. Reassurance is vitally important, for the patient often fears that he may have a cerebral tumour. Moreover, since migraine is not infrequently a reaction to fear, it is always wise to try to discover what the patient actually fears. This information can often be readily obtained from questioning, either in the waking or in the hypnotic state. The complete disappearance of the complaint should never be promised, but diminution of the severity and frequency of the attacks can reasonably be expected. Nevertheless, the relief from tension and anxiety that hypnosis can afford is often followed by remarkable improvement. In these cases, whenever sufficient depth can be obtained, the teaching of auto-hypnosis can be of great value, as in asthma, in enabling the patient to treat a threatened attack at its onset and inhibit its further development.

Once again, speed is essential and a quick method of induction is required.

With the patient in as deep a hypnotic state as possible, I begin treatment with the full ego-strengthening suggestions, and proceed with those directed toward symptom removal immediately after the section quoted below:

Every day . . . *you* will become . . . and *you* will remain . . . *more and more completely relaxed . . . both mentally . . . and physically . . . even when you are no longer with me.*
And . . . *as* you become . . . *more and more relaxed . . . and less tense . . . so* . . . you are beginning to feel *more and more comfortable.*
As this relaxation increases . . . so . . . *your pain is becoming easier and easier* . . . and presently . . . *you will feel so completely relaxed and comfortable* . . . *that the pain will disappear completely.*

At this point, I get up and stand behind the patient's chair, and gently stroke his forehead and the side of his face, using both hands alternately:

As I stroke your forehead and face . . . you can feel a *feeling of warmth* . . . *spreading all over your head . . . face . . . and neck.*
That feeling of warmth is increasing . . . with every stroke of my hands.
As soon as you can feel this warmth . . . please lift up your hand.

I continue to stroke the forehead, slowly and gently, until I see the patient raise his hand:

Good!
Now . . . put it down again.
And as this feeling of warmth increases . . . with every stroke of my hands . . . *so* . . . *your head is beginning to feel more and more comfortable.*
As the warmth increases . . . so . . . *the pain is becoming less and less.*
All pain . . . all aching . . . all feelings of discomfort . . . are gradually disappearing . . . *and in a few moments . . . your head will feel so warm and comfortable* . . . *that all the pain and aching will have disappeared completely.*
Your head will feel quite clear and normal . . . and you will feel quite free from all pain . . . aching . . . and discomfort.
As soon as you feel that all the pain and aching have disappeared . . . please lift up your hand.

Once again, I continue the stroking until I see that the patient has raised his hand.

Now, put your hand down again!
And, as I continue to stroke your head . . . *the warmth is still increasing* . . . *and it is spreading into the nerves of your head and face.*

As a result of this . . . *the nerves will become stronger . . . much less easily irritated . . . much less sensitive to pain.*
As this happens . . . *and as you become emotionally much more settled . . . much less easily disturbed . . . so . . . your attacks will become much less severe . . . much less frequent . . . until finally, they will disappear completely.*
Moreover . . . *since pain . . . even migraine . . . is often caused . . . and is always aggravated by tension . . . so . . . as you become, and remain . . . more relaxed and less tense each day . . . these attacks will become much less likely to occur . . . and will fade away completely.*
In a few moments . . . when I count up to *seven* . . . you will open your eyes . . . and be wide awake again.
You will wake up . . . *feeling perfectly fit and well . . . with your head completely clear and comfortable . . . without the slightest trace of any pain . . . aching . . . or discomfort.*

Wherever possible, it is most advantageous to teach the patient auto-hypnosis. Since, in order to inhibit the development of a threatened attack, speed of induction is all-important, I use exactly the same technique already described in connection with asthma whereby the patient is enabled to put himself into a trance state on counting up to five. I then re-hypnotize the patient, and give him the following instructions:

Whenever you feel that an attack is beginning . . . *stop whatever you are doing . . . lie back in a chair . . . and put yourself in a deep sleep by counting up to five.*
As soon as your eyes have closed . . . *start stroking your forehead and face . . . slowly and deliberately.*
You may use either hand, alternately.
Say to yourself . . . over and over again . . . ' As I stroke my forehead . . . *I can feel a feeling of warmth . . . spreading into my head and face.*
That warmth is increasing . . . with every stroke of my hand.
As the warmth increases . . . so . . . the pain is becoming easier and easier . . . and, in a few minutes . . . *my head will feel so warm and comfortable . . . that all the pain . . . all the aching . . . all the discomfort will disappear completely.*'
Continue to stroke . . . and go on repeating these suggestions to yourself until your head does feel so warm and comfortable, that the pain has disappeared.
Then waken yourself up . . . by counting up to *seven* . . . telling yourself that you will wake up . . . *without the slightest trace of pain . . . aching . . . or discomfort.*

Migraine is a difficult condition to treat, no matter what methods are adopted, and some failures are bound to occur with hypnosis as with any other means, but I have found that the above techniques have been extremely effective in many cases. Most of them seem to experience varying degrees of improvement (more, in fact, than they have previously experienced) and some even lose their migraine completely. I can recall several patients who had suffered severe attacks once or twice a week for years, who responded so well to hypnosis that they have remained entirely free from trouble for periods of three to five years after the conclusion of treatment.

The same techniques can often be adopted with success in dealing with other forms of headache, whether organic or psychogenic in origin. Naturally, the latter will usually respond more readily than the former. It may, of course, be necessary to make suitable modifications of the wording, in accordance with the particular type of case.

Hypnosis in Insomnia

Insomnia causes a great deal of distress and anxiety and is very commonly encountered in general practice. The amount of sleep required will vary with the age of the individual. Infants require much more sleep than the adult, probably up to 15 or 16 hours, and older children or adolescents, up to 10 hours. Adults, however, are more dependent upon their individual peculiarities. The idea seems to be prevalent amongst the general public that a minimum of 8 hours sleep a night is essential if health is not to be impaired. This is far from being the case for many habitually poor sleepers, *who do not worry about it*, seem to suffer neither in health, nor in comfort. Indeed, most of us can remember how, during the period of nightly air-raids, the amount of sleep we had was severely curtailed for weeks on end without serious consequences to our health, or our ability to carry out our daily duties.

It is what the individual is accustomed to under ordinary conditions that really matters. If he is in the habit of having 8 hours sleep a night, and some ordinary situation or worry causes him a few sleepless nights, he begins to become afraid of the consequences. He might imagine that if this state of affairs continues, he will suffer mental harm, brain damage, or even insanity. This immediately sets up nervous tension, often accompanied next day by psychogenic headaches. These not only confirm his worst fears but also cause him to dread going to bed the next night in case he will be unable to sleep. Naturally enough he fails to do so. The harder he tries, the more wide awake he remains and the more worried he becomes. In this way the vicious circle is established and his condition gradually worsens day by day.

The chief causes of insomnia may be broadly classified under four headings:

1. Psychical.
2. Pain and discomfort.
3. Febrile conditions.
4. Organic brain disease.

Since insomnia arising from the last three causes will usually be dealt with in the course of treatment of the underlying condition, I do not propose to discuss it in this chapter. We are concerned with the insomnia that is caused by psychical factors, which is one of the most important and commonest symptoms of functional nervous disturbance. There are two questions to be answered:

1. What is the precise nature of the sleeplessness?
2. What is it that is keeping the patient awake?

In the first instance the patient may complain mainly of an inability to get off to sleep at all. On the other hand, he may be troubled by broken or interrupted sleep or, whilst having little difficulty in falling asleep, he invariably wakes up at about 3 a.m. or 4 a.m. in the morning, and cannot get any more sleep that night.

In the second instance, the patient may find it impossible to sleep through over-anxiety and worry. Sufferers from insomnia of this type will constitute far the largest group. Then the sleeplessness may be due to bad habits of thought. The patient remains too pre-occupied with his daily affairs. He continually visualizes the events of the day, or even goes over conversations that have taken place. Finally, he may be unable to sleep solely because he has become obsessed with the idea of sleeplessness.

No matter how bad the insomnia the patient actually gets more sleep than he thinks, but it is impossible to convince him of this. People who sleep badly almost invariably exaggerate the symptom. ' I never closed my eyes all night.' ' I never had a wink of sleep—I heard the clock chime, every hour.' This is not difficult to understand, since lying awake for one hour in the middle of the night seems as long as two or three hours in the daytime, particularly when the mind is beset with worries and anxieties. The brief periods in which sleep intervenes seem so insignificant in comparison that it is hardly surprising that they become overlooked. In many cases the sleep that is obtained is restless and disturbed by distressing dreams, so that the patient often wakes up feeling more tired and exhausted than when he went to bed. Sometimes insomnia can be caused by phobias related to sleep. The patient may be literally afraid to go to sleep. This may be because he dreads regularly occurring nightmares, but is more commonly associated with an unconscious fear of death which he knows occurs frequently in the early hours of the morning.

The first and most important task in the treatment of insomnia is to try to discover the cause. Only then can attention be directed towards the correction of the conditions or attitudes underlying the sleeplessness. Almost invariably, the patient is over-interested in whether he is going to be able to sleep or not, and it is precisely this fact that tends to keep him awake. I find that the best approach is to talk to him frankly on the subject of sleep in general. I begin by trying to get his ideas on sleep, and how much he thinks he requires each night in order to remain fit and healthy. I then ask him what he thinks is likely to happen to him if these requirements are not fulfilled. His replies are often both surprising and illuminating. Anything from a general deterioration in mental and physical health, to such graver conditions as brain damage or even insanity may frequently be anticipated. This is because of the general conception, almost universally held, that the main function of sleep is to rest the tired brain. Although there is certainly some truth in this, it cannot represent the whole story by any means. For instance, it is curious to note that most brain workers seem to thrive on much less sleep each night than people engaged in heavy manual employment. Biographies of famous novelists, scientists and philosophers often reveal the fact that they would work into the small hours of the morning, having only 4 or 5 hours sleep, and that this could continue indefinitely without any apparent deterioration in their health. On the other hand, it would be virtually impossible for an agricultural labourer to do the same thing and to continue to carry out his duties efficiently the next day.

T. A. Ross considers that one important function of sleep lies in the withdrawal of interest. As he points out people will often fall asleep in church during a dull and uninspiring sermon, yet they will seldom do so in a theatre. I find it useful to point out such facts as these, in an effort to calm the patient's fears and offer him reassurance. But no matter what form of treatment is ultimately decided upon I never under any circumstances promise that sleep is going to be restored either quickly or easily. Rather do I encourage the patient to believe that at the moment his sleeplessness doesn't matter very much, and that sooner or later as a result of treatment sleep will be restored. In the meantime, nothing very dreadful or serious is likely to happen to him.

Hypnosis can prove very useful in the management of insomnia, and it is surprising how readily the milder types of case will respond to hypnotic suggestion. The chronic case who has relied upon drugs for a long time and in whom emotional disturbances and tension predominate is, however, much more difficult to deal with. Nevertheless, with perseverance, the dependence on drugs can be gradually broken since it is usually a purely psychological dependence.

People suffering from insomnia are not usually very good hypnotic subjects. For one thing, they find it extremely difficult to relax, and many resistances may arise in the process of induction. They are often over-sensitive to the word *sleep*, the mere mention of which immediately causes them to become more wakeful.

When attempting to hypnotize a patient suffering from insomnia, you should always avoid the use of the word sleep, in the course of your induction.

The word *sleep*, by association of ideas, will immediately revive in the patient's mind exactly the same doubts, fears and anxieties that prevent him falling asleep each night, and will thus paralyse his ability to respond to the induction. Fortunately this difficulty can easily be met by the substitution of the words *tired*, *relaxed* and *drowsy*, in whatever method of induction may be used.

Acute Insomnia

When the insomnia is acute and of short duration, hypnosis may succeed in a direct attack upon the symptom. In this case the patient is induced into as deep a state as possible. The usual ego-strengthening suggestions are administered, and the patient is told that, *as he becomes more able to cope with, and face up to the situations that have been causing him anxiety, so he will begin to sleep more easily and more soundly.*

Chronic Insomnia

Treatment of chronic insomnia is much more difficult but still well worth while. The patient will usually be extremely agitated, tense and literally frightened to death of the consequences of his inability to sleep. Some take large quantities of drugs each night, with gradually decreasing effect. Others are terrified of the continued necessity to rely upon hypnotic drugs, as they dread the possibility of developing an addiction. In people who are emotionally disturbed in this way reassurance is obviously of the greatest importance, and until this has been accepted to some extent, not only is trance induction likely to be difficult, but depth will prove almost impossible to achieve. Even should a trance be achieved, it is only rarely that direct suggestions of the restoration of a natural sleep rhythm will be successful.

It is not solely the inability to relax that makes these patients difficult hypnotic subjects. Although relaxation constitutes an integral part of most methods of induction, it is by no means essential for the production of the hypnotic state. After all, many stage performers hypnotize their subjects whilst they are standing upright, under which circumstances they can certainly not be in a relaxed state. By far the most important drawback is the patient's emotional disturbance and instability, which often renders it impossible for him to concentrate sufficiently. Because of this, it pays to go slowly and I *never* attempt to induce hypnosis in the course of the first interview. Neither do I try to secure depth quickly, as I find it much more effective to spread it over 3 or 4 sessions. In the chronic insomniac patient, the agitation is usually accompanied by a varying degree of underlying depression, and this in itself renders the induction and deepening of hypnosis more difficult. In such cases I often find it extremely helpful to reduce their tension and emotional instability to some extent by using phenelzine, 15 mg. and perphenazine, 4 mg., three times a day for a week or two before commencing hypnotic treatment; this combination has proved most effective in agitated states even when no obvious signs of depression could be observed. Sargent, Hare and others have pointed out that the beneficial effects of phenelzine and other mono-amine oxidase inhibitors in depressive illnesses is due more to their sedative action in relieving anxiety than to any specific antidepressive action. This has been borne out by my own clinical experience, and it is surprising how often this premedication will prove successful and facilitate hypnosis.

The bad sleeper invariably begins to worry long before bedtime. He is only too well aware that he has utilized all the usual remedies time and time again without avail. Reading books until the early hours of the morning, or counting sheep, are both completely futile and ineffective. A proper routine is essential. The patient should be encouraged to take sufficient exercise and fresh air each day. Hot drinks and hot baths last thing at night can be of great assistance, and it is important that *the patient should be instructed to retire to bed at the same hour, each night.* Preliminary questioning should already have shed a great deal of light on the nature of his particular fears and anxieties, to which attention can be paid in the course of his treatment.

My own procedure is to put the patient into as deep a hypnotic state as possible, gradually over a period of 3 to 4 sessions. I am in the habit of varying the method of induction, according to the particular patient with whom I am dealing, but *I almost invariably refrain from using any relaxation suggestions at all until the hypnotic state has been achieved.* One typical and effective routine is as follows:

> Lie back in the chair, and stretch your legs out in front of you.
> Make yourself as comfortable as possible.
> Now, I want you to fix your eyes on the tip of this pencil.
> Try not to let them wander . . . just keep staring at the pencil.
> And whilst you are doing this . . . start counting slowly backwards from 300 . . . mentally, to yourself.
> Go on counting . . . until you hear me tell you to stop.
> You'll hear everything that I am saying . . . but try not to listen to me . . . any more than you can help.
> Just you stick to your counting.
> Breathe quietly . . . *in* . . . and . . . *out* . . . *in* . . . and . . . *out.*
> And . . . *whilst you are looking at the pencil . . . your eyes are beginning to feel very, very tired.*
> *They may feel a little watery . . . your sight may become a little blurred.*
> *You are beginning to feel drowsier and drowsier.*
> *You can feel a feeling of heaviness in your legs . . . in your arms . . in your body.*
> *Your eyelids are beginning to feel heavier and heavier . . . so heavy, that they are wanting to blink.*
> *Just let them blink . . . as much as you like . . . and, as they do so . . . your eyelids are beginning to feel so very, very heavy . . . that they are wanting to close.*
> *As soon as they feel they want to close . . . just let them close . . . on their own.*
> *They're wanting to close, now . . . closing . . . closing . . . tighter and tighter . . . let them go . . . . . . let them close completely.*
> Now that your eyes have closed . . . you will not want to open them, until I tell you to. You are feeling more and more comfortable . . . and I want you to let all the muscles of your feet and ankles relax completely.

From this point onwards, I use the usual sequence of relaxation suggestions, coupling these at each stage with suggestions of increasing depth. You will notice that, in the induction routine, the word *sleep* is never employed. Once the trance has been achieved and the relaxation suggestions administered, I awaken the patient and do no more on this occasion. During subsequent sessions, I gain the greatest depth that I can by using the usual sequence of graded responses.

In as deep a trance as possible, I tell the patient that one of the main causes of his sleeplessness is the fact that he worries about the consequences of not sleeping. I once again point out to him that if he doesn't sleep nothing serious is likely to happen, and that worry will cause far more trouble than the insomnia. In other words, I do my best to instil the following ideas into his mind: ' *If you do fall asleep . . . so much the better !* *If you don't . . . it doesn't matter, because sooner or later, you will.*' Whilst all this has already been said in the waking state, it is of the utmost importance that it should be repeated in the trance state.

I then follow with the customary ego-strengthening routine, laying particular stress on those passages directed towards relaxation and the relief of tension. I find that, in the course of a few sessions, as the patient begins to feel that the hypnotic relaxation is actually relieving and diminishing his tension, he tends to respond more and more to the suggestion that, as he becomes able to relax in bed, the main cause of his sleeplessness has been removed, and he will consequently fall asleep more easily, more quickly, and will sleep more soundly.

Usually the patient has been taking sedatives in various combinations and increasing doses over a long period during which his tolerance has gradually become greater. He himself is well aware of this fact, which worries him considerably. It would be a grave mistake to try to deprive him of sleep-inducing drugs. The primary objective is that of re-establishing a regular pattern of sleep by whatever combination of means that can serve this purpose. Then, under hypnosis, a gradual diminution in the amount of drugs required can be suggested. I usually point out that the reason that the sedatives were effective was because they diminished anxiety and thus promoted sleep. Now that the tension has been reduced by treatment, and he can relax more easily, he will be able to sleep with smaller doses. When he is ready for this I suggest that he should begin by taking only half his usual dose when he goes to bed, and the rest when he wakes up in the middle of the night, but only if absolutely necessary. In my experience, most of these patients dislike having to depend upon drugs so much that they are only too pleased to be able to reduce them once they have gained the confidence to do so.

Immediately following the ego-strengthening suggestions, I proceed with precise instructions regarding a nightly routine:

As a result of this treatment . . . you will feel *more relaxed . . . less tense and anxious . . .* each day.
As bed-time approaches . . . you will feel *more and more pleasantly tired.*
You will go to bed *at the same time, each night . . .* and *. . . as soon as you put your head on the pillow . . . you will begin to relax . . . exactly as you do, whilst you are in this chair.*

You will no longer worry as to whether you are going to sleep or not . . . you will devote the whole of your attention to allowing your whole body to relax.
As it does so . . . you will feel a feeling of heaviness in your body . . . as if it is beginning to feel just as heavy as lead . . . as if it is sinking down . . . deeper and deeper . . . into the mattress.
And, as it does so . . . you will feel drowsier and drowsier . . . and presently . . . your eyes will close . . . and you will fall into a natural, healthy sleep . . . which will last throughout the night . . . until your usual time for getting up in the morning.
If . . . for any reason, you should wake up in the night . . . you will not be worried.
You will fix your eyes on the ceiling . . . and concentrate upon producing that same relaxation . . . heaviness . . . and drowsiness . . . once again.
And . . . within a very short time . . . your eyes will close . . . and you will fall into a natural sleep again . . . which will last . . . quite undisturbed . . . until your usual time for getting up in the morning.

The efficiency of the above routine can be greatly increased by rehearsal. Whilst in the hypnotic state, the patient's attention can be called to the fact that his body is actually feeling heavier and heavier, and is sinking down, deeper and deeper into the chair. He can then be told that, when he gets into bed at night, he will experience *exactly the same feeling of heaviness as he is doing at the moment.* Precisely the same feeling of drowsiness will arise in his mind, and before long, he will fall asleep. Not only this, but breathing and relaxing exercises can also be taught in the trance state, and the patient rehearsed in his ability to reproduce them after waking up.

Wolberg describes an additional technique in which he induces the hypnotized patient to picture himself relaxing in the sun, in pleasant surroundings, with his mind calm and unworried, feeling progressively drowsier and drowsier. Once this has occurred, the patient is told that he will picture the same peaceful scene every evening when he is in bed, and experience the same feelings of relaxation and drowsiness.

Auto-hypnosis, taught through post-hypnotic suggestion, is of the greatest value in these cases.

As soon as you put your head on the pillow . . . you will count slowly up to five.
Immediately you reach the count of five . . . your eyes will close . . . and you will fall into a sleep . . . just as deep as this one.
Your body will become completely and utterly relaxed . . . your mind will become calm and relaxed . . . and . . . very, very quickly . . . this sleep will merge into

ordinary, healthy, natural sleep . . . which will last throughout the night . . . until your usual time for getting up in the morning.

Insomnia in Children

Whilst the same general principles apply to the treatment of this complaint in children, advantage can be taken of the fact that they can usually be deeply hypnotized, many being able to achieve somnambulistic trances with little difficulty. The following technique depends entirely upon the ability of the patient to open his eyes without waking up from the trance. I have used this method with great success, not only in children, but also in adults, whenever somnambulism could be secured.

I prepare a postcard in advance upon which the following instructions are typed:

As you are reading this card . . . your eyes are beginning to feel very, very tired. You are feeling drowsier and drowsier . . . your eyes are wanting to close . . . and, in a few moments . . . when you have finished reading it . . . your eyes will close immediately . . . and you will fall, immediately, into a sleep, just as deep as this one.

The patient, in a deep somnambulistic trance, is then told to open his eyes without waking up.

You are now so deeply asleep . . . that, in a few moments . . . when I count up to *five* . . . *you will open your eyes* . . . *without waking up from this deep sleep.*
Your eyes will open . . . *you will be able to see, quite clearly* . . . *but you will not wake up from this very deep sleep.*
Now . . . *open your eyes!*

As the patient does so, the characteristic far-away, rather vacant expression in his eyes shows that he has not awakened from the trance. I then hand him the card that has been prepared.

I want you to read this card . . . *slowly and deliberately.*
And . . . after I have wakened you up . . . *when I give you the card* . . . *and ask you to read it* . . . *you will obey every instruction on the card* . . . *and* . . . *the moment you have finished reading it* . . . *your eyes will close immediately* . . . *and you will fall, immediately, into a sleep, just as deep as this one.*

Following this, I waken him up, and after talking to him briefly, I hand him the card and ask him to read it. As he does so, his eyelids begin to flicker and close, and he falls into a deep sleep.

From now on . . . as soon as you have undressed, and got into bed at night . . . *you will pick up this card, and read it.*

As you are reading it . . . your eyes will become more and more tired . . . and . . . the moment you have finished it . . . they will close . . . and you will fall immediately into a sleep, just as deep as this one.

Within a very short time . . . this sleep will change into normal healthy sleep . . . which will last throughout the night . . . until your usual time for getting up in the morning.

If . . . for any reason . . . you should wake up in the middle of the night . . . you will not be worried.

You will pick up the card again . . . and read it . . . and once again you will fall immediately into a deep, deep sleep.

This will only happen when you are undressed, and in bed.

If you read the card at any other time . . . it will have no effect upon you at all.

But . . . whenever you are undressed and in bed . . . you will always obey its instructions, faithfully.

It is vitally important to place restrictions upon the use of the card, and to define accurately the conditions under which it will prove effective. To a child I usually say, during the trance, that *the card will only take effect at night, when he is undressed and in bed, and the card is handed to him by his mother.* There is not the slightest doubt regarding the efficacy of this procedure, for I can recollect one instance where it worked admirably under the conditions specified, yet on an evening when the mother was out, and the father handed the card to the child, it failed to have the slightest effect.

The technique is just as successful in adults as in children, provided that a somnambulistic trance can be achieved. Although complete amnesia is not essential, it is always advantageous whenever it can be secured.

CHAPTER 18

Speech Disorders, Tics and Other Nervous Habits

Hypnosis in Speech Disorders

When problems of speech are purely functional in character, the normal speech rhythm becomes both inhibited and interrupted. This is particularly likely to occur in certain social situations which tend to produce shyness, embarrassment and uneasiness. The patient dreads having to speak in the presence of other people, and seems to look upon speech as an act through which he is bound to reveal himself and his own shortcomings. Most stammerers are of the dependent type, lacking in self-assurance to an extent that makes it extremely difficult to assert themselves in the company of others. Curiously enough, they are usually able to talk to themselves, to sing, or to talk to animals without difficulty.

Sometimes stammering is precipitated by a shock or traumatic emotional experience. In children, especially, it may be connected with emotional conflicts centred upon the parents, brothers or sisters, which, if treatment is to succeed, will often have to be revealed and explored. Le Cron and Bordeaux state that 80 per cent of cases appear before the age of 6 years, and that the incidence in boys is approximately nine or ten times greater than in girls. They consider stammering to be a neurosis, possibly of the compulsive type, and emphasize the difficulty of cure after the age of 30. It is generally acknowledged that a stammer *must* be treated as early as possible, since once a deep-seated habit pattern and conditioning has been established it is exceedingly hard to break and cure not only becomes difficult, but the treatment becomes tedious and is often ineffective. Indeed the shorter the duration of the stammer the greater will be the prospect of success. The prognosis also tends to be more favourable when the stammer is associated with subjective feelings of anxiety, for individuals who stammer badly, without becoming unduly anxious or embarrassed, rarely seem to improve to any marked extent. The prospect is also much worse in the case of children who have never learned to speak properly. Those who once spoke normally and subsequently developed a stammer, usually do much better under treatment.

Stammering varies greatly in its intensity and may be mild or exceedingly severe, accompanied by spasms of various muscles, twitching, or even blinking. Nervousness, shyness, embarrassment and fear lead to tension, which usually affects the muscles of the larynx, throat, face, tongue and lips. Even the diaphragm and respiratory muscles may become involved. The harder the patient tries to overcome the speech defect, the more muscular inco-ordination seems to occur, with the result that the spasm becomes greatly intensified.

It is not always realized what agonies of mind the stammerer experiences, especially when the difficulty threatens to prejudice his career or prospects of advancement. His feeling of inferiority becomes greater and greater. Talking becomes more and more associated with anxiety, his speech mechanism becomes momentarily paralysed, and his uncertainty is manifested in stammering. He dreads having to speak to other people. He becomes more and more self-conscious and embarrassed. He becomes increasingly afraid of failure, of being criticized, and of appearing conspicuous. He is unable to think clearly, whilst he is talking to others, since he is constantly on the look-out for words which he thinks he will be unable to pronounce. He tends to develop phobias designed to extricate him from difficult situations, and to withdraw from people more and more as a result of his difficulty in talking; this leads to a progressive loss of self-esteem. His speech defect will be less marked when he is amongst friends or acquaintances who are aware of it, and much more pronounced when he is with strangers. He is likely to be much worse when he is in the presence of people in authority, and upon occasions which are of some importance to him. He may experience difficulty and hesitation in starting to speak, or his speech may become interrupted by his inability to pronounce certain words or consonants, and he will be unable to continue. The harder he tries, the worse his stammer becomes. In many cases, stammerers tend to think faster than they can speak, and their attempts to catch up only lead to increased difficulty.

Treatment, particularly under hypnosis, is likely to be of the greatest value in young children: in older people results are extremely inconsistent. In cases which fail to show any material improvement, hypnosis is more effective when combined with speech-therapy by a recognized speech therapist.

Treatment

Schneck points out that the treatment should be aimed at the underlying neurosis. From the general practitioner's point of view, direct symptom removal combined with suggestive psychotherapy under hypnosis will usually prove the best method of approach. Direct symptom removal should include specific suggestions of easier speech. Some patients can talk quite easily in the hypnotic state, without the slightest suspicion of a stammer, whereas others continue to stammer however deeply hypnotized they may be. Since, by the time treatment is begun, the complaint is a *habit* in which the original emotional conflict is no longer active, the formation of substitute symptoms is most unlikely to happen.

Ambrose finds that children who stammer are usually tense, anxious and dependent, and that they are often both highly strung and difficult before the onset of the complaint. He emphasizes the importance of investigating, and if necessary correcting, the parents' attitude towards the difficulty. Sometimes, simple questioning under hypnosis will reveal some emotional incident in early life which precipitated the onset of the stammer. In more obstinate cases, age regression under hypnosis may be required provided that the necessary depth can be achieved.

In planning systematic therapy, certain fundamental principles should be borne in mind, and some important explanations given, both in the waking and in the hypnotic state:

1. Where it is suspected, emotional trauma should be investigated, and any relevant conflicts explained and resolved.

2. Environmental disturbances must be dealt with and, in the case of children, parental attitudes explored and adjusted.

3. General suggestions of calmness, physical and mental relaxation, increased confidence and reassurance should be given.

4. Feelings of equality should be encouraged, and any sense of inferiority removed.

5. The patient should be told that he will become so deeply interested in what he has to say, that he will develop complete confidence in his ability to say it.

6. It should be explained to him that he pays far too little attention to what he has to say, and far too much to how he says it.

7. He must face the fact that he has this difficulty, and be prepared to admit it, not only to himself, but to others, who will take far less notice of it than he thinks.

8. He must be told that, in everyday life, he will form the habit of

speaking more slowly and more deliberately, and that this will help considerably with his speech.

As deep a hypnotic state as possible is always desirable, and when this can be obtained, certain desensitization techniques can be most advantageously employed.

Technique 1. Wherever possible, it should be proved to the patient that, when he is completely calm and relaxed under hypnosis, he can speak quite easily without stammering at all. The depth of hypnosis can then be gradually reduced until the patient does not stammer when in the hypnoidal state. This not only leads to increased confidence, but also tends to overcome self-consciousness, and thus breaks the established habit pattern and conditioning.

Technique 2. The patient is shown that he can speak quite clearly without stammering whilst he is in the hypnotic state. He is then told to visualize himself speaking to a group of people with whom he usually experiences difficulty. As his stammer returns, it is pointed out to him how his speech has become affected by the emotional factors in the imaginary situation, causing him to become tense and anxious and to lose his previous feelings of calmness and relaxation. Whilst still in this fantasied situation, it is suggested to him that he is once again becoming calm and relaxed, and that as this happens his stammer will disappear, and he will continue to talk without difficulty.

It will be seen that the real basis of treatment lies in persuasion and re-education, whereby the patient learns to display more tolerance towards himself and others, and to accept his own limitations. He should be encouraged to practise regularly, and in this respect, self-hypnosis when taught can be of great assistance.

Wolberg holds the opinion that some forms of speech-training do as much harm as they do good, and often have a bad psychological effect. He considers that through emphasizing will-power and control, they concentrate the attention too much on the mechanics of speech, rather than upon what is said. Because of this, the patient becomes more and more conscious of his difficulty.

Routine Hypnotic Treatment

Having induced as deep a hypnotic state as possible, I find it most effective to begin with the standard ego-strengthening suggestions, up to, and including the section on relaxation and increased confidence. I then proceed as follows.

As you become . . . and as you remain . . . more relaxed, and less tense each day . . . *so you will become . . . and will remain . . . more relaxed, and less tense when you are in the presence of other people . . . no matter whether they be few . . . or many . . . no matter whether they be friends . . . or strangers. You will be able to meet them on equal terms . . . without the slightest feeling of inferiority . . . without becoming confused, self-conscious, or embarrassed . . . without feeling conspicuous . . . without worrying in the slightest, as to what they may think.*

You will become so deeply interested and absorbed in what you are actually saying . . . that you will no longer pay the slightest attention to how you are saying it. Consequently, you will become much less aware of the presence of other people . . . they will no longer bother you . . . and you will gain much more confidence in your ability to speak clearly and distinctly.

In everyday life . . . you will cultivate the habit of speaking more slowly and deliberately . . . so that, as you begin to speak . . . you will become completely relaxed, both mentally and physically . . . quite calm and composed . . . and so you will be able to start to speak without the slightest hesitation . . . and will be able to continue with less and less difficulty.

If . . . at any moment . . . you should begin to feel any difficulty with a particular word or consonant . . . *you will never try to force it out* . . . that will only make matters worse . . . and will always aggravate the stammer.

You will stop speaking immediately . . . for a moment or two . . . and during that brief period of silence . . . *the muscles of your face . . . your throat . . . your tongue and lips . . . even the muscles of your chest, which control your breathing will all relax completely* . . . so that when you start to speak again . . . the difficult word will slip out quite easily . . . and you will be able to continue with much less difficulty. In fact . . . the pause will be so brief that it will hardly be noticed by other people . . . much less, in fact, than the stammer. As a result of this . . . your speech will steadily improve . . . and will become easier and easier.

Treatment, particularly in adults, is frequently both difficult and prolonged. It is even likely to be unsuccessful in those cases where the personality disorder cannot be corrected. Curiously enough, however, I have encountered a number of cases in which I have only noticed relatively slight improvement, yet the patient stoutly insists that he has been much better. Since I can only judge progress objectively from the way he speaks in my presence, it is possible I suppose that he may still be better in his everyday life than when he is with me. What seems much more likely is the probability that, although he continues to stammer in the presence of other people, it no longer bothers him or distresses him as it used to do, and consequently he is able to ignore it to a much greater extent.

Hypnosis in the Treatment of Tics

Tics are repetitive, habitual, involuntary muscular movements usually of a purposeless type. They may begin as automatic or voluntary reactions to a local stimulus or external situation, and subsequently develop into a habit which becomes perpetuated into a compulsive symptom. They appear to afford some sense of relief to the sufferer since any effort to inhibit them seems to result in emotional distress. The patient is usually fully conscious of the movement which is both uncomfortable and uncontrollable, and the condition is generally associated with feelings of inadequacy and inferiority. He is usually quite unable to give any explanation of his insistent need to carry out the movements, but will admit that he feels more and more discomfort until he yields to it.

Tics are more common in children than in adults. They can occur in either sex, and are most frequent between the ages of 7 to 12 years. Such children are usually normal and intelligent, but highly strung, restless, over-active and excitable, similar in every way to those that develop asthma, bed-wetting and stammering. Heredity may be important and occasionally tics may be imitative. They may be initiated by some external stimulus such as a local inflammation. Blepharitis or conjunctivitis may produce a ' blinking ' tic which persists long after the local condition has subsided. Much more frequently, however, anxiety plays a major part and the tics are the outward expression of psychic conflicts. Indeed, they always indicate the need for some form of psychiatric investigation since they so often present themselves in a picture of general, psychopathic maladjustment.

The most commonly observed tics are those involving the facial muscles. They usually appear as grimacing, incessant blinking, frowning, or twitching of the mouth. Continual clearing of the throat, jerking of the head or arms, and shrugging of one or both shoulders may also occur. Sometimes they are much more complicated. Respiratory tics include sneezing, coughing and hiccups, and multiple tics may even involve the limbs and the whole body.

Since the compulsive character of the movements is so distinctive, the diagnosis is usually easy. The involuntary movements, however, must be distinguished from those of organic origin, especially those of chorea. Typical features to be noted are the repetitive nature of the movements in the simpler tics, and the complexity and elaboration of the movements in the more severe ones.

The prognosis is variable. Many children recover completely, whereas a few will continue to twitch throughout their lives. Sometimes they have even been known to subside and disappear completely if their presence has been entirely ignored and no reference has been made to them. When tics are maintained by habit, if little or no anxiety is present, the prognosis is likely to be poor. Indeed, the presence of anxiety greatly enhances the possibility of successful treatment. Tics of which the patient seems to be unaware are much more resistant than those of which he is fully conscious.

The Treatment of Tics

Whether they cause the child discomfort or not, tics are invariably extremely annoying to other members of the family. Superficial questioning will usually establish the fact that they first appeared at a time when the patient was emotionally disturbed and that only at a later date did they become habitual.

It is a commonly held, yet entirely mistaken idea that tics are easily treated by hypnosis. They are certainly almost invariably due to psychological conflicts, often arising from environmental difficulties, but as long as these conflicts are still active and the environmental troubles still operative, it is most unlikely that they will yield to direct hypnotic suggestion, and some form of full-scale psychotherapy or 'insight therapy' will be required. If, on the other hand, the original causal factors have long since disappeared and the tic has persisted solely as a habit or conditioned reflex, then the prospects of successful hypnotic treatment are greatly improved.

The task, then, is that of enabling the child to come to terms with his environment and to overcome his emotional difficulties. These may arise from an inability to adjust himself to his home or to his school surroundings. Tics are often a direct reaction to such difficulties, and represent a direct expression of the child's unconscious feelings of disgust and hostility to things or persons. The child's home life must consequently be closely investigated and his relationships with its parents, particularly the mother, also explored. Tics have often been known to start as a result of quarrels in the home or the loss of one or other of the parents. School difficulties must also be enquired into. Whenever possible disturbing factors should be corrected and treatment directed towards altering the child's attitude to them.

Schneck points out that tension is at the root of most childish ills, and that conflict, repression and frustration result in the production of anxiety which first results in tension and subsequently in neurosis. Hypnosis can be used to remove the tension and will allow the physician to re-educate both the child and its parents. In this way it will eventually dispose of the conflict, repression and frustration, and the tic will be likely to disappear.

When using hypnosis, I find that the deeper the trance the more successful treatment is likely to be. Fortunately in most children this presents no real problem. As for enuresis and asthma, I always precede any direct suggestions with the modified ego-strengthening routine (p. 199), to which I usually add suggestions of relaxation that will persist after the child has awakened. I then gradually introduce direct suggestion by coupling this relaxation with the disappearance of the tic in the following manner:

> *As* you become . . . and *as* you remain . . . *more and more relaxed*, each day . . . even when you are no longer with me . . . *so* . . . *the muscles of your face* (*neck, shoulders, arms, etc.*) *will remain more relaxed each day* . . . *and will stop twitching.*
>
> In a few moments . . . I am going to count slowly up to *five* . . . and *as I count up to five* . . . *your face will stop twitching* . . . *and the muscles will remain completely relaxed* . . . *completely still.*

I then count slowly up to *five.*

> You see . . . *your face has stopped twitching completely* . . . *and it will not start again after I wake you up.*

Naturally if there are environmental difficulties I include suggestions that the child will be able to cope with them.

Hypnosis in the Treatment of Nail Biting

This is an extremely common habit which occurs most frequently during childhood and adolescence. Whilst in itself it is of no great importance, it often serves as an outlet for tension. In many instances it is an anxiety reaction, associated with feelings of insecurity and sometimes repressed hostility directed against an over-dominant parent. It consequently represents a combination of oral gratification and self-punishment, the aggression being masochistically turned back on the child's own body. The oral satisfaction is identical with that gained by the baby from its comforter, or later on, the adult from the pipe, cigarette or cigar.

Nail biting is generally much more distressing to the parents than it is to the child itself. Nevertheless, it should always be regarded as an indication for enquiring into the child's emotional problems. Sensible parents can often tell you exactly when the habit started and may even be able to suggest the possible cause. The birth of another child—going to school for the first time—an illness—or admission to hospital may all be instrumental in starting the habit. Sometimes it has been known to start after only a few days' separation from the parents, and in such cases it usually responds extremely rapidly to direct hypnotic suggestion. However, when nail biting is associated with continuing emotional conflicts or maladjustments, direct suggestion will rarely succeed and hypnosis must also be used to resolve the conflicts, to relieve the tension, to re-establish a feeling of security, and to re-educate the child.

The Treatment of Nail Biting

Occasionally, if the habit can be completely controlled for a continuous period of 48 hours, this will prove quite sufficient to break the conditioning. In every case, however, an attempt should be made to discover the cause and to deal with the root of the trouble, despite the fact that symptomatic treatment will often be successful.

Adults and adolescents generally seek relief solely from the embarrassment of their habit. They cannot understand the persistence of the urge to bite their nails, and have no idea that they may need psychotherapy. Whenever children are concerned, it is always wise to interview the parent, usually the mother. She must be told that her own attitude will greatly influence the success or failure of the treatment. She must try to ignore the habit altogether since constant nagging will only result in the prolongation of the trouble. Sympathy and constant reassurance to the effect that it really doesn't matter, because presently the habit will cease, may even induce the child to reveal the nature of its worries.

I have found that one of the most important factors in successful treatment is to be found in strengthening the patient's desire and motivation to stop the habit. This is equally essential in child, adolescent or adult, first in the waking state, and subsequently repeated during hypnosis. Once again, the deeper the trance, the more rapid and effective treatment is likely to be. The procedure seems to be particularly successful when the patient is female:

> As you grow up . . . you will become more and more attractive.
> You will not want your appearance to be spoilt by ugly hands.

Nice hands and shapely nails will make you even more attractive . . . and you will want to make every effort to stop biting your nails, and spoiling them.
With my help . . . you will be able to stop biting them altogether . . . and then they will soon begin to grow.

I start treatment with the routine ego-strengthening suggestions and then proceed in the following manner:

As your nerves become stronger and steadier . . . as you become calmer and more relaxed, each day . . . so, there will be no reason for you to go on biting your nails.
You will no longer *want* to bite them . . . you will *stop* biting them.
If at any time you do start to bite them, without realizing what you are doing . . . *the moment your fingers touch your mouth . . . you will know immediately what you are doing . . . and you will be able to stop yourself right away . . . before you have done any damage at all.*
From now on . . . you will stop biting your nails . . . they will begin to grow . . . and you will begin to feel proud of your hands.

Strong, authoritative, direct suggestions under hypnosis will often succeed in stopping the habit altogether. Where a very deep trance, or somnambulism can be obtained, the prohibition may be rendered much more effective by telling the patient that he will experience a strong feeling of distaste whenever he puts his fingers in his mouth:

Whenever you start biting your nails . . . the moment you put your fingers in your mouth . . . you will get a horribly bitter, nasty taste in your mouth.
This will become stronger and nastier . . . and will make you feel sick.

Conditioning a feeling of nausea to the habit in this way may help greatly in establishing control. When this particular method is used, however, fairly frequent sessions will be necessary, and even when the nails begin to grow the suggestions may need to be reinforced about once a fortnight, for a time. In my opinion, increasing motivation is a much superior method and the results are likely to be much more permanent.

An alternative method is to *permit the biting of one or two nails, whilst allowing the others to grow.* Once this succeeds, it is surprising how often and rapidly the habit is abandoned altogether.

I have often noticed that whilst the patient has actually stopped biting his nails after one or two sessions, he seems to substitute a habit of picking them instead. This occurs more in adults and adolescents than in the case of children. It is not difficult to deal with, since the inclusion of specific suggestions prohibiting this as well will usually cause it to stop.

Hypnosis in Thumb-sucking

This is a very common childish habit which seems to provide comfort through oral gratification in much the same way as nail biting. If it persists into adolescence, it may well result in deformity of the palate and mal-occlusion of the teeth. The parents usually become very worried about the prospect of the child developing unsightly teeth. In most cases it seems to continue simply as a habit which is not as frequently associated with emotional conflicts as in nail biting, but when it is, an antagonistic child-parent relationship may be the cause and greatly reduces the chance of successful treatment.

Treatment of Thumb-sucking

The parents should always be interviewed and warned not to discuss treatment with the child. They must do their best to ignore the habit completely, and refrain from scolding or nagging.

As deep a trance as possible is always desirable, and the approach should be persuasive. Once again, the establishment of adequate motivation is of the greatest importance.

> When you grow up . . . you want your teeth to look nice and attractive, don't you?
> If you do . . . you will have to do your best, with my help, to stop sucking your thumbs and fingers.
> I can help you to stop.
> If you go on sucking your thumb, your teeth will become crooked and ugly as they grow.
> This won't happen if you stop sucking your thumb now . . . and I am going to help you to stop.

As in nail biting, in deep-trance subjects it is possible to condition a bitter, unpleasant taste to the act of sucking the thumb or fingers, and this may accelerate the breaking of the habit. In this case the fingers and thumbs of *both* hands should always be included.

An interesting and original approach is that of Erickson. After insisting that the parents do not interfere with his treatment of the child in any way, he proceeds to obtain his co-operation by saying that he would under no circumstances consider stopping the child sucking his thumb. He gets him to agree, however, that one of the most important lessons he had to learn when he went to school was that of sharing things with other children. Erickson then points out that, in sucking one thumb only, he is hardly being fair to his other thumb and eight fingers, each of which is entitled to a share. He proceeds to get the child to promise that every time he sucks his thumb, he will not only suck the other one as well, but also each individual finger. In carrying this out, the child soon tends to give up the habit altogether since, instead of continuing to give him pleasure, it has become converted into a intolerable nuisance.

Hypnosis in the Treatment of Blushing

This is a nervous habit which causes great distress to those who suffer from it. Although blushing is quite trivial in itself, the misery it causes to the unfortunate victim of the habit is wholly out of proportion to the severity of the actual complaint. The small blood-vessels in the skin of the neck and face become dilated, and it is this increased rush of blood which causes the heightened colour to appear. This common skin reaction, together with pallor and sweating is functionally related to the psychological emotions of fear and embarrassment.

Most people blush at some time or other, particularly when they are young, but do not worry about it and the incidents are soon forgotten. Later they seem to gain more control over their blood-vessels and lose the habit of blushing. In other people, however, blushing makes a deep impression and becomes associated with a host of unpleasant memories. They consequently begin to dread the habit, and the more they worry, the more likely they are to bring about the very thing that they fear. It is difficult to realize the agonies of mind such people experience whenever they have to appear in public, at meetings, conferences or even social events. In some cases, they go to extreme lengths to avoid them and cease to mix, almost entirely.

The Treatment of Blushing

With the patient in as deep a hypnotic state as possible, I always begin treatment with the usual ego-strengthening routine, and then continue in the following manner:

> As you become more relaxed . . . and less tense each day . . . *so . . . you will remain more relaxed . . . and completely at ease . . . when you are in the presence of other people . . . no matter whether they be few or many . . . no*

matter whether they be friends or strangers.
You will be able to meet them on equal terms . . . to talk to them quite easily
. . . without feeling self-conscious . . . without feeling embarrassed . . . without
becoming confused . . . without feeling conspicuous in any way.
You will be more self-confident . . . more self-assured . . . and so deeply interested
in what you have to say . . . that you will be much less conscious of yourself . . .
and of your own feelings.
And because you will remain emotionally calm and undisturbed . . . you will no
longer blush nearly so easily . . . or as frequently.
If you do feel yourself beginning to blush . . . you will not become worried, uneasy
or confused . . . you will be able to ignore it completely . . . and carry on the
conversation without letting it disturb you in the least.
And because of this . . . it will die away, very very rapidly indeed . . . so that
it will pass almost unnoticed by others.
The less notice you take of it . . . the less frequently and intensely it will occur
. . . and with each treatment . . . it will happen less and less . . . until, eventually,
it will no longer happen at all.

I have found that this method is very effective, and often produces
successful results. Therapy may have to be prolonged for 10 to 12
sessions or more in severe cases if the trouble is to be completely
eliminated.

The Hypnotic Treatment of Lack of Confidence and Stage Fright

This is usually characterized by an outbreak of acute anxiety whenever
the individual has to perform, make a speech or deliver a lecture in
front of an audience. Under such circumstances he always under-
values and depreciates himself, expects disapproval, and fears adverse
criticism. He may be a neurotic with strong over-perfectionistic traits
who sets himself far too high a standard. In everyday life he is likely
to feel uncomfortable and ill at ease in the presence of people in authority,
or those he believes to be superior to himself. Conversely he will always
be able to express himself without fear or anxiety whenever he feels
his own superiority.

When lack of confidence arises as the result of deep-seated personality
defects, nothing less than the analytical approach is likely to be successful,
but if the patient has a reasonably well-integrated personality a more
direct and persuasive hypnotic approach will often produce remarkable
results. My own experience in such cases has led me to believe that
the restoration of self-confidence is one of the easiest and most rapid

results that can be achieved by hypnotherapy. The full ego-strengthening routine, suitably reinforced by specific suggestions appropriate to each individual case, has proved invaluable in the treatment of this condition. I always begin with this, and then proceed in the following manner:

> As you become . . . *more relaxed* and *less tense*, each day . . . *so* . . . you will remain *more relaxed* . . . and *less tense* . . . when you are in the presence of other people . . . no matter whether they be few or many . . . no matter whether they be friends or strangers.
>
> You will be able to meet them on equal terms . . . and you will feel much more at ease in their presence . . . *without* the slightest feeling of inferiority . . . *without* becoming self-conscious . . . *without* becoming embarrassed or confused . . . *without* feeling that you are making yourself conspicuous in any way.
>
> You will become . . . *so deeply interested* . . . *so deeply absorbed in what you are saying* . . . *that you will concentrate entirely upon this to the complete exclusion of everything else.*
>
> Because of this . . . *you will remain perfectly relaxed* . . . *perfectly calm and self-confident* . . . *and you will become much less conscious of yourself and your own feelings.*
>
> *You will consequently be able to talk quite freely and naturally* . . . *without being worried in the slightest by the presence of your audience.*
>
> *If you should begin to think about yourself* . . . *you will immediately shift your attention back to your conversation* . . . *and will no longer experience the slightest nervousness* . . . *discomfort* . . . *or uneasiness.*

When the patient is likely to be called upon to appear upon the stage, to make a speech, or to deliver a lecture, the above may well be modified in the following manner.

> *The moment you get up to speak* . . . *all your nervousness will disappear completely* . . . *and you will feel* . . . *completely relaxed* . . . *completely at your ease* . . . *and completely confident.*
>
> *You will become so deeply interested in what you have to say* . . . *that the presence of an audience will no longer bother you in the slightest* . . . *and you will no longer feel uncertain* . . . *confused* . . . *or conspicuous in any way.*
>
> *Your mind will become so fully occupied with what you have to say* . . . *that you will no longer worry at all as to how you say it.*
>
> *You will no longer feel nervous* . . . *self-conscious* . . . *or embarrassed* . . . *and you will remain throughout* . . . *perfectly calm* . . . *perfectly confident* . . . *and self-assured.*

Whenever a speech or talk has to be given, or a stage appearance made, the patient must be impressed with the importance of making thorough preparation. The feeling that he has mastered his subject or become word-perfect in his lines will help him enormously. It is always essential to rehearse it thoroughly before the actual performance. He should be instructed to speak slowly, clearly and deliberately, and to concentrate entirely upon what he is saying.

The teaching of self-hypnosis, whenever possible, can prove invaluable in these cases. Not only can the patient be taught to visualize himself addressing an audience without difficulty, but he can also suggest to himself, during hypnosis, that he will gradually be able to do this without nervousness, self-consciousness or apprehension *in real life*.

I have helped many patients with this technique, which seems to be extraordinarily effective. Indeed, some months later they have told me that, whenever they have to make a speech or give an address, they make a habit of arriving early and finding a quiet place where they can spend five minutes or so before entering the meeting. Here, they induce a self-hypnotic trance, in the course of which they suggest to themselves that *the moment they start to speak,* all nervousness will disappear completely, that they will feel completely calm and relaxed, and will become so interested and absorbed in what they have to say that they will remain quite confident and self-assured.

Notice how these self-suggestions tend to act post-hypnotically upon the signal *the moment I begin to speak*.

The Use of Hypnosis in the Academic Field

Hypnosis can often be used most effectively to help students to gain more efficiency in their studies. Many fail to realize all their natural capabilities because so many factors tend to interfere with the efficient use of the mind. Lack of attention, distraction, the inability to concentrate sufficiently, and even a dislike for the subject to be studied, can all cause the student to fall behind with his work, and become over-anxious and discouraged.

When hypnotic treatment is contemplated, the first step to be taken is to discuss the situation fully with the student himself, to discover the precise nature and, if possible, the cause of the difficulties he is experiencing. He should be closely questioned about his home life, his working conditions, his habits, his interpersonal relationships, his attitude to his teachers, and his particular worries and anxieties. As a result of this, disturbing emotional factors (which are seldom deeply seated) may often be brought to light, and appropriate advice may be given both in the waking and in the hypnotic state which will help him in coping with these.

In the case of school-children, it is always essential to talk to the parents as well. Only too often they are so over-anxious for their children to succeed that they unconsciously press them too hard or, with the best of intentions, repeatedly stress the importance of passing an examination and the disastrous results of failure; the child becomes resentful and develops a feeling of inferiority with excessive anxiety and a complete lack of confidence. Whenever this is so the parents must be encouraged to alter their own attitudes and behaviour if a successful result is to be obtained. Where the child has become disheartened in its efforts to keep up with the others, or when its difficulties seem to arise as a result of disturbed relationships with certain teachers, a change of class or even of school may sometimes be necessary as a preliminary step. Each individual case must be carefully considered on its merits.

Treatment must necessarily be rather prolonged, but the results are usually most rewarding. Obviously the deeper the hypnotic trance and the more frequently treatment can be given, the more rapid and efficient it will be. I have found that in my successful cases some 12 to 18 weekly sessions have been required. This may seem a long time until one realizes that the essence of this treatment is the inculcation of a habit. Before starting treatment, one should always find out the most convenient hours to allot to study each day, so that a regular programme of work may be arranged and adhered to. One of the advantages of this lies in the fact that the precise times agreed upon can be incorporated in the suggestions that will be made, and are then likely to be observed post-hypnotically.

I always begin with the usual ego-strengthening routine and incorporate any specific suggestions that seem appropriate to the individual's particular difficulties. I then follow with more strongly directive suggestions aimed at correcting the student's attitudes and regularizing his habits. These are most important since they act post-hypnotically, and are greatly strengthened by each successive treatment.

> Every day . . . [at such and such a time] . . . you will get into the habit of working for at least two hours or so . . . without fail.
> You will be able to *think more clearly* . . . you will be able to *concentrate much more easily*.
> You will become . . . *so deeply interested and absorbed in what you are studying* that you will be able to *give your whole attention to what you are doing* . . . *to the complete exclusion of everything else*.

Because of this . . . you will be able to *grasp things and understand them more quickly . . . more easily . . . and they will impress themselves so deeply upon your memory that you will not forget them.*
With every treatment that you have . . . *your memory will improve enormously . . . and your work will become easier and easier.*
You will not only be able to remember what you have learned . . . but you will be able to recall it without difficulty . . . whenever you need to do so.

Many students and school-children fail to do themselves justice during examinations. No matter how thoroughly they may be prepared, they become so nervous and apprehensive that their minds seem to go blank and they are unable to remember things that they know quite well. They consequently put up a much poorer performance than might reasonably have been expected from them, and fail examinations which they ought to have passed without difficulty. In such cases hypnosis can be of the greatest possible assistance.

The moment you enter the examination room and pick up your paper to read the questions . . . you will become completely calm and relaxed . . . and all your nervousness and apprehension will disappear completely.
No matter how difficult the questions may seem at first sight . . . or how little you seem to know . . . *you will not panic . . .* because you will find that things are not as bad as they seem.
You will *read all the questions carefully and deliberately . . . you will decide upon the one that you can tackle best . . . and answer that one as fully as you can . . . without worrying about the others until you have completed it.*
As you do this . . . *you will find that you will actually remember far more than you originally thought you would.*
When you have put down all you know about this first question . . . *choose the next easiest to answer . . . and tackle that in exactly the same way.*
Continue in this way with the rest of the questions until you have written all that you can remember . . . or until the time is up.
When you have finished . . . you will find that you have remembered far more than you thought possible when you first read the questions.

I have found the combination of the two techniques just described to be extremely successful in the many cases I have treated; the two which follow are representative of the main types of problem with which one has to deal.

Case 1. The matron of a hospital asked me to see if I could help one of her student nurses, a girl aged 22 years. She was apparently a most promising nurse but had already failed her final examination twice. She was allowed to sit for it once again, in three months' time, but if she failed on this third attempt she would have no alternative but to give up nursing altogether. I was only able to treat her once a week for about 12 weeks, but fortunately she was a reasonably good hypnotic subject and began to gain steadily in confidence. After the first few sessions she told me that she was not only finding that her work and studies were becoming much easier but that her memory was certainly improving. As the date of the examination drew near she remained much calmer and less apprehensive than on any previous occasion, despite the important issue that was involved. She passed the examination quite easily, her marks averaging between 70 and 80 per cent.

Case 2. A very worried father consulted me about his son, a boy aged 12 years, who was in the junior house at a public school. The headmaster had told him that he should make arrangements to transfer the boy to another school as he was not prepared to keep him after the next term. Apparently he stood not the slightest chance of passing the Common Entrance examination which was essential before he could enter the senior school. He was not only far below the average standard of his form, but took little or no interest in his work and was inclined to be both unruly and difficult in his behaviour. The father had asked for his son to be kept in the junior school for a further 12 months to give him a last chance, but the headmaster was not disposed to grant this request.

The boy was quite bright and intelligent and proved to be extremely co-operative since he did not want to be sent to another school. He was only able to see me during the Easter holidays before returning to school, so I arranged to treat him three times a week (approximately 12 sessions in all). Since it was obviously impossible in this short period for him to recover the ground he had lost, I concentrated upon stressing the importance of working really hard and trying to do his best, in the hope that the headmaster might appreciate the difference in his attitude and allow him to stay on in the junior school for another year in order to try for the Common Entrance examination. At the end of the summer term, his school report had improved remarkably: although his placing was not much better, it was noted that in almost every subject he had worked hard and had obviously done his best. As a result of this performance and his change in attitude, he was permitted to stay on for a further year.

During the summer vacation I treated him twice a week (a total of 9 sessions). The treatment was now directed at improving his powers of concentration and capacity for learning, improving his memory and fostering a desire and determination to continue to work really hard. By Christmas this was reflected in his school report again, but this time his position in his form had noticeably improved. In the course of this holiday I saw him once a week (3 sessions only) and continued with the same treatment. His Easter report showed further improvement, and the headmaster told his father that he seemed to stand a reasonable chance of passing his Common Entrance in June. I saw him on only 4 further occasions, on each of which I included (for the first time) instructions relating to the examination itself. The ultimate result was extremely gratifying since he passed the examination without any difficulty, and was accepted in the senior school.

CHAPTER 19

Miscellaneous Conditions

Organic Diseases

Whenever a patient becomes physically ill, it is inevitable that certain emotional factors also enter into the picture. These will tend both to influence his symptoms and, in many instances, to retard his recovery. The extent to which they do this will depend largely upon the way in which the patient regards his illness, and if such factors are also taken into account and treated adequately, a great deal can be achieved in increasing the patient's resistance and accelerating the process of healing.

People respond to illness in many different ways. Some look upon it as something to be ashamed of or as a sign of weakness and try to hide it both from themselves and others. Others will admit their incapacity and react to their illness with a considerable amount of tension and anxiety. Hypnosis can be extremely useful in chronic, incapacitating diseases in persuading the patient to accept both his illness and his limitations philosophically. He can be induced to accept the fact that whilst there are certain things that he may not be able to do again, there are others that he will be able to achieve successfully despite the handicap imposed by his illness. Even when little more than this can be accomplished, the resulting improvement in his morale and general outlook will prove most gratifying.

In incurable, painful and ultimately fatal illnesses, hypnosis may often be used advantageously to alleviate pain and suffering in addition to helping the patient to accept his illness. When employed in this way the greatest success is likely to be achieved when the depth of hypnosis is sufficient to secure complete analgesia. Unfortunately this can only rarely be obtained; even so, a considerable degree of relief from pain can often be secured as a result of which the amount of analgesic drugs administered can frequently be substantially reduced. Even in cases of inoperable cancer, hypnosis can sometimes augment and prolong the action of the milder analgesic drugs and thus delay considerably the need to resort to morphia.

In our approach to this type of case I am afraid we often tend to adopt too perfectionistic an outlook, and the fact that the pain seems so intense and the possibility of securing any significant degree of analgesia so remote only too frequently discourages us from even considering the use of hypnosis. Such an attitude is entirely wrong, for we should always remember that there are two major components in any pain:

1. The actual pain itself.
2. The distress that it causes.

Consequently, even when hypnosis can only be used to minimize the distress suffered by the patient, the pain itself tends to become rather less severe and more easily tolerated. Relaxation and the reduction of tension, worry and anxiety, all of which can be achieved in the light or medium stages of hypnosis, can afford some relief to the sufferer and, in many cases, actually reduce the amount of medication he requires.

Quite apart from analgesia itself, there are a number of other methods that will sometimes succeed under hypnosis. ' Distraction ' will sometimes succeed for we all know that it is possible to forget pain, just as we can forget a headache whilst watching an exciting film. We should also be more willing to settle for things than *can* be endured, rather than to fail to change things that cannot otherwise be changed. Indeed, one of the things we can sometimes do is to *substitute or replace pain by a lesser or altered sensation*. It may be possible to transform a distressing pain into a feeling of unpleasant, but not painful, warmth which is much more easily tolerated and infinitely preferable to the original pain. Indeed in a receptive patient in a reasonably deep trance, pain can be ' displaced ' for it need not necessarily be experienced at the site of the lesion or disease. After all, a gall-bladder pain is felt between the shoulders, and a cardiac pain in the upper arm. Under these circumstances, under hypnosis, a patient can be told that the pain he is feeling in his stomach, he would be able to tolerate much better if it were in his left hand, and you proceed to induce it in the latter as a replacement of the former. In certain instances, ' time-distortion ' can afford relief from pain. When friends visit you time passes quickly, but when unwelcome visitors arrive you wonder whether the day will ever end. This is an everyday example of ' time-distortion ' or subjective time. Using this principle, you can teach a patient how to experience 20 minutes of pain in only 10 seconds of actual time, thus shortening its duration to such an extent that the painful periods appear very short in comparison with the time he is pain-free.

It may also be suggested to the patient that he can achieve a *slowly progressive diminution of his pain.* In this case, you tell him that if the 100 per cent of pain he is suffering were reduced to 90 per cent he would hardly be able to notice any difference. That the level might even drop to 85 per cent . . . or 80 per cent . . . 75 per cent . . . or even 70 per cent . . . and so on, and the patient will often go along with you because you have not asked of him a major task. In deeper hypnosis of course ' dissociative ' procedures may be most effective. For these brief references to various possible methods of dealing with chronic pain, I am deeply indebted to a paper given on this subject by Milton Erickson at the International Congress of Hypnosis and Psychosomatic Medicine in Paris, April 1965, which concluded with the following observations.

' *In all such hypnotic procedures, you must speak to the patient with an utter intensity and belief. You should also realize that maybe not all of these things will work in any particular patient, but surely since he is a human being, he will respond to some of them. It is consequently your duty as a clinician, to be sure to present to him these ideas, some of which he may be able to accept and act upon.*'

Ulcerative Colitis

Ulcerative colitis is a chronic disease in which periods of quiescence tend to be followed by acute exacerbations. The latter, not infrequently, are found to coincide with the occurrence of emotional disturbances. In the course of this illness, the patient's mind and attention becomes more and more fixed upon his bowels to such an extent that they eventually become his sole topic of interest and conversation. Hypnosis can often be very useful in influencing this state of mind, and should be employed in addition to the usual medical procedures. It is sometimes surprising to note the symptomatic improvement that takes place once a state of mental calm, tranquillity and relaxation has become established.

If hypnotic treatment is contemplated it is always wise to begin by enquiring into the nature of any emotional disturbances to which the patient may be subjected. Marital conflicts, bereavements, even such emotions as anger and resentment may produce excessive activity on the part of the colon. Where family ties are excessively strong, the threat of having to break them that is implied by an engagement and prospective marriage can often result in exacerbations of the illness. Should any disturbances as these be discovered, appropriate steps may be taken to adjust the patient's attitude towards them in the course of his hypnotic treatment.

Since the results of both medical and surgical treatment of ulcerative colitis are frequently unsatisfactory, suggestive therapy may well be considered at a relatively early stage. There is everything to gain and nothing to lose. Some cases respond very well indeed, and should failure occur, it cannot interfere in any way with any further treatment which may be required.

Meares advises that, since most patients who react to stress with disordered bowel-function exhibit marked obsessional traits, hypnosis should always be induced in a very precise manner.

Nervous Dyspepsia

Disturbed emotional states lead far more frequently to alterations in the normal functioning of the gastro-intestinal tract than almost any other system in the body. Many expressions commonly used in every-day life such as ' I can't swallow his attitude ', ' She makes me sick ' or ' I can't stomach this much longer ' illustrate this tendency only too well. Anxiety, fear, anger or disgust will often inhibit stomach activity and lead to chronic indigestion, nausea and flatulence, or to excessive secretion of hydrochloric acid that may even cause peptic ulceration. Indeed many gastro-intestinal disorders, nervous dyspepsias and even gastric and duodenal ulcers are classified amongst the stress diseases. The symptoms often seem to represent a defence mechanism designed to protect the individual from his environmental difficulties, his feelings of resentment and his frustrated ambitions.

Most individuals who work extremely hard and undertake consider-able responsibilities are prone to develop this type of complaint. Doctors and highly placed business executives tend to fall into this category. Long hours and heavy responsibility, particularly if associated with irregular meals and habits, lead to a constant state of worry, anxiety and tension which, if left untreated, will inevitably result in eventual breakdown. This deterioration will be greatly accelerated if there are also unconscious feelings of inadequacy, fears of losing the job, or frustrated ambitions, all of which provoke an acute mental conflict against which the patient constantly struggles in vain.

Hypnotic treatment can often afford invaluable assistance in such cases, particularly if the emotional difficulties of the patient are first exposed and then explained to him, and if he is helped to re-adjust his attitude towards them and to correct his faulty habits. The mental and physical relaxation that hypnosis can produce will benefit such patients enormously.

The ego-strengthening routine forms a sound basis for the hypnotic treatment of these cases, incorporating as it does suggestions of personal well-being, mental and physical relaxation and increased confidence, for many of these patients suffer additionally from subjective feelings of inferiority, self-consciousness, shyness and embarrassment, and tension is almost always present. It is not to be expected, however, that a condition for which the patient has been treating himself for years with innumerable patent medicines, pills and powders, is going to clear up either quickly or easily. Considerable patience will be required, for the most difficult task will be that of dispelling the patient's constant expectation of dyspepsia.

Essential Hypertension

The fact that disturbed emotional states can affect the blood-pressure has long been recognized. Indeed if a patient becomes aware that he has a high blood-pressure, he may worry about it and dread the consequences, with the result that his condition tends to become progressively worse. Even when attending the surgery for a routine medical examination, the nervous patient will develop an increase in his blood-pressure. If it is taken at the beginning of his interview and retaken just before the examination is concluded the blood-pressure will often be found to have dropped to an appreciable extent since the individual will have become much calmer and more composed, and will have lost his initial apprehension.

The basic causes of essential hypertension are still not fully understood, but it is well known that the condition frequently occurs in people who are anxious and over-excitable, and who worry excessively and take life far too seriously. It is yet another complaint that falls into the category of ' stress diseases ', so it is hardly surprising that the complete mental and physical relaxation that can be achieved in the hypnotic state can often benefit the hypertensive patient to a considerable extent. The condition is insidious in onset, and may have been present for long periods before it is ultimately discovered.

The physiological mechanism underlying essential hypertension seems to be the constriction of the smaller arteries as a result of nervous impulses. During natural sleep, when the body and mind are completely at rest, these impulses become greatly reduced, as a result of which the blood-vessels tend to relax, and the blood-pressure falls. This sheds a good deal of light on the reason why hypnotic treatment can so often succeed in alleviating the condition; it also underlines the advantage of allowing the patient to remain in the trance state for prolonged periods, whenever possible.

The presenting symptoms are both many and various. Throbbing headaches, attacks of vertigo and bouts of flushing are exceedingly common. These are frequently accompanied by lack of concentration, defective memory and mental and emotional instability.

Hypnosis can often prove extremely valuable in the treatment of these cases. Provided that a medium or deep trance can be obtained, direct suggestion will often secure a surprising improvement in the patient's condition. Naturally it cannot be expected to cure long-standing cases of high blood-pressure, but the regular use of the ego-strengthening routine, with particular stress laid upon rest and relaxation and the importance of 'taking things more easily', will usually succeed in alleviating the patient's suffering to a considerable extent, and render his life more tolerable.

The benefit of continuous hypnotic sleep has already been briefly mentioned. Once the trance has been induced, the patient can be told that he will wake up in several hours time, feeling completely relaxed, mentally and physically. Alternatively, he may be told that his hypnotic sleep will gradually merge into normal sleep, from which he will wake up in the usual manner.

Hypnosis in Anorexia Nervosa

This distressing and serious condition is almost invariably confined to females, usually girls and young women. Cases generally have a simple beginning, the initial restriction of diet being entirely voluntary. Later, all desire for food is completely lost, and the patient refuses to eat since she has no appetite whatsoever. Emotional factors are always involved. In many cases, the patient begins to diet because she fears that she is putting on weight, and has a horror of becoming too fat. In others, the starvation represents a rebellion against a dominating or over-solicitous parent, usually the mother, and as in the case of a hysteric, the symptom is used as a weapon with which to influence the parents.

Food is constantly refused, and the patient loses weight with alarming rapidity. An extraordinary degree of emaciation is often reached, the patient becoming reduced to a mere skeleton. If forcibly fed, against her will, by spoon or tube, she will generally take the first opportunity, when unobserved, of making herself vomit. Despite this extreme emaciation, however, the patient will usually display almost tireless activity. If not arrested in time, the mortality rate is high, many of these patients succumbing to pulmonary tuberculosis.

Various secondary symptoms occur. In addition to the progressive loss of weight, constipation is commonly found, and the pulse is often slow. The condition is associated with amenorrhoea, depression and restlessness, although actual gastric symptoms are usually slight. The most careful investigations reveal no organic cause.

Treatment

It is obviously important that treatment should be started as soon as possible, once a diagnosis has been made. The first question to be decided is whether the patient should be treated at home, or whether she should be admitted to hospital. Where the condition has become severe, and the loss of weight and emaciation considerable, there is little doubt that the dangers will be minimized by hospitalization. Similarly, when strong emotional attitudes, centred upon the home and parents, constitute a causal factor, removal from these environmental influences has much to commend it. Should such advice be necessary, it will often be found that the parents are most difficult to convince, and a great deal of persuasion is required.

Irrespective of where treatment is undertaken, however, it should always be conducted in accordance with certain basic principles. Superficial questioning will often succeed in revealing some of the originating ideas, which are frequently fully conscious. This enquiry is extremely important since it convinces the patient that her motives are fully understood, and thus helps in securing her confidence.

Where fears of fatness exist, it should be pointed out that under no circumstances will she be expected to eat to such an extent that she will put on too much weight, so there will be not the slightest reason to fear adiposity. Indeed, the most solemn assurances must be given that, under no circumstances whatever, will this be allowed to happen. So much pressure has been brought to bear on the patient in the past, that it is far from easy to reassure her in this way. I usually tell her that I am in a position to prescribe drugs which will easily reduce weight, and that if she will only co-operate with me, and try her best to eat more of the right kinds of food, I will promise her that, should her weight tend to become excessive, I will take the necessary steps to reduce it to the correct level. In making such a promise, it is essential that you should be prepared to carry out your part of the bargain, should it become advisable to do so, to obviate any anxiety that arises. In all my cases so far, I have never been called upon to implement this guarantee, which has proved an invaluable step in the removal of the patient's fear and dread.

Food should never be deliberately pressed upon the patient. Increase will have to be very gradual, and it may take several months before the patient can take a perfectly normal diet. It is most essential to interview the parents, in order to explain the gravity of the situation fully, and to adjust their attitudes towards it. They should be told that, whilst the patient is under treatment and trying to co-operate, she must not be worried by them, and no attempt should be made to force food upon her. If her condition is such that this becomes a necessity, then it is much better and safer to admit her to hospital, where isolation and special feeding can be undertaken. In such cases, this should begin at once, and not wait upon the results of psychotherapy. In many instances, the closest supervision will be necessary to avoid deception as to the food intake.

The voluntary dieting at the beginning of an anorexia nervosa never represents an ordinary attempt to reduce weight. There is always some associated psychological disturbance such as fear and anxiety, or some emotional conflict, usually centred upon the mother. The patient often displays defects of personality, not infrequently hysterical in nature, that existed long before the illness arose. Amongst these, the need to attract attention to herself is one of the most significant. Once the illness has become established, as the patient's condition deteriorates, so her personality tends to disintegrate to a greater and greater extent.

Here, hypnosis can prove exceedingly valuable and effective in helping to re-integrate the patient's personality. The standard ego-strengthening routine, suitably modified to fit existing circumstances, is most successful in achieving this object. Simple questioning under hypnosis will generally succeed in elucidating the relevant fears and emotional conflicts when these are not conscious, and they can then be dealt with, and the patient's attitudes gradually re-adjusted by the incorporation of the necessary suggestions.

The first, and most important use of hypnosis in these cases, is to establish an emotional relationship with the patient, in order to enlist her willingness to co-operate. Any promises or reassurances that are given should be regularly repeated in the hypnotic state. The instillation of confidence, the removal of anxiety, and the gradual re-education of the patient are of primary importance. An infinite amount of patience and understanding is necessary, but the results will prove well worth while.

Direct suggestions alone that the appetite will increase, are of very little value, and will seldom succeed. Indeed, under certain circumstances they can even be harmful, for if accepted, they may precipitate an acute attack of anxiety. Such suggestions are best directed towards increasing the patient's desire and will to gradually eat more of the right kinds of food, and her determination and wish to co-operate to the best of her ability. She should also be encouraged to keep a weekly chart of her weight.

Many of these cases, particularly in the earlier stages, can be dealt with most successfully by the general practitioner. The more severe ones, however, that exhibit deep-seated emotional conflicts or gross hysterical features, should be referred for psychiatric treatment without delay, since they can deteriorate to an alarming and even dangerous degree, very, very rapidly indeed.

Hypnosis in the Treatment of Obesity

It has customarily been considered that this common condition is caused by taking food in excess of normal dietary requirements, and the various methods of dealing with this depend upon the same principle—that of increasing the body's consumption of calories until it exceeds the daily intake. This object has usually been achieved in several different ways:

1. By increasing daily exercise.
2. By the use of drugs such as thyroid extract.
3. By restricting the diet.
4. By reducing the appetite with appropriate drugs.

In recent years, however, our attitude to this problem has been changing, and we no longer necessarily assume that, in the overweight patient, the accumulation of fat roughly equals the amount of calories he has consumed over and above the number expended in daily activities. Formerly, we used to regard most of these patients as 'compulsive eaters', but we now know that this is not invariably the case. Many people over-eat, yet some remain moderate in weight, some are underweight and others overweight, so it is certainly not correct to regard every overweight person as a compulsive eater.

At times, we also encounter the patient who has indulged in over-eating as a means of reducing tension. In this case, it represents a form of 'oral gratification' which arises when childhood has been associated with insecurity and illness. Eating then seems to produce feelings of peace and contentment, and represents a regression to the soothing and comforting effect of breast-feeding in infancy. Yet once again it is wrong to generalize. As we look around, we can see plenty of people with pipes, cigarettes or even pencils in their mouths from which they are gaining some oral-gratification, but it would be absurd to assume that all such individuals had unhappy, insecure and possibly love-less childhoods. Naturally both the above assumptions of 'over-eating' and 'oral gratification' are sometimes true, but they are certainly not applicable in all cases of obesity and can only be definitely established by careful history-taking.

We are only just beginning to understand something of the physiology and pathology of obesity, and to recognize the fact that the common types of obesity are *not* due to over-eating. In fact, in obesity there is a metabolic defect closely resembling that in diabetes, so that the obese person is really a sick individual.

You will find that most obese patients have previously consulted several doctors, and have tried all sorts of diets, losing weight repeatedly only to regain it after a few weeks. Consequently, they have become more and more frustrated and are constantly seeking methods of dealing with excess weight which do not depend upon abstemiousness. This, of course, is an impossibility and you should make it quite clear from the outset that, whilst hypnosis will be able to help them considerably, treatment is bound to take time and that no rapid or magical cure will take place. I usually tell my patient to imagine that we are both standing at the foot of a very steep hill, with a heavily loaded hand-cart. It is far too heavy for him to push it to the top of the hill by his own unaided efforts. It is also too heavy for me to pull it up to the top on my own. *But if only he will push whilst I pull, it will go up quite easily.* In other words, he will no longer have to make the necessary effort to adhere to a diet without help, and that through hypnosis I can increase his ability, not only to make that effort but also to be able to maintain it. But, hypnosis or no hypnosis, unless he is prepared to co-operate with me and undertake his share of this task, failure will once again be inevitable.

I also consider it important to let your patient know that his obesity is not necessarily his fault, and that in many instances it is due to a disturbance in metabolism. It is extraordinary how much this encourages the patient when he realizes for the first time that there is something wrong. He has already been castigated so much, and has blamed himself to such an extent that he has a very poor self-image and feels that other people look down on him. Thus, if his condition is due to some disturbance for which he, himself, cannot be held responsible, he need no longer feel ashamed. Indeed, once the obese patient is receptive to the idea that his trouble is due to faulty metabolism and can be helped to maintain a suitable diet with the use of hypnosis, then we are in a favourable position to proceed with hypnotherapy.

Treatment

I usually begin by telling my patient that I am not in the least interested in the number of calories in his food, but that I am very interested in the type of food he eats. A proper diet is essential and should be chosen to conform with the beliefs and experience of the therapist. Personally, I like to recommend a high-fat, high-protein, low-carbohydrate diet—the so-called ' unlimited calorie ' diet. The patient is always most relieved to find that, under this régime, he no longer has to weigh his food, to measure his food or to calculate the number of calories in his food. It is usually best to start on a diet which includes little or no carbohydrate and eliminates starches and sugars, particularly sucrose and fructose. Occasionally a little carbohydrate may be permitted in the form of a limited amount of potatoes, and the patient will still lose weight but all others are strictly forbidden.

And here we encounter our principal difficulty. No matter what diet is prescribed, our main problem, and a very frustrating one, is *how to change our patient's eating habits*. It is in tackling this task that hypnosis can prove invaluable. But let us make no mistake about one vitally important fact. Direct suggestions to the effect that the patient will not want to eat as much, that he will be satisfied with much smaller quantities of food or that he will shed as much weight as he wishes within a month or two will fail miserably. Hypnosis will never succeed in altering a person's personality or habit-formation in this way. We have to develop more realistic goals and use it to re-educate him in his eating habits. For instance, *instead of merely using suggestion to help him in his determination to avoid undesirable foods, we can use it to enable him to begin to really enjoy the foods that are permissible*, and thus greatly diminish his feeling of deprivation and craving.

In explaining this to the patient, I find it most useful to enlist his imagination, a technique I learned from Dr Herbert Mann of California, to whom I am also indebted for my present approach to the problem of obesity. I ask the patient to visualize a ' wine-taster ' who pours a little wine into a glass, spends a few moments looking at its colour and clarity and then lifts the glass to his nose and smells it, enjoying the aroma and ' bouquet ' before actually tasting it and fully enjoying its flavour. He is then to compare this with the man who opens a bottle of wine and drinks it up immediately, and to ask himself which of the two is getting the greater enjoyment. I then tell him that with the help of hypnosis he can be taught to enjoy the sight and smell as well as the taste of well-prepared, nicely served food, and that he will learn to savour it more fully by eating more slowly. Above all, he will begin to appreciate more and more the flavour of the foods which are permitted, so that his craving for those he must avoid will gradually diminish and disappear.

I frequently find that the trance relationship in itself seems to satisfy the patient's longing for dependency and begins to lessen his craving for food. Consequently, I believe the effect of my suggestions is heightened if they are given firmly and with a certain amount of authority, once the preliminary explanations have been made. After beginning with the usual ' ego-strengthening ' routine which, in my opinion should never be omitted, once I have reached the section dealing with relaxation, I proceed in the following manner:

Remember the four important things that are going to happen.

First of all . . . *relaxation.*

Every day . . . you will become . . . and will remain more relaxed and less tense.

That relaxation will lead to greater *calmness.*

Every day . . . you will become calmer . . . and more composed.

That increased feeling of calmness will result in greatly increased *confidence.*

Every day . . . you will feel more confident . . . more self-assured.

And that confidence will lead inevitably to much greater power of *self-control.* You will gain much more control over the way you think . . . over the way you feel . . . over the way you behave.

Day by day . . . you will find it much less difficult to keep to the diet I have given you.

You will begin to enjoy more and more the sight . . . the smell . . . as well as the taste and flavour of the foods that are good for you . . . so that you will gradually lose your craving for those which you cannot metabolize properly and will consequently lead to the accumulation of fat.

In the particular diet that I have prescribed for you . . . you will begin the day by having a little breakfast . . . say, one fried or scrambled egg and one slice of bacon.

You will also get into the habit of having smaller meals . . . more frequently . . . because when people eat a little, more often . . . they tend to lose weight faster than if they only eat once or twice a day.

Even when you cut out carbohydrate foods (including cakes and pastries) . . .
foods rich in starch . . . sweets etc. . . . there are still plenty of appetizing
foods. . . salads, meats etc. . . . which will begin to appeal to you more and
more . . . as you eat more slowly . . . thus really enjoying the sight . . . smell
. . . and flavour. Consequently . . . you will no longer be tempted into eating
between meals . . . and will have less and less difficulty in avoiding foods
which are fattening.

You will begin to take more exercise each day . . . and as you gradually lose
weight . . . you will become much healthier and fitter . . . and your personal
appearance will improve.

Every day . . . your desire and determination to stick to your diet . . . and
change your former eating habits will increase . . . to such an extent that it
will completely overwhelm any temptation to depart from it . . . which will
eventually disappear.

Teaching the patient ' auto-hypnosis ' can also be extremely helpful
and, in certain instances, ' group hypnosis ' lends itself admirably to the
treatment of obesity provided that the groups are not too large—say
some 8 to 10 people. This not only reduces the cost to the patient but
also introduces the competitive element in addition to proving time-
saving for the therapist.

Wolberg points out that in deep trances, an urge to over-eat can often
be converted into some other form of activity, and considers that the
dangers and risks of obesity should also be brought to the patient's notice.
It is most important that full details of the diet should always be supplied—
what foods may be taken, and what must be avoided.

Hypnosis in the Treatment of Constipation

For many years the general public have held the firm conviction that
if they fail to have a regular bowel-action every day and waste products
are allowed to accumulate, their health will inevitably suffer and poisoning
of the whole system will be bound to occur. They consequently indulge
in the most strenuous efforts to secure a complete ' clear-out ', in order
to get rid of the poisons they assume to be the cause of their lethargy
or loss of appetite.

Generally speaking motions are passed at regular times of the day,
which vary greatly in different individuals and even from time to time
in the same person. If for any reason the act of evacuation is postponed,
the urge will usually pass off, and it will often not be experienced again
until the corresponding time on the following day. In the meantime,
the motions will have become harder and more difficult to pass. Greater

muscular efforts will be called for to secure evacuation, and these may even be accompanied by pain. This implies that constipation has occurred. Forel points out that the ultimate cause of constipation is stagnation of faecal material in the bowel, no matter how it is brought about. He considers that, in most instances, habitual constipation is simply a chronic ' cerebral neurosis '.

The causes of constipation are many. If organic disease has been eliminated the causes of simple, uncomplicated constipation can be considered under two main headings:

1. *Errors of diet*

   (*a*) Too-bland food, deficient in vegetables and coarse residue.
   (*b*) Too-rough or irritating food, causing spasm.
   (*c*) Too-dry food with deficient fluid intake.
   (*d*) Insufficient food, deficient in vitamins.

2. *Other causes of defective peristalsis*

   (*a*) Sedentary habits.
   (*b*) Depressing emotions, anxiety and worry.
   (*c*) Prolonged disregard of the call to defaecate.
   (*d*) Poor general tone and weak abdominal muscles.

Even in healthy individuals, the frequency and consistency of the motions varies enormously from time to time. Sometimes they are soft, sometimes formed and sometimes hard. Certain foodstuffs are often said to be constipating. On the whole fruit tends to produce a softer motion, yet only too frequently the food which constipates one person will purge another. It is important that the food should provide ample coarse residue for the bowel to push along, and in this respect, green vegetables such as cabbage or french beans should always form an integral part of the diet. Oatmeal, whole-meal or brown bread, raw vegetables, onions, figs, prunes and ripe fruits should all be taken in sufficient quantities. The fluid intake can often be increased with advantage, and a tumbler of cold water sipped slowly first thing in the morning and last thing at night is frequently extremely helpful. Large quantities of milk should be avoided. A sedentary mode of life is much more likely to produce constipation than an active one, so that it is important that regular exercise should be taken.

The action of the bowels is particularly prone to be influenced by the emotions, especially those of fear and expectation. Examples of this can often be observed in everyday life. The desire to defaecate frequently tends to present itself when one fears that it will, for instance, in trains that have no corridors or toilet accommodation. Apart from this, spasm of the colon can occur as a result of mental irritation, resentment and anger. Wolberg points out that in the psycho-analytic field, certain individuals seem to have a reluctance to give out anything because of a fear of losing their own intactness. The unconscious conviction behind this seems to be that, since they expect nothing from others, they have no obligation to give anything in return. This mental attitude is often symbolized by faecal retention and constipation.

General Principles of Hypnotic Treatment

Chronic constipation will sometimes respond extremely well to direct hypnotic suggestion, and its duration seems to be no bar to improvement and recovery. Treatment should always be preceded by a full explanation in the waking state, including the removal of ill-founded fears of the serious consequences of constipation. Advice should be given regarding the regulation of faulty diets and the greatest importance laid upon the inculcation of regular daily habits. Even although there may be no inclination to go to stool, the patient should be encouraged to try to open the bowels for at least ten minutes by the watch at precisely the same hour daily. Instructions should be given, however, not to strain hard enough to produce abdominal pain or headache.

As deep a hypnotic state as possible is always desirable. Whilst it is true that in some instances a considerable degree of improvement can be secured in medium depth I have found that, generally speaking, the greater the depth, the more satisfactory the results are likely to be, especially in long-standing cases.

The initial suggestions should be general in character. Feelings of hope and confidence in ultimate recovery should be instilled, and suggestions made to the effect that not only will the urge to evacuate become more frequent and powerful and the abdominal muscles contract more strongly, but that the nervous impulses will also become greatly increased and the peristaltic movements of the bowel greatly strengthened. The effect of these suggestions can be considerably enhanced by stroking the abdomen. The older hypnotists used to lay a good deal of emphasis on the importance of this procedure. Wingfield considered that it aroused in the patient's mind the conception that something is actually being done to the abdomen, and Moll believed it to be so significant a factor in treatment that he advised that, whenever necessary, the suggestions should be strengthened by touching the naked abdominal wall. I have never found any necessity for this, possibly because whilst stroking the abdomen through the clothing I invariably induce a feeling of warmth in the stomach and bowels, and couple the appearance of this with the suggestions already mentioned:

> As this feeling of warmth spreads into your stomach and bowels . . . the muscles in your bowel walls will become stronger and stronger, and will contract much more powerfully and efficiently.
> The nervous impulses that control the contractions of your bowels will become greatly increased . . . the sluggishness of the bowels will consequently disappear definitely and permanently . . . and the urge to open your bowels will become much more frequent and powerful.

More specific suggestions should then be made to the effect that, at a fixed hour *every second or third day*, upon arising in the morning the patient will get the desire to go to the toilet *whilst he is dressing*. This is a most convenient signal for the post-hypnotic suggestion to take effect. He will try to take no notice of this, *but the more he tries to ignore it, the stronger and stronger the urge will become*. Ultimately, the urge will become so great that he will be compelled to go. Wolberg states that this technique is often effective even when no amnesia has been secured, but there is no doubt whatever in my mind that when amnesia is present, success will always be much more rapid and certain. Usually it is best not to try for a *daily* action of the bowels at first. It is much wiser to start with a suggested action *every two or three days*, and then gradually to decrease the interval.

The precise degree of success achieved through the hypnotic treatment of chronic constipation will vary greatly from case to case, but in my opinion it is always well worth trying whenever deep hypnosis can be secured, particularly if it is accompanied by amnesia. Occasionally the results can be really dramatic. The case is quoted of the businessman who, through hypnotic treatment succeeded in establishing a regular toilet habit at 7 o'clock each morning. He was subsequently compelled to revisit the hypnotist in a hurry to get the time altered as he was going away on holiday, and 7 o'clock would have been most inconvenient.

Hypnosis in the Treatment of Excessive Smoking

Excessive smoking is a very popular method of dealing with nervous tension that arises from fear, worry and strain. Nicotine certainly seems to have a sedative effect at first, but this soon passes off and leaves the patient with the craving to smoke more than ever. Heavy smokers are often unable to break the habit through their own efforts, and attempts to do so may mobilize a great deal of anxiety.

It is quite possible to abolish the smoking habit altogether by the use of hypnotic suggestion, but there are two important provisos:

1. The patient must have a strong motivation for giving up the habit. It is not sufficient that his doctor has advised it (except in real emergencies) nor that he wishes to do so to please his wife and family. He must wish to give it up of his own free will.

2. *He must be prepared to give up smoking altogether.* Unfortunately very few people are anxious to give it up completely. All they wish you to do is to help them to reduce it to reasonable proportions, say from 40 to 10 cigarettes per day.

This is a hopeless task from the start, and you will be well advised to have nothing to do with it. I believe that just as to the alcoholic one drink is too many, and twenty are not enough, so to the habitual cigarette smoker one cigarette is too many, and twenty are not enough. Consequently, unless I am satisfied that the patient is anxious and willing to make every effort to give up cigarettes completely, I always decline to undertake treatment, which would necessarily be prolonged, and the results both impermanent and unsatisfactory.

I usually find that the two strongest motives for completely abandoning the habit are first of all the financial one, and secondly the fear of consequences when the patient has some serious physical condition which is aggravated by smoking. Even when true motivation is inadequate, the initial recovery rate with hypnotic treatment is high; unfortunately so is the relapse rate, both in individual and group therapy. Treatment is bound to be prolonged and at least 12 sessions are likely to be necessary.

I consider it quite useless to adopt the much publicized method of causing the cigarettes to taste unpleasant. It is true that in deep hypnosis this is quite easily accomplished, and produces both rapid and dramatic results. Within a short time, however, the effect of the suggestion wears off and a complete relapse occurs unless the treatment is continued indefinitely. Even should an occasional cure occur, it is not likely to be permanent for nothing has been done to alter the underlying tensions, to increase the patient's self-control, or to teach him how to face up to his problems.

The Hypnotic Treatment of Smoking

The only rational and successful way to tackle the problem lies in the skilful use of suggestion to build up and strengthen the determination and desire not to smoke, until this becomes powerful enough to overcome completely the craving to smoke.

As deep a hypnotic trance as possible is always desirable, and a persuasive approach is usually the best. Under hypnosis, the patient should be quietly told of the harmful effect of nicotine on his system, and the advantages, financial and otherwise, of giving up the habit constantly stressed. Every effort should be made to enable him to build up his own will-power to resist the craving successfully. In achieving this, the standard ego-strengthening routine, slightly modified where necessary, will prove extremely helpful in dealing with the underlying tensions.

Whilst still in the trance state, the patient should be asked to express in his own words his desire to overcome his urge to smoke. Strong suggestions may then be made that his craving for tobacco in any form will gradually disappear, and he will even begin to develop a distaste for smoking. He should be told, with conviction, that his powers of control will increase progressively until he can give up smoking completely. His desire and determination not to smoke will become so strong that it will overwhelm entirely his craving for tobacco.

Although sometimes effective, this procedure is far from being universally successful so that, since the public demand for assistance in tackling this problem under hypnosis seems to be increasing, one or other of the following techniques may be adopted.

Von Dedenroth has devised a totally different method of approach with great success. He begins by inquiring how long the individual has smoked, whether he recalls why he began, whether he has ever tried to stop smoking, why he desires to stop now, what benefit, if any, he derives from smoking, at what specific times does he most feel the need (after meals, before breakfast etc.), and finally, how much does he smoke? Answering these questions not only tends to increase rapport but also sheds some light upon the smoker's own feelings regarding his smoking and his reasons for wanting to give up the habit.

At the second session, therapy begins and the patient is told that 21 days from this day will be 'Q Day' or 'Quitting Day'. Next, he is instructed to change his favourite brand of cigarettes and determine never to go back to them again. Then, smoking is to be eliminated altogether:

1. *Before breakfast.*
2. *For one half-hour after each meal.*
3. *For 30 minutes before retiring.*

At these times, he is to get into the habit of going to the bath-room, gargling with mouthwash and cleaning his teeth. He should have a glass of fruit-juice available upon awakening. He is to notice particularly the fresh feeling of his mouth in the morning and following each of these routines. After his breakfast, he again cleans his teeth and uses the mouth-wash, paying close attention to the clean feeling in his mouth. In one half-hour's time he may have a cigarette, but not before. This tends to break the association between the taste of food and the inevitable cigarette that usually follows a meal. He is also told to get a small note-book to carry with him, and to write down, from time to time, his reasons for giving up smoking (physical, financial and personal).

Then a trance state is induced and the above suggestions, given in the waking state, are repeated and consequently greatly reinforced. Following the trance, the patient is encouraged to ask questions, and the next appointment arranged.

The second therapeutic session follows one week later, two weeks prior to ' Q Day '. The patient is told once again to change his brand of cigarettes, preferably to one that he does not particularly care for. All the other instructions are repeated and the contents of his note-book inspected and discussed. It is then suggested that:

1. *He should refrain from smoking for ONE HOUR after meals.*
2. *He should not smoke for ONE HOUR before going to bed.*

and once again these directions are repeated in the trance state.

The third session occurs one week later, seven days before ' Q Day '. He should now either refrain from alcohol altogether, or at least restrict himself to meal-time drinking only. This is intended to break the association between the occasional drink and its accompanying cigarette. A trance state is again induced and all the previous instructions reinforced. It is also suggested that cigarette-smoke will no longer be enjoyed—that the first puff may be enjoyable, the second less enjoyable, and the third, possibly irritating to the linings of the nose, throat or chest. By the time ' Q Day ' has arrived, the individual is usually only taking 10 to 12 puffs per day.

The fact that smoking can be reduced and stopped—and by the individual himself—in this manner affords him tremendous relief and a great feeling of self-accomplishment. Moreover, the lack of conscious and subconscious frustrations is emphasized. ' Q Day ' itself is begun by the immediate induction of a trance state, and the fact that good habits have replaced bad ones, stressed and re-stressed. It is also emphasized that for several weeks, cigarettes have become more and more unpleasant. In conclusion, it should be noted that in this particular type of case, suggestion and persuasion are quite efficient in light or medium trance states, without there being a need for deep trances. A more detailed account can be found in Von Dedenroth's original paper in the *American Journal of Clinical Hypnosis*, Vol. 6, No. 4, April 1964.

Another interesting and effective method of tackling this problem is that used by Calvert Stein. He approaches it from a totally different angle, that of cultivating a compensatory displacement technique for inhalers—how to attain more smoking satisfaction without absolute prohibition. Light or medium depth trances only are required. He points out that smoking is meant to afford pleasure or satisfaction and to relieve tension and that denial accentuates desire, whereas permission to smoke ' *as much as you may need* ' tends to reduce the quantity or degree of associated anxiety. An essential basis for this treatment lies in the teaching of the subject to relax by other means. The subject learns how to relax also by experiencing the tension that is built up in his chest, neck, and head when he holds his breath for a slow count of ten. As he lets his breath out slowly, his attention is called to the degree of relaxation that follows the expiration of ordinary smokeless air.

The subject is then invited to follow this particular technique when he smokes a cigarette, since it is designed to enhance his smoking pleasure whilst also affording increased relaxation. Whenever he takes a cigarette from the packet, he is to pause and notice the whiteness of the paper, the filter or cork-tip, the natural fragrance of the tobacco, the feel of the cigarette between his fingers and his lips. Also, the flame of the light, the satisfaction of watching and extinguishing it, the aroma of the burning tobacco, the taste of the smoke in one's mouth, the importance of seeing the smoke rising slowly in the air, and the pleasure of blowing smoky air from the mouth. The smoker is told *to fill his mouth only with smoke, to keep the smoke in his mouth as he would a mouthful of water whilst filling his lungs with clean soothing air by breathing in deeply through his nose. Then slowly to exhale through his mouth as he blows out not only the mouthful of smoke but also the lungful of clean soothing air.* The effect of this is not only to convert smoking into a deliberate conscious process instead of an unconscious habit, but also to enable the smoker to gain satisfaction *without inhaling.* Stein also rightly points out that adequate psychotherapy for compulsive smokers must often include adequate investigation and discussion of other causes of anxiety such as domestic and personal tensions, occupational stress etc.

In some smokers there is a rapid response to the suggested technique for displacement of the pleasure zones from the lungs to the mouth, eyes and fingers. In others, there is a delayed response to the implied suggestion that inhaling is unnecessary to smoking pleasure. In most cases, however, there is a prompt reduction in the total quantity of smoking and a lessening of other signs of emotional tension. Indeed, some patients voluntarily give up smoking altogether after a week or two under the new regime, whilst others shift to pipes and cigars. The technique is more fully described in Calvert Stein's book *Practical Psychotherapy in Nonpsychiatric Specialities* (Springfield, Ill.: Thomas).

Hypnosis in the Treatment of Alcoholism

Drinking is one of the most universal of human habits, but fortunately few drinkers become true alcoholics. Alcoholism is not a disease in itself but a symptom of a disordered personality—a person who cannot face reality and turns to liquor as an alternative. Because of the narcotizing effect alcohol exercises on the higher brain centres, it will temporarily alleviate tension, increase self-confidence and produce a general sense of well-being. It consequently reduces anxiety, overcomes phobias and causes obsessional fears to recede for the time being, so it is hardly surprising that it is used as a means of escape from suffering and that certain people with grave emotional problems come to depend upon it. These effects, however, are only transitory and are usually followed by heightened depression which increases the craving, and causes the unfortunate patient to seek relief in larger and more frequent doses.

Alcohol removes inhibitions, and shy and reserved individuals find that a few drinks remove their fears and enable them to meet people with more confidence. It lessens feelings of hostility and antagonism, overcomes inferiority and lends spurious courage and strength. It helps certain individuals to escape from feelings of isolation and loneliness.

The alcoholic is usually an over-sensitive, dependent, lonely type of individual who finds it difficult to tolerate frustration and is lacking in self-esteem. Self-pity is often a prominent characteristic, and unconscious feelings of hostility are frequently present. As a child, he was over-protected by his parents and consequently grew up ill-equipped to face responsibility. Later in life, unfavourable social conditions, family and domestic troubles or business and financial worries may well cause him to seek consolation in alcohol, which ultimately blunts his critical judgement and renders him incapable of resisting urges and cravings he would normally be able to suppress. If he continues to drink, he begins to deteriorate morally and tends to avoid his former friends, seeking companionship in bars and public houses. During his drinking bouts he becomes vain, boastful and sentimental. At first, he is able to exercise some control over the frequency and amount of his drinking, but as his tolerance gradually becomes reduced, this control is ultimately lost. The alcoholic often feels extremely guilty about his drinking and becomes ashamed of it. He fully realizes the harm that he is doing both to himself and to his family, and despises himself on that account. None the less, he is utterly incapable of controlling his craving.

The Treatment of Alcoholism

Just as the cigarette smoker seeks treatment to cut down his smoking to reasonable proportions, rather than to give up the habit altogether, so the alcoholic who applies for treatment usually clings to the hope that he will 'learn to drink normally and in moderation' and 'be able to hold his liquor' like most people. In the true alcoholic this is an absolute impossibility. The use of alcohol in any form must be altogether prohibited and completely eliminated from his regime, once and for all. This is aptly expressed by *Alcoholics Anonymous* in the following phrase: to the alcoholic—one drink is too many—and twenty are not enough.

Treatment is only likely to succeed if it is instigated as a result of the patient's own wish. If, on the other hand, he is brought by despairing friends and relatives, he rarely possesses any real desire or incentive to give up drink, and will consequently fail to respond. By far the most favourable moment for the initiation of treatment is when the patient has just recovered from his intoxication and is in a state of remorse and regret.

The therapist must always have certain well-defined objects in view:

1. To establish an understanding and sympathetic relationship with the patient.
2. To encourage the patient's self-esteem.
3. To induce him to undertake outside interests.
4. To help him to be able to cope with frustration.
5. To help him to stop drinking.
6. To assist him in making more social contacts.

In undertaking the treatment of an alcoholic, you must never, under any circumstances, condemn his habit. Your attitude must always remain both tolerant and sympathetic. This is often far from easy, since the patient is quite likely to put you to the test by indulging in a further bout of heavy drinking, just as he seemed to be making some improvement. Despite your natural disappointment, you must never allow yourself to become embittered by this, and must continue to deal with the situation with understanding and sympathy.

You should begin by trying to get the patient to realize that not only does he know how important alcohol is to him, but that he is also fully aware of the reasons for this. That your intention is to enable him to cope with the reasons in a different way, without the need for resorting to alcohol in the future. You must try to rid him of the idea that he is a hopeless case, and emphasize the many good qualities that he has that have been obscured by his habit. You should do your best to encourage him to take up hobbies and indulge in outside interests. One thing, however, is vital right from the start: *he must, once and for all, abandon the idea that he will ever be able to drink in moderation like other people.* Only when he is prepared to give up alcohol altogether, on his own account, will you be prepared to do all you can to help him. If treatment is only sought on behalf of his suffering parents or relatives, then it is far better that he should be treated institutionally.

The analytical approach is usually quite useless since the patient's ego is too immature. The object of treatment, as already described, is to wean him from alcohol, to strengthen his personality and to enable him to adjust to his surroundings. Every effort must be made to convert the patient's attitude that he cannot face life without alcohol into one in which he loses the desire for alcohol since he has learned how to face his problems without it.

Sometimes it is possible to start treatment by directing it at the basic cause. People drink excessively for a number of different reasons. The shy individual drinks in order to overcome his self-consciousness and be able to mix more easily. The depressive drinks in order to dispel his melancholy and gloom; the business man to forget his financial problems, and the married man to seek escape from his domestic difficulties. If the cause can be remedied, or if you can help the patient to be able to cope more adequately with these conditions, the chance of successful treatment becomes greatly improved. In this case, however, some kind of insight therapy will be required.

One of the usual methods of treating alcoholism depends upon establishing a conditioned reflex in the patient which causes him to experience a feeling of nausea each time he drinks. This is often achieved by the use of drugs such as apomorphine, emetine or disulfiram (Antabuse), followed by the administration of the coveted drink. The drugs cause the patient to feel violently nauseated, and the repetition of this procedure eventually establishes a conditioned reflex which can be indefinitely prolonged; indeed the patient's stomach will revolt every time he tries to drink. With a good hypnotic subject capable of achieving a deep enough trance, all this can easily be produced as the result of post-hypnotic suggestion. Every attempt should be made to bring the patient to the point where he either refuses to drink, or is actually unable to drink without considerable discomfort.

Fortunately alcoholics, provided that they are sober at the time, are usually extremely susceptible to hypnosis and often turn out to be very good subjects. Only when disintegration of the personality has taken place does hypnosis become either very difficult or even impossible. Even if light hypnosis only is attainable, some of these patients can be helped to a considerable extent. In this instance, however, it will not be possible to obtain a cure by ordering the patient to give·up drink, or by telling him that drink will make him feel sick. Ego-strengthening suggestions will help to dispel his nervous tension, to stabilize him emotionally, and to increase his self confidence. Discussion of his problems combined with a certain amount of re-education will often help him to tackle them more efficiently and systematically without having to seek refuge in alcohol. All this can frequently be achieved in light hypnosis.

Wolberg describes two excellent conditioning techniques which can be used most effectively whenever a deep enough trance can be obtained. The first depends upon a substitution of oral craving.

> As soon as you wake up, you will have an irresistible longing for a drink. This will be so strong that it will occupy your mind completely, and you will be able to think of nothing else. Although you will realize that drink is poison to you, your craving will become stronger and stronger.
> You will notice that there is a bag of sweets lying on the table.
> You will help yourself to one of these sweets, and as soon as you start to suck it . . . the craving for drink will disappear . . . and you will gradually become quite calm and relaxed.

Naturally this is much more likely to succeed when a complete amnesia can be produced. In any case, it should be repeated on many subsequent occasions.

From now on . . . you will want to give up drink altogether.
Your desire and determination to give it up will become so strong . . . so
powerful . . . that it will completely overwhelm your craving to drink.
You will begin to feel a strong dislike for alcohol in any form.
Every day . . . your craving will become less and less . . . weaker and
weaker . . . utnil presently it will disappear completely.
You will realize . . . more and more . . . that alcohol is a poison to you.
Whenever you feel that you simply must have a drink . . . sucking a sweet
will immediately remove that urge . . . and you will quickly become
both relaxed and comfortable.

The second technique involves conditioning, in which the actual drinking
of alcohol becomes associated with feelings of nausea and disgust.

The moment you drink any alcohol . . . your stomach will begin to feel
more and more uncomfortable . . . and you will begin to feel really sick.
This will become worse and worse . . . and if you actually swallow your
drink . . . you will be quite unable to keep it down . . . and will immediately
vomit it back.

Obviously conditioning of this kind will need regular reinforcement,
daily if possible at first. Once it begins to act satisfactorily, it can be
reduced to once a week until the habit has been kept under control for
several months. From then on, fortnightly or even monthly treatments
will be quite enough to strengthen and maintain control.

Quite apart from conditioning, owing to the intimate doctor-patient
relationship that occurs in hypnosis, the satisfactory rapport that so often
develops can be itself manipulated to assist the treatment. Under these
circumstances, little is said about the actual drinking, but the good
relationship that is eventually formed is utilized to demand more adult
and mature behaviour from the patient. Meares stresses the importance
of this, and considers it to be a valuable, educative, emotional experience.

The general consensus of opinion seems to be that hypnosis can often
yield most gratifying results in the treatment of this very distressing
condition. Gindes points out that the effects of alcoholism can often be
removed even though the exact cause of the trouble remains undiscovered.
He considers that the fact that the patient is enabled to return to his job,
his family and society, and manages to adjust to them, fully justifies
hypnosis as the therapy of choice.

Drug Addiction

The drugs which most commonly lead to addiction are opium and its
derivatives, morphine and heroin, *cannabis indica*, cocaine, barbiturates

and amphetamine. In Great Britain addiction to *Cannabis indica*, barbiturates and amphetamines is much more common than addiction to opiates.

The personality structure of the average addict shows the same fundamental defects as those of the chronic alcoholic (p. 259), and two distinct types of addiction can usually be recognized:

1. That which occurs in people suffering from neurosis who try to control their tension and anxiety with drugs.

2. That which occurs in people who resort to drugs for the ' uplift ' and feelings of euphoria that they induce.

In either case, once addiction has developed, a physical dependency upon the drug rapidly follows as the result of biochemical changes which produce an incessant craving for the drug. Total withdrawal of the drug can make the patient very sick and ill indeed, so much so that the withdrawal symptoms may even be severe enough to cause death.

It must be admitted that hypnosis is often less successful in dealing with drug addiction than it is in the case of alcoholism. In the less severe, more chronic cases of alcoholism, some authorities consider that no actual *physiological* bodily craving develops in which the body demands and must be supplied with the one particular drug, so that severe withdrawal symptoms are not so likely to occur. If he is totally deprived of alcohol, the patient will certainly be exceedingly depressed and unhappy, but he will probably not become *physically* sick, or in danger of death. But *once alcoholism has become acute and has progressed to delirium tremens, the withdrawal symptoms do become physiological,* and the patient can then be in very genuine danger through toxic reaction, dehydration and shock. Under these circumstances the results of the total withdrawal of alcohol, or of the drug of addiction, will be exactly the same: the patient will become very gravely ill to the extent that his life may even be seriously endangered.

In cases of drug addiction, it is almost always advisable to insist upon institutional treatment in the first place, for a period of not less than six months.

There is no doubt that hypnosis can be extremely helpful to the patient in alleviating the rigors of the withdrawal period. The mental and physical relaxation that can be achieved and the reassurance that can be afforded in deep trance states will often prove an invaluable adjunct to other forms of treatment. When total withdrawal has been successfully achieved, hypnotic treatment should be continued on the lines described in the treatment of alcoholism (p. 281). The patient can never be considered as being completely cured until his craving has completely disappeared and he can resist the temptation to take drugs even when they are available.

CHAPTER 20

Menstrual Disorders, Dermatological Conditions and the Use of Hypnosis in Surgery

Hypnosis in Menstrual Disorders

Many menstrual disorders prove to be largely psychogenic in origin, so that hypnosis can often play a highly effective part in the treatment of these conditions. It is, of course, all the more likely to succeed in those menstrual disturbances in which the emotional factors are of recent origin. Most hypnotically orientated psychiatrists advise the use of hypno-analysis in these cases, but this is by no means necessary as a routine procedure. Consequently, the general practitioner need not feel discouraged, since in many instances remarkably satisfactory results can be achieved by the combination of direct symptom removal and simple psychotherapy.

The three commonly occurring disturbances of menstruation which lend themselves particularly to hypnotherapy are:

1. Functional uterine bleeding.
2. Amenorrhoea.
3. Functional dysmenorrhoea.

Functional Uterine Bleeding

Whilst it is well known that this condition often results from worry, shock or anxiety, it is essential that before any psychotherapeutic measures are adopted, an adequate physical examination of the pelvis should be undertaken to exclude any organic factors.

The psychological causes may be extremely varied. In the case of a newly married woman, for instance, the symptom may arise as an unconscious defence against the sexual act. Alternatively, it may some-times represent an unconscious fear of pregnancy.

Many of these cases of psychogenic uterine bleeding will completely clear up as a result of direct hypnotic suggestion alone. For this, however, a reasonably deep stage of hypnosis will usually be necessary. Such direct symptom removal will be all the more likely to succeed if it is combined with explanation and reassurance. When menorrhagia is treated in this way, suggestion may either be made to eliminate the periods altogether for a time to allow the patient to recuperate, or directed towards slowing the flow, and reducing the amount of blood loss.

Sometimes it will happen that treatment on this superficial level is insufficient to effect a cure. If the relevant emotional conflicts are not too deeply seated, questioning in the hypnotic state, when they can quite frequently be disposed of by explanation and reassurance, may succeed in exposing them. If this is not possible, hypno-analysis will be required, provided that adequate depth can be secured.

Functional Amenorrhoea

This may vary from a total cessation of the menses to a decided scantiness of the blood flow. Amongst the psychogenic factors frequently involved are shock, anxiety, fear of pregnancy, faulty attitudes to sex, deprivation of male society and even changes in environment. Direct suggestion under hypnosis will often succeed remarkably well, indeed cases have been reported in which a complete cure has been effected in one single session. This is hardly surprising, since instances have occurred in which the condition has cleared up solely as the result of a long talk with a sympathetic and understanding doctor.

The suggestion should always be made that, within a given period of time, the menstrual function will be restored both normally and painlessly. It can always be suggested that menstruation will occur every 28 days without fail, and sometimes the precise date, time and duration of the period may be specified with success.

In obstinate or difficult cases some degree of analysis, however superficial, may be necessary in order to give the patient some insight into her condition. The unconscious emotional conflicts involved are not usually very deeply rooted, so that the general practitioner who is experienced in hypnosis is usually quite able to deal with these himself. Only in relatively few cases will a more profound form of hypno-analysis be required.

I should like to stress the value of starting the treatment of all menstrual disorders with the standard ego-strengthening suggestions, before proceeding to embark upon direct symptom removal, as I am convinced that the efficiency of the latter procedure is thereby greatly enhanced. It is important, however, before hypnotic treatment is started, that steps should be taken to exclude any possibility of pregnancy to avoid wasting the therapist's time.

Functional Dysmenorrhoea

When this condition has been successfully treated by orthodox methods, the result obtained has often seemed to be more due to the influence of unintentional suggestion than to the particular form of medication that has been employed. Consequently, hypnosis affords a particularly efficient means of combating this distressing and frequently disabling complaint.

In the majority of cases menstrual pains are largely functional in origin. In fact, dysmenorrhoea often arises solely as a conditioned response, without any underlying emotional conflicts whatever. Many girls learn either from their mothers, sisters or friends that the act of menstruation is almost invariably accompanied by pain and discomfort in addition to the blood loss. They consequently expect to have pains— and get them—and the pains are certainly real, and in no sense imaginary. This tendency to over-emphasize the expectation of pain when explaining menstruation to their daughters is particularly likely to happen when the mother herself displays any neurotic trends. No wonder the unfortunate girls react with pain when they experience their first periods.

In other cases psychogenic factors play a very significant part, indeed some sudden emotional stress may often precipitate the condition. Meares points out that psychosomatic dysmenorrhoea may be a response to an anxiety state arising from conflicts in any area, genital or not. Feelings of guilt connected with masturbation, fears of marriage, of sexual intercourse and even of pregnancy are not infrequently involved. Domestic conflicts and difficulties can also constitute an underlying cause. Most women, in fact, are much more susceptible to pain whenever emotional instability is present.

Dysmenorrhoea is an exceedingly common complaint. It occurs in both girls and young women more frequently when they are unmarried. In those instances when it first appears following marriage, it may well be a sign of marital tension and disharmony. It varies greatly in degree. Some girls experience pain for a day or two but are still able to carry on with their work, whilst in others it is so severe as to disable them completely, and cause them to have to take one or two days off each time a period occurs.

The first step in the treatment of this condition is the elimination of any organic cause. But even should such be discovered, hypnosis can still play a valuable part in dealing with the associated psychogenic overlay. Hypnosis, in fact, can often succeed when all other measures (including curettage) have utterly failed.

The ordinary methods of pain removal by direct hypnotic suggestion, already described, will frequently prove remarkably successful, particularly if combined with suggestions aimed at the removal of fear, anxiety, tension and expectancy. As one would expect, this approach is most likely to be effective when the main cause of the dysmenorrhoea is to be found in previous conditioning. It will also succeed in many cases where the milder types of emotional conflict only are involved, without the need to resort to analytical methods.

Kroger and Freed consider that, since the emotional conflict expressed as painful menstruation is not resolved and may seek another physical outlet, much more gratifying and permanent results are likely to accrue from the use of hypno-analysis. Although hypno-analysis is superior, in my experience this anticipated conversion from one symptom to another rarely takes place, even when direct symptom removal alone has been employed. Even so, since many of these emotional conflicts are far from being deep-seated, they can often be brought to light by simple questioning in the hypnotic state, a procedure that falls well within the scope of the general practitioner. When deeper forms of emotional conflict exist, hypno-analytical methods aimed at the re-integration of the patient's personality will undoubtedly be needed whenever sufficient depth can be obtained. Such cases, however, I consider as coming into the category of psychiatric, rather than general problems.

Treatment does not usually have to be unduly prolonged. Complete and often permanent relief may be obtained sooner than one might expect, even in long-standing cases. Fortunately, such cures are not usually followed by relapses, and the patient remains quite free from pain. In several of my own cases, after many years disability, the patient has no longer needed to take the usual day or so off from work at the height of each period.

Hypnosis in Dermatology

Many skin conditions that are seen almost daily in the general practitioner's surgery can be treated effectively under hypnosis. Moreover, since he usually sees them first during the acute stages, he should be in the most favourable position to prevent the disease from becoming chronic, at which stage treatment is bound to be much more difficult and prolonged.

The true study of dermatology involves not only the pathology of the skin itself, but also an accurate assessment of the emotional factors underlying the somatic reaction observed.

Such a relationship is not surprising when one realizes that in embryology, both the skin and neural systems spring from a common ancestry—the ectoderm—and this, in itself, partly explains the close connection between the cutaneous and nervous systems. Then again, the skin is in contact with both the individual and his environment, and is consequently readily influenced by both, through its neural, vascular and glandular components. In fact, it often acts as a medium through which strong emotions can be expressed.

Normally healthy individuals will flush when they are angry, become pale when they are afraid, blush when embarrassed or confused, and even itch when their desires are frustrated. Indeed, the skin reacts very quickly to stimuli of itching, touch or temperature, and being so readily available, it easily enables patients with unconscious aggressive or masochistic tendencies to ' take it out on their skin '. In this way, it acts as a defensive and protective agent for the mind as well as the body, in times of stress and strain. For instance, it has been observed that in psoriasis, the waxing and waning of the rash often coincides with varying emotional situations, and that eczema not infrequently masks unconscious aggressive tendencies which cannot be openly displayed.

As one might expect, the converse of this is equally true. Skin disorders in themselves often produce mental and emotional disturbances. And since the co-existence of such disturbances as anxiety, tension and fear can both increase the severity and prolong the duration of many somatic skin diseases, a vicious circle becomes so easily established. The following is a typical example:

As a result of emotional tension the patient's skin becomes excessively moist. This renders it extremely vulnerable to secondary infection with the production of such symptoms as pruritus and insomnia. These in turn aggravate the mental tension, the vicious circle becomes set up, and it consequently becomes our main therapeutic task to break it as best we can.

In considering the usefulness of hypnosis in the field of dermatology, we should always bear in mind one vitally important fact. *Hypnotherapy does not remove the need for conventional dermatological therapy, but can be most profitably employed in conjunction with it.* Under these circumstances it will often succeed when all other methods have failed. Many details may have to be taken into account. It may be necessary to adjust the patient's diet, to change the soap that he uses, to eliminate external causes of irritation, to help him with unconscious psychological problems in addition to the application of local treatment to the skin.

From my own experience in this field, I would classify the main methods of dermatological hypnotherapy as follows:

1. *Supportive therapy.*
2. *Direct suggestion* (including *post-hypnotic suggestion*).
3. *Symptom substitution.*
4. *Hypno-analysis.*

The choice of therapeutic technique to be employed in any given case should be governed by the duration of the symptoms, the severity of the symptoms, the personality of the patient, and the depth of hypnosis attainable.

1. Supportive Therapy

In my opinion, this is an absolute necessity in every case, and you should never omit its use in conjunction with any of the three alternative methods. It is certainly essential that it should precede any attempt at symptom-removal by direct suggestion. After inducing as deep a hypnotic trance as possible, I always begin treatment with the standard sequence of ' ego-strengthening ' suggestions, no matter what the precise skin condition may be, or what particular form of therapy I propose to adopt. I am convinced that this practice has contributed greatly to any success I may have achieved.

2. Direct Suggestion

You should never allow yourself to be deterred from using direct suggestion in dermatological cases on the grounds that you are treating the symptom instead of the basic underlying cause. Is it reasonable to expect a patient to put up indefinitely with intolerable itching on the grounds that his basic problem is a psychological one? Or that he should continue to endure an unsightly and irritating dermatitis just because it is considered to be the result of deep-seated personality conflicts. Remember how easily a vicious circle can become established. In actual fact, many patients who are found to be poor subjects for any form of insight therapy can often be treated successfully by direct suggestion alone, particularly when this is preceded by ego-strengthening.

I find direct suggestion most useful for the relief of symptoms such as itching, burning, anxiety and insomnia. It can also help a patient to restrict himself to a particular diet he finds difficulty in maintaining for any length of time. Moreover, hypnotic analgesia (when attainable) can be of the greatest possible assistance. You should, however, avoid suggesting that the patient will feel *no* itching or discomfort. Tell him instead: ' *No matter what sensations you feel, you will find that they will not bother you so much* '. Similarly, in dealing with pruritus I often say: ' *You may still feel some slight itching, but you will no longer have any desire to scratch* '.

I think this is highly important for I do not consider the control of itching by direct suggestion to be as easy as some of the less critical authorities have reported. Despite his protestations of inconvenience, the patient rarely has the necessary motivation, as he is usually gaining some pleasurable, if morbid, satisfaction from the act of scratching. It represents to him an easy way of relieving unpleasant tension. In point of fact, the key to success in most dermatological conditions lies in the diminution or abolition of scratching, so that the deeper the trance, the more rapid and satisfactory the results are likely to be. Somnambulism, preferably with complete amnesia, is always desirable though certainly not essential, and instruction in auto-hypnosis can be of the utmost possible assistance.

In many dermatological patients, a sound basis is the production of really good relaxation. No matter what their complaint may be, if only you can secure a sufficient degree of relaxation, this in itself will often afford considerable relief from the itching and irritation. Never forget, however, that it is vitally important to treat the whole patient and not to confine your attention to the itching, scratching, or whatever the primary complaint may be. *The symptom alone should never be your sole objective.*

The significance of the symptom to the patient is also frequently of the greatest importance. Whenever an originally psychologically based symptom ceases to serve any useful purpose, direct suggestion is an ideal way of getting rid of it. The symptom may, however, still be fulfilling an unconscious emotional need, and therefore I consider that the approach should be largely permissive and certainly not authoritarian. *In some cases, the patient may still need some type of defense mechanism, and one should not summarily deprive him of it.*

This is where the value of an efficient ego-strengthening technique becomes apparent. Not only does it enhance the patient's general feeling of well-being, apart from his symptom, but it also gradually strengthens his ego-defences so that his need for an emotional crutch will diminish and thus facilitate the removal of the symptom.

Never tell the patient then that his itching is going to cease. Suggest instead a gradual diminution of the symptom. In this way, you can notice and avoid any adverse reaction that might have occurred had you succeeded in depriving him of it completely. Occasionally, it may even be wise to leave him with a residual amount of pruritus, discomfort or even eczema. I can remember one case of disfiguring eczema of the face, hands and body which eventually I succeeded in clearing up completely. However, in view of a series of relapses, I found that the only way to prevent these was to leave him a small patch between his shoulder-blades. Whilst causing him a minor degree of irritation and inconvenience, it was apparently sufficient to satisfy his emotional needs, for the rest of his body remained clear.

Dr Michael Scott, an eminent dermatologist in America, describes a very effective use of direct suggestion. In dealing with cases of intolerable itching, he offers the following advice which I have adopted successfully in a number of cases. *In the first instance, try removing the pruritus from one small area of the body, beginning with a distal phalanx, then a whole finger, followed by the hand.* In some individuals, and in the deeper stages of hypnosis, it may be possible to start with a whole limb, an arm or a leg. In either case, the patient is permitted to scratch the rest of his body to his heart's content, provided that he leaves the designated part strictly alone. *If only you can succeed in securing one small area of unscratchable skin you can subsequently extend this and make slow but steady progress.*

Dr Scott also describes another technique in which, in a deep-trance subject it may be possible to· induce the patient to scratch or mutilate some small object of his choice, *and to derive the same satisfaction from doing so that he obtains from scratching his skin.* The object should always be small enough for him to bring it along for inspection at his next session, and may prove most illuminating. Dr Scott gives an example in which a patient, given this instruction, brought along a family photograph of a group, one individual of which was almost completely obliterated by scratches. It transpired that this was his mother-in-law, and this inform-ation proved most helpful in elucidating the basis of his problem.

I cannot overemphasize the fact that relief from scratching is one of the most important factors in effecting a cure, and that direct symptom-removal will seldom succeed until scratching has been brought under some degree of control.

A typical series of suggestions that I often use for this particular purpose is as follows:

As a result of this treatment . . . you are going to feel stronger and fitter in every way.
Your circulation will improve . . . particularly the circulation through the little blood-vessels that supply the skin.

Here, I usually specify the precise areas most affected by the rash.

Your heart will beat more strongly . . . so that more blood will flow through the little blood-vessels in the skin . . . carrying more nourishment to the skin. Because of this . . . *your skin will become much better nourished . . . it will become healthier . . . more normal in texture . . . and the rash will gradually diminish . . . until it fades away completely . . . leaving the underlying new skin perfectly healthy and normal in every respect.*

And . . . *as your circulation improves . . . and your nerves become stronger and steadier . . . so . . . they will become much less sensitive . . . much less easily irritated.*

Consequently . . . *the itching and irritation of your skin will gradually subside . . . and disappear.*

It will become less and less each day . . . and you will no longer have any desire to scratch.

If . . . at any time . . . unknowingly, you do begin to scratch . . . the moment your fingers touch your skin . . . you will immediately know what you are about to do . . . and you will be able to exercise sufficient self-control to stop yourself . . . before you have done any damage at all.

Because of this . . . you will not only feel much less irritation and discomfort . . . but your skin will begin to heal . . . and your rash will begin to disappear much more rapidly.

Even if you should start to scratch . . . in your sleep at night . . . the moment your fingers touch your skin . . . you will wake up immediately and realize exactly what you are doing . . . and will be able to stop yourself.

And . . . because of this treatment . . . you will be able to exercise enough control to stop scratching at all times . . . before you have done any damage to your skin.

You will notice here the valuable use that is being made of post-hypnotic suggestion.

A suggestive routine such as this is equally applicable to the treatment of all dermatological conditions. It will naturally need augmenting by suggestions designed to deal with the distinctive features of each individual case, and to conform with the particular therapeutic method of approach you intend to adopt. Where discharges are present, it can be suggested that they will gradually diminish and dry up. Where the skin is dry and cracks continually, suggestions can be made that the skin will become more normal and flexible, and that the dryness will disappear.

3. Symptom Substitution

This involves trying to re-educate the patient's unconscious mind, during a trance state, to replace one habit pattern with a more desirable and constructive type of behaviour. We seek, in fact, to replace some undesirable mental or physical outlet with a more acceptable one.

In this approach, there are two important facts which should be borne in mind. In the first place, the substituted activity should have the same significance to the patient as the one it replaces, and secondly, the new pattern must be logical enough to destroy the earlier one in the patient's mind. Preferably, it should have the same symbolical significance as the original symptom. *If the original symptom expresses underlying aggressive or even masochistic tendencies, we should try to select a substitute symptom of a more desirable nature that would provide an alternative outlet for the expression of the same tendencies.*

For instance, the act of scratching often satisfies unconscious aggressive impulses. Consequently, one can suggest to the athletically minded patient that he will derive greater satisfaction from hitting a tennis-ball or golf-ball than from continuing to scratch. Many alternatives can be found, particularly in the field of arts and crafts such as painting etc., and once you know your patient and his complaint, it is not difficult to select one to suit his individual needs. This selection can be greatly facilitated by making the following suggestions, during the trance state:

> I am going to ask your unconscious mind . . . whether it will accept some form of physical exercise (or whatever alternative may seem desirable) . . . as a fully adequate and satisfying outlet for your tensions . . . in place of your scratching.
> If your unconscious mind is willing to accept this . . . it will cause your *right* fore-finger to rise.
> If not . . . then your *left* fore-finger will rise.

Used in this way, the 'ideomotor finger-signalling technique' will often simplify the task of securing an acceptable symptom-substitute.

4. Hypno-analysis

Where unconscious psychological factors are involved, they can often be exposed and their significance explained during hypnosis. Fortunately, in many disorders of the skin falling into this category, the unconscious mental and emotional conflicts involved are relatively superficial and connected with the patient's current environmental circumstances, and thus not too difficult to expose. In fact, I have occasionally found that simply placing one's hand on the patient's forehead during a medium depth trance and instructing him that he will be able to go back in time and remember clearly and review in his mind exactly what was happening in his domestic or business circumstances, together with the worries he had at the time his skin condition first appeared, has produced a surprising amount of valuable information.

In other cases, such uncomplicated investigatory procedures as *Wolberg's* ' *theatre-visualization technique* ' (page 352) and *Redlich's* ' *jig-saw puzzle technique* '(page 353) can prove extremely effective and useful, particularly in general practice. Neither require more than an average depth of trance (although the deeper the trance, the more rapidly they will succeed) and only in the more obdurate, chronic psychosomatic types of neuro-dermatitis are the more involved hypno-analytical techniques, often necessitating somnambulism, likely to be required.

In these cases, a great deal of patience is necessary both on the part of patient and therapist, for deep fundamental conflicts are never easily uncovered. And, although the recall of such repressed conflicts often results in an amelioration or even cure of the skin condition, this does not always occur. Consequently, we should always remember that *it is not just what is recalled that is of primary importance, but the use we make of it in order to benefit the patient*. Also, that in many cases *it is the patient's own reaction to stress that is most significant, rather than the actual stress itself*.

Occasionally in such conditions as pruritus, the mere elucidation of the unconscious mental conflict and its significance to the patient can result in the dramatic disappearance of the symptom. The following case is an excellent example of this:

Mrs X, a young married woman aged 34 years, was referred to me, suffering from a severe pruritus vulvae. The consultant dermatologist concerned, told me that the condition had failed to respond to all forms of treatment, and asked if hypnosis could offer some degree of relief. She was getting little or no sleep, and the labia were both inflamed and deeply excoriated as a result of the incessant scratching. The trouble had first appeared some 9 months previously.

Two years ago her husband had left her for another woman and she had heard nothing of him since. There were no children and she continued to live on her own but had to go out to work in order to maintain her home.

Despite this emotional disturbance, she remained quite well for the next 15 months, after which she gradually developed a severe pruritus of the vulvae, which worsened to such an extent that she was unable to continue with her work. She could not account in any way for the onset of this trouble, and stated that her circumstances had not deteriorated at all, neither had she been subjected to any additional worry or stress during this particular period. She got on extremely well with all her relatives and neighbours, and was quite happy in her work. This corresponded in every way with the information I had already received. I decided, therefore, to try to afford some relief by attacking the symptom directly, under hypnosis, in the manner already described. Although she attained reasonable depth, and was able to enter the hypnotic state readily, upon word of command, all attempts proved completely unsuccessful, and the itching and irritation continued unabated.

I then told her, under hypnosis, that she would be able to go back 9 months or so, to the time that the condition first appeared, that she would be able to remember accurately everything that had happened at this period, particularly those which were connected with the cause of her trouble.

She immediately began to show signs of emotional distress, and gradually the whole story emerged. Twelve months after her husband had left her, she found it difficult to maintain her home, and consequently took a lodger. Within a very short space of time, they became attracted to each other, and fell in love. She and her husband were both strict Roman Catholics, so that divorce was out of the question. Obviously, continuing to live under the same roof in the existing circumstances was gradually imposing an intolerable strain upon both of them, since her rigid moral upbringing rendered it impossible for her to contemplate living with him as his wife unless such union were sanctified by marriage. The intense feeling of guilt and fear of yielding to ever-present temptation had become repressed and consciously forgotten. Such feelings, however, were far too powerful to be held permanently in check, and consequently when they threatened to break through into consciousness, became converted into a physical symptom, the defensive nature of which was immediately apparent, for as long as the condition remained, even normal marital relations would have proved too painful, and a physical impossibility.

Upon awakening, since there was no amnesia present, I discussed the matter fully with the patient, giving whatever explanations were necessary to convince her of the true state of affairs. She seemed to accept these quite readily, and when I saw her a week later, she said that the itching and irritation had completely disappeared, and that she had been sleeping well for the first time for many months. She said voluntarily that she fully realized the need to change existing circumstances, but whether she ever did so or not, I never found out, for she failed to keep her next appointment. I heard subsequently that she had left the district.

Numerous skin diseases respond favourably to hypnotic techniques.

Schneck considers that the relative significance of organic or psychological factors in the causation of the disorder have little bearing on the prognosis. This is a conclusion with which I cannot agree since I have found that, as in asthma, the more the psychological or emotional factors predominate, the more successful the results of hypnotherapy are likely to be.

Amongst the various dermatological conditions which often respond well to hypnotherapy are *alopecia areata, eczema, hyperhidrosis, neuro-dermatitis, pruritus, psoriasis, rosacea, urticaria,* and *warts.* I append a few notes arising from my own experience.

1. *Alopecia areata.* The few cases that I have treated, eventually did extremely well. Treatment, however, is necessarily prolonged, and directed primarily towards the correction of the underlying nervous factors, and associated worries, rather than against the symptom itself.

2. *Eczema.* Some cases respond most satisfactorily, many others experience varying degrees of relief, whilst some seem to remain entirely unaffected. It is extremely difficult to give a prognosis. Generally speaking, the more acute and recent the condition, the better is the prospect. Also, cases in which underlying psychological conflicts and attitudes are present, are likely to improve more readily under hypnosis.

3. *Hyperhidrosis.* Since the increased sweating is usually ascribed to central nervous system activity, hypnotic treatment of this condition is often very successful. Direct methods will sometimes suffice, although the elucidation of emotional factors will always facilitate matters.

4. *Neuro-dermatitis.* These cases are always associated with unconscious psychological disturbances, and it almost invariably follows that the discovery and correction of these will result in most gratifying improvement. Symptom alleviation and general psychotherapy under hypnosis can also play an important part.

5. *Psoriasis.* Many authorities have described the connection between acute outbreaks of the eruption, and existing emotional disturbances, the adjustment of which is usually followed by rapid improvement. Whilst in some cases, my own experience has tended to confirm this, hypnotic treatment does not seem to eliminate the occurrence of intermittent relapses, so that, whilst useful under certain circumstances, I cannot regard it as being a curative agent.

Hypnosis in the Treatment of Warts

This condition is seen so regularly in the average surgery, and responds so well to hypnotic treatment, that from the general practitioner viewpoint, it is worth considering it in some detail.

It has long been known that warts not only tend to disappear spontaneously, but that they are also susceptible to the influence of strong suggestion. Indeed, many methods of ' charming warts away ' can be found in folk-lore, together with much evidence to prove their efficiency. A number of patients, all suffering from warts, were given X-ray treatment, and a control group, who thought they were receiving the same treatment, was compared with them: the warts disappeared just as rapidly and completely in the second group as in the first. Suggestion had induced in these patients' minds a thorough conviction that they would be cured, and surely enough, the warts vanished. Since suggestion acts so much more powerfully in the hypnotic, than in the waking state, its effect upon warts becomes quite understandable.

In the actual treatment of this condition, it is always advisable to induce as deep a hypnotic trance as possible. Whilst by no means essential, the deeper the hypnosis, the more rapid will be the results. Most children, except the very timid and nervous, can be induced into deep or somnambulistic trances, but probably no more than 20 per cent of adults, even with training, will be able to achieve such depth. Consequently the treatment of an adult is likely to require far more time and patience than that of the average child. Another significant factor is the frequency of the treatment. Owing to pressure of work, I am seldom able to give treatment more than once a week, although I am convinced that two or three attendances per week, at least in the early stages, would secure quicker and more satisfactory results.

Once adequate depth has been obtained, I lightly stroke the affected areas, and proceed as follows:

> As I stroke your hand . . . *you can feel a feeling of warmth, spreading into the skin of your hand.*
> As I go on stroking . . . *that feeling of warmth is increasing . . . so that you can now feel it quite clearly.*
> *As soon as you can feel this sensation of warmth . . . please lift up your other hand.*

I continue to stroke, and to suggest the sensation of warmth, until I see the hand rise.

> Good!
> Now put it down, again!
> And now . . . I am beginning to stroke the warts, themselves.

And . . . as I stroke each of these warts . . . you will feel that the warmth is becoming concentrated in the warts . . . and that the warts are feeling warmer than the rest of your hand.
As soon as you can feel this warmth . . . in each of the warts . . . please lift up your other hand.
Very good!
Put it down again!
As that warmth spreads into your warts . . . they will gradually become smaller . . . they will begin to shrink . . . they will become flatter . . . and will gradually disappear.
With every treatment . . . your skin will become healthier . . . the roots of the warts will shrivel . . . and the warts, themselves, will gradually wither away.

Since my cases have been limited to the common multiple warts that usually appear on the hands, limbs and face, I cannot express an opinion as to the usefulness or otherwise of this treatment in allied conditions, such as verrucae on the soles of the feet.

As a somewhat typical example of successful response to hypnosis, when all other methods of treatment had failed, the following case is worth quoting.

The patient was a boy in his late 'teens, who was employed as a butcher's assistant. He was referred to me by a consultant dermatologist in June 1956, and had large and numerous warts on both hands. These varied considerably in size, and their proximity was such as to render any ordinary method of treatment a matter of considerable difficulty. He had been attending the dermatological department of a general hospital for a long period without showing any marked improvement. Since it was impossible to see him more than once a week, it was obvious that even hypnotic treatment would necessarily be prolonged. Had more frequent attendances been possible, there is no doubt that a much quicker result would have been obtained.

The technique employed was the one already described, and in three sessions the patient was induced into a somnambulistic trance. Within six weeks, many of the smaller warts had disappeared completely, some of the others had flattened and shrunk, whilst the largest remained apparently unaffected. By early November, the warts had practically all vanished, only two particularly large ones remaining on his right hand. It was also noticeable that, whereas upon his first visit he was a rather nervous, untidy boy, obviously lacking in self-confidence, he had become brighter, more cheerful, neater in personal appearance, and more confident in every way.

The last two warts proved extremely resistant, but treatment was continued, and by the end of February 1957 these too had disappeared, and he was discharged completely cured.

Over six years have now elapsed, and he has not had to report for any further treatment.

In this case, at no time was any method other than hypnotic suggestion employed, and even his weekly treatment was far from being continuous. On various occasions, it was interrupted for periods of two to three weeks, on account of holidays and illness.

Hypnosis in Surgery and Anaesthesia

In surgery, hypnosis is usually employed for one or other of the two following purposes:

1. To produce anaesthesia or analgesia.
2. To free the patient from anxiety and to produce mental and physical relaxation prior to operation.

Hypnosis possesses all the pre-requisites of the ideal anaesthetic agent. When complete anaesthesia can be secured hypnosis involves no dangers at all and can be induced in the operating theatre by the surgeon or his assistant. However, it must be admitted that such depth is only rarely attainable and, in so far as major surgery is concerned, hypnosis offers certain grave disadvantages compared with chemically induced anaesthesia:

1. Except in those cases where the patient has been previously trained and conditioned, hypnosis is certainly neither as quick nor as easy a method of inducing anaesthesia.

2. It is rarely possible to secure the deeper stages of somnambulism which are essential before major surgery can even be considered.

3. Hypnosis is necessarily more time-consuming than any existing orthodox procedure.

4. The induction and deepening of hypnosis for anaesthesia is an art which has to be learned and mastered, and should consequently only be undertaken by a specialist experienced in the subject.

Even when complete hypnotic anaesthesia is possible, the best results will only occur in those operations that do *not* require a very deep state of surgical anaesthesia.

It is important to appreciate exactly what can reasonably be expected in each of the three main stages of hypnosis:

Light trance. Only seldom is it possible to produce the slightest degree of analgesia. Nevertheless fear and anxiety can be alleviated, and the psychological overlay of pain reduced.

Medium trance. At this stage, varying degrees of analgesia can be produced in some 30 to 40 per cent of patients. Hypnosis can consequently be usefully employed to reduce discomfort in painful surgical procedures that have to be repeated, such as painful dressings which normally do not justify the use of a general anaesthetic. It can facilitate lumbar punctures and similar investigations, and even certain painful manipulations necessitated in physiotherapy can be undertaken under hypnosis with a minimum of discomfort.

Deep trance. No more than 15 to 20 per cent of patients can be induced into the deepest somnambulistic trances in which considerable degrees of analgesia become possible, and of these probably even less than 15 per cent can achieve the complete surgical anaesthesia that is essential for major operations. When this does occur, however, such surgical procedures as amputations of limbs, mastectomies, Caesarean sections and appendicectomies can be performed quite painlessly. Hypnotic anaesthesia offers certain distinct advantages:

1. Pre-operative fear and anxiety can be almost completely removed.
2. There is a complete absence of toxic effects from anaesthetic drugs.
3. Shock is greatly diminished.
4. The cough reflex is not interfered with.
5. Post-operative pain, discomfort and sickness can all be controlled.

Once the somnambulistic stage has been successfully achieved, direct suggestions are usually made to the effect that the patient will become completely relaxed, both mentally and physically, and will enter so deep a sleep that he will feel no pain or discomfort whatever, and will subsequently remember nothing that has taken place. More often than not, however, *anaesthesia* such as this cannot be produced and yet a complete *analgesia* may still be possible. In such cases some sensation (without pain) may be permitted, and painful stimuli allowed to reach consciousness as non-painful experiences. The advantages of this procedure will be enlarged upon in the section on the use of hypnosis in obstetrics (p. 319).

Apart from its limited use in the production of surgical anaesthesia, hypnosis can prove extremely useful to the anaesthetist in his routine work. Any method that can overcome fear, conscious or subconscious, can afford considerable assistance and hypnosis is the ideal agent for this purpose. It is a relatively easy task to secure both mental and physical relaxation under hypnosis, and once this has been achieved much less chemical anaesthetic will be required to produce and maintain the depth at which surgery becomes possible. Moreover, if it is used pre-operatively for several days, hypnosis can ensure restful sleep and can allay the fear of pain, fear of the operation itself, and of untimely death. Needless to say, such reassurances as these will enable the patient to face his operation with much more confidence and in a much calmer and more relaxed frame of mind. Indeed, as an introduction to general anaesthesia, hypnosis offers all the advantages and none of the dangers or disadvantages of Thiopentone.

In children hypnosis can be an invaluable asset since it can usually be induced both easily and quickly, and fairly deep trance states secured without much difficulty. In both children and adults, an appropriate dose of secobarbital given last thing at night, and about half that dose repeated about two hours before the operation, can render the induction of hypnosis much easier.

Whenever medium or deep stages of hypnosis can be attained and a considerable amount of analgesia secured, it is often to be preferred to the use of general anaesthetics in minor surgical or dental operations, particularly in children. Even these minor procedures often cause a great deal of fear and anxiety, and since hypnosis is so successful in controlling and eliminating this, it offers many advantages over the use of orthodox chemical anaesthesia.

Goldie's valuable investigation into the usefulness of hypnotic anaesthesia or analgesia in emergency work in casualty departments has already been referred to (p. 204). His claim that hypnosis can be advantageously used in casualty departments as an adjunct to the more orthodox anaesthetic facilities deserves the most serious consideration, for he has demonstrated conclusively how effective the technique can be in untrained subjects, reducing to an appreciable extent the number of general anaesthetics that would otherwise have been required.

The conclusion may fairly be drawn that whereas hypnosis can be of considerable assistance to the anaesthetist in his work, in so far as hypnotic anaesthesia itself is concerned it can in no way be considered as a serious rival to the efficiency, simplicity and ease of administration of modern pharmacological anaesthetics.

CHAPTER 21

Hypnosis in Obstetrics

Many of the ailments from which human beings suffer arise solely through belief, suggestion and expectation. It is generally believed that women necessarily suffer great pain and discomfort during childbirth. Indeed, the average woman has had this fact dinned into her so consistently throughout the years, that she is bound to suffer pain at her confinement because her mind has been conditioned to expect it.

Grantley Dick-Read's recognition of this fact, and his explanation of the *fear-tension-pain* syndrome, have done much to alter the whole approach to obstetrics. The methods which he employed so successfully to deal with this, consisted of education, relaxation and suggestion. Although he described a ' trance-like ' state which occurred in some of his patients during labour, he stoutly denied that hypnosis played any part in the techniques he evolved. Nevertheless suggestion forms such an integral part of the Dick-Read procedure that there is not the slightest doubt that hypnosis can greatly enhance the use and effectiveness of his methods.

Since the causes of pain during childbirth are largely psychological, it is obvious that the most effective methods of dealing with them must also be psychological. It must be remembered, however, that the hard work and effort connected with labour cannot be avoided, but the pain and mental anxiety can. Training in the hypnotic state can teach the expectant mother to exercise a remarkable degree of mental control over her bodily functions.

The general practitioner who uses hypnosis and suggestion will find that his efforts are amply repaid in the field of obstetrics alone. It is not nearly as time-consuming as he might imagine, and whilst results vary from patient to patient there are few who fail to benefit to a considerable extent. Hypnosis is also helpful to the single-handed general practitioner obstetrician, particularly if some form of anaesthesia is required.

In obstetrics there are three essential requirements that the ideal anaesthetic agent should fulfil.

1. It should be capable of affording complete relief from pain, however severe.

2. It should not interfere with the normal mechanics of labour.

3. It should not depress either the respiration or the circulation of the child.

Whereas the best chemical anaesthetic agent is at the best a compromise, hypnosis fulfils all these conditions, and has been rightly called the ideal anaesthetic agent in midwifery.

The pain that is commonly experienced during labour is always caused by two main factors:

1. The physical contractions of the womb and the distension of tissues as the baby is born.

2. The psychological overlay of fear, anxiety and tension, arising from expectation and belief.

Every dentist knows to what extent anticipation increases pain and tension. The pregnant woman's ability to relax depends not only upon the extent of her suggestibility, but also upon her attitude to pregnancy, her emotional reaction to the event, her previous conditioning to pain, the level of her threshold of pain, and whether she is primiparous or multiparous. All the emotional factors, which play such an important part in influencing labour pains, can be controlled by hypnosis.

Whereas hypnosis has a great deal to offer as an obstetric analgesic, two objections are usually put forward:

1. The time required to induce hypnosis, to produce depth and to train the patient in readiness for her confinement is considerable.

2. The degree of analgesia that can be obtained in any given case is unpredictable.

Now hypnosis itself is far from being a complicated or difficult procedure; moreover, since no apparatus or expense is involved, it is ideal for use in either home or hospital. Considerable depth is, of course, necessary to ensure complete anaesthesia and freedom from pain, but even if this is aimed at, since pregnancy affects mainly the younger age groups, in which hypnotizability is at its greatest, and the motivation for it is usually very strong, a sufficiently deep state can fairly easily be obtained, and even somnambulism is likely to occur in 20 to 25 per cent of cases.

As far as the training and preparation of the patient for her confinement is concerned, fortnightly or three-weekly sessions of 20 to 30 minutes' duration are all that are required in the early stages, and even these may be extended to longer intervals, if necessary, until shortly before term. To ensure the best results, I generally see the patient weekly for about the last 6 weeks. At this stage, each individual treatment can be completed in approximately 15 minutes, and whilst it is true that the patient will have to be seen rather more frequently than under ordinary conditions, there is no doubt whatever that the extra trouble involved will be found to be well worth while.

The objection regarding the unpredictability of the degree of analgesia that can be secured is certainly not valid since that is far from being the main objective of hypnotic treatment. Abramson and Heron consider that the greatest value of hypnotic training lies in its ability to achieve the following:

1. The eradication of erroneous ideas by the use of counter-suggestion.
2. The teaching of relaxation.
3. The teaching of auto-hypnosis to the patient and the ability to produce such relaxation whenever required.

In their view, the induction of hypnotic anaesthesia is of secondary importance since relaxation itself will always automatically raise the threshold of pain. When the patient receives proper psychological preparation for labour, it is questionable whether induced anaesthesia is necessary since labour will tend to proceed with a minimum of discomfort except for that associated with hard work.

It is certainly true that if the expectant mother can be taught to relax, to feel confident, and to look forward to her confinement with pleasure as a most rewarding and satisfying experience, her labour is likely to be shortened in duration, much easier and far less distressing. Fortunately this can be achieved without deep hypnosis or somnambulism. Early training in both mental and physical relaxation can be achieved even in the lighter or medium stages of hypnosis, and can prevent a great deal of anxiety, apprehension and tension. Moreover, the increased confidence acquired will minimize the amount of anaesthesia required, should this have to be reinforced in the later expulsive stage. Abramson and Heron reported an average reduction of 20 per cent in the length of the first stage of labour in women who had had prenatal hypnotic training, and some 20 per cent of their patients were able to achieve the deepest hypnotic states with spectacular results in the complete elimination of pain. Probably 90 per cent of all pregnant women can achieve some degree of hypnosis, depending largely upon the skill of the operator and the personality of the individual patient. This always has to be taken into account, for the woman who has responded to menstruation, marriage or motherhood with fear and apprehension, will naturally tend to feel over-anxious, tense and apprehensive during pregnancy and labour. The great value of hypnosis is amply confirmed by the patient's subjective reactions to the experience when questioned post-natally. Almost invariably the reply will be that future confinements will hold no terrors whatever, and that the patient will even look forward to having another baby under similar circumstances.

The Advantages of Hypnosis in Obstetrics

1. *It can greatly increase the patient's ability to relax, both mentally and physically.* Under hypnosis, the patient will readily accept the fact that there is nothing to fear, and that since she will be able to relax completely, the tension and pain will disappear, and her labour will become very much easier. She is easily taught to gain much more control over her bodily functions.

2. *It produces no depression of the respiratory or circulatory functions, in either mother or child.* Most chemical anaesthetic agents, and analgesic or sedative drugs tend to produce anoxaemia. This is particularly likely to occur when morphine or the barbiturates are employed. Not only is this danger avoided in hypnosis, but there is much less need for the use of drugs, and consequently much less risk of foetal damage.

3. *Hypnosis usually effects some shortening of the first stage of labour.* Evidence has shown that this reduction will generally amount to at least 2 hours in the case of multiparae, and possibly to between 3 and 4 hours in primiparae.

4. *Hypnosis increases the patient's resistance to obstetric shock.* The risk of shock is greatly diminished since the mother becomes much less exhausted during the first stage. Under hypnosis, she can eat, drink, sleep and attend to her natural functions. She is able to co-operate fully with both doctor and midwife, even when the contractions are strong and frequent. The mother is also enabled to relax her muscles so completely that the danger of foetal injury is also much reduced.

5. *Hypnosis does not interfere in any way with the normal mechanics of labour.* Both general anaesthetics and analgesic or sedative drugs have the dis-advantage of exercising a depressing action upon uterine contractions. They consequently tend to delay and to prolong labour. Under hypnosis

drugs may often be dispensed with altogether, and even when some supplementary medication is required the effective dosage will be much reduced.

6. *In the lighter and medium stages hypnosis greatly reduces the liability to pain by relieving the fear-pain-tension syndrome, and substituting the ability to relax, both mentally and physically.* Even in the second stage, when the contractions become stronger and more frequent, the patient who has been taught in hypnosis to couple suggestions of increasing relaxation with deep, rhythmic breathing, can greatly relieve, and sometimes even remove all feelings of pain. It is only as the head descends and the perineum becomes distended that pain is likely to be felt, and supplementary measures are needed to keep it under control. In the course of her prenatal training, the patient should always be told that ' gas and air ' and analgesic drugs will be readily available should she require them. Whether they are actually used or not should be left to the mother herself. Some women resent a general anaesthetic as they feel they have missed the delight of hearing the baby's first cry; for this reason alone the mother's wish should always be respected.

7. *In the somnambulistic stages of hypnosis partial or complete analgesia and anaesthesia may be produced in any part of the body by direct suggestion.* The patient's ability to produce complete muscular relaxation is tremendously increased and the perineum can often be rendered completely insensitive during the second stage. Acute pain is most likely to be felt as the head crowns, but direct suggestion can greatly lessen its intensity and may sometimes succeed in removing it altogether.

In complete somnambulism, particularly if amnesia has been obtained during prenatal training, labour can usually be rendered completely painless. Kroger points out that the subjective pain element need not be completely lost. In his view, the pain of childbirth is a necessary psychological experience, and he therefore considers it important that the patient can be awakened at any time to feel the contractions and to see the birth of her baby.

Somnambulistic patients always enter deep hypnosis immediately upon a prearranged signal. They can be told that whenever the contractions occur, no matter how heavy or frequent they may be, no pain will be felt. The only sensations experienced will be those of a certain amount of discomfort and pressure, and even this will be rendered much less uncomfortable by bearing-down when instructed to do so. The behaviour of somnambulistic patients is remarkable as they remain calm, quiet and relaxed throughout their labour.

8. *In these stages, hypnosis affords almost complete control over the rate of expulsion of the head and shoulders.* As the head is about to emerge, the uterine contractions become so powerful, frequent and urgent that the mother feels it impossible to stop pushing, even when told not to do so. The perineum is consequently given no opportunity to stretch and tears. However, the moment that the hypnotized patient is told to stop pushing she will obey implicitly and so allow her abdominal muscles to relax completely leaving the contractions to do their own work, and when she is told to push, she will do so most effectively. The obstetrician therefore has complete control over the rate of delivery, and perineal tears are much more likely to be avoided.

9. *An episiotomy can be performed quite painlessly, under hypnosis alone.* If perineal repair is required, it can easily be done without pain and without anaesthesia. The third stage and the expulsion of the placenta usually proceeds quite normally under hypnosis, although the average blood loss seems to be appreciably diminished.

10. *Post-operative recovery is usually both smooth and uneventful.* Most women feel remarkably fit and well after hypnotic delivery and show much less physical and mental exhaustion. The fact that they can move their legs freely and exercise their muscles immediately following the birth, greatly diminishes the risk of any subsequent venous thrombosis. Other complications also seem much less likely to occur, and there is much less danger to both mother and child.

11. *Lactation can be stimulated, and breast-feeding facilitated by direct suggestion under hypnosis.* This is hardly surprising, for it is well known that the physiological process of lactation can often be seriously influenced by conscious and unconscious emotional disturbances.

In brief, the greatest value of hypnosis in the field of obstetrics lies in its ability to produce complete mental and physical relaxation, together with the relief of fear and anxiety. Once the element of fear is removed the patient will approach her confinement with confidence, and consequently only a minimum of analgesia is likely to be required. It is important that the general practitioner should remember that even when the depth of hypnosis is insufficient to remove all pain, repeated suggestion, with or without supplementary medication, can still render labour a great deal easier by abolishing the *fear-tension-pain* syndrome.

The Disadvantages of Hypnosis in Obstetrics

1. *Prejudice against the idea of hypnosis itself.*

2. *The time and effort required to produce and deepen the trance and to give adequate prenatal training.*

3. *The variability of degrees of susceptibility to hypnosis.*
These three objections have already been fully discussed.

4. *Lack of co-operation and understanding on the part of trained personnel.*
The patient may lose whatever composure she has acquired during her prenatal training if she is admitted to a ward where other women, in various stages of labour, are causing disturbances. In domiciliary midwifery, this difficulty will not arise, but the practitioner may have to work with a midwife who fails to understand or is totally unsympathetic to the idea of hypnosis. Even during the early stages of labour, it is essential that the patient should remain quiet, and be allowed to relax and sleep. She should be aroused only when necessary. In too many instances, the midwife fails to grasp this fact, and often disturbs and worries the patient by rousing her and talking to her unnecessarily.

The Technical Application of Hypnosis in Obstetrics

The most successful results will always be obtained when the obstetrician undertakes the induction of hypnosis and the prenatal training of the patient, and is subsequently present to conduct the confinement. Consequently, the general practitioner is in a much better position to use it successfully than anyone else. Hypnosis can be undertaken by a professional colleague, and provided that both are present at the confinement and working as a team, excellent results will be obtained.

Hypnosis is not necessarily contra-indicated when the patient is to be delivered by a midwife alone. Provided that the mother has been adequately prepared, she will still be able to relax completely and greatly diminish her discomfort, particularly if she has been taught how to put herself into a trance whenever she wishes to do so. She can then be put ' en rapport ' with the midwife, whose instructions she will be told to follow exactly as if they were given by the obstetrician himself. The midwife must naturally be fully instructed as to the conduct of the labour, and must co-operate fully in complying with any special conditions that need to be observed. For instance, no matter how successful the patient may have been throughout the earlier stages of labour, she is quite likely to break down and lose control as the actual delivery becomes imminent. At this point, she should certainly be given some form of supplementary analgesia such as gas and air should she desire it. *It is essential that the patient should receive adequate preparation for her confinement during the prenatal period.* Only rarely will hypnosis achieve any degree of success if the first induction has to take place whilst labour is in progress. I consider it wise to see the patient for the first time as soon as possible after the pregnancy has been confirmed, although some authorities defer this until just before the seventh month of gestation. The sooner misconceptions, fears, anxieties and tensions are removed, the more quickly the patient can be trained to look forward to her confinement rather than to dread it. Moreover, the necessary contact can be made with the midwife, and early discomforts such as morning-sickness, heartburn or flatulence can be dealt with.

I see the patient once a week for a few weeks in the course of which I establish as deep a state of hypnosis as possible, deal with any existing disturbances, and proceed with the initial training and conditioning of the patient's mind. Very often, depending upon the personality of the individual, these preliminary sessions may be extended to fortnightly intervals. As soon as I am satisfied that sufficient progress has been made, I tell the patient to return between the seventh and eighth month or, should she so desire, I continue to see her at monthly or six-weekly periods in the interim. I believe it to be most important to see the patient once a week for the last six weeks of her pregnancy.

Hyperemesis Gravidarum

This is a very common problem which is considered to be psychogenic in origin and to represent a conscious or unconscious wish to get rid of the pregnancy. It has also been suggested that the customary disappearance of the symptom between the third and the fourth month occurs because foetal movements compel the mother to accept it as a separate individual. Other psychological factors may lie behind this symptom: disturbed marital relations, a craving for or even lack of affection, and fears concerning the birth and subsequent rearing of the child may all play a part. Sometimes vomiting is regular and really severe, in other instances there is nothing more than nausea. No matter how severe the case hypnosis can always prove extremely useful, even when it is combined with other therapeutic measures. Direct suggestion under hypnosis, constantly repeated and re-inforced, is capable of curing over 50 per cent of cases. In resistant cases treatment should also be directed towards the patient's emotional attitudes and not aimed at the symptom alone.

My own method, which cannot be quoted in its entirety since it is bound to vary from case to case, consists essentially of a modified version of the routine 'ego-strengthening' suggestions, followed by direct symptom removal:

As I stroke your stomach . . . you will begin to feel a feeling of warmth, spreading into your stomach.
That feeling of warmth is increasing . . . with every stroke of my hand. As soon as you feel that warmth . . . please lift up your hand.
That's right.
Now, put it down again.
And as your stomach feels warmer . . . it is beginning to feel more normal . . . more and more comfortable.
All feelings of sickness are passing away completely . . . you no longer feel at all sick.
Your stomach feels perfectly normal . . . and comfortable, in every way.
And in a few moments . . . when I count up to *seven* . . . you will open your eyes, and be wide awake, again.
You will wake up . . . with your stomach completely comfortable . . . without the slightest feeling of sickness or discomfort . . . and you will find that . . . when you wake up, each morning . . . you will not feel the slightest trace of sickness whatever . . . your stomach will remain perfectly normal . . . without the slightest discomfort of any kind.
And, with every one of these treatments . . . this trouble is going to disappear . . . more and more quickly . . . more and more completely.

Heartburn and Flatulence

Causation is most frequently psychogenic, and a great deal can be achieved simply by the alleviation of anxiety and tension. The condition usually subsides quickly under direct hypnotic suggestion, if this is combined with a full discussion and explanation of the harmlessness of the symptom.

Many other prenatal symptoms such as backache, pruritus and insomnia can be greatly relieved by hypnosis.

Prenatal Training

This is by far the most important part of the patient's preparation for her confinement, and has two main objects:

1. To teach the patient to relax, both mentally and physically, to the greatest possible extent in order to ensure as easy a labour as possible.

2. To teach the patient to gain increased control over her body-functions by achieving a positive and healthy attitude of mind.

There can be no doubt that by far the best and easiest way of securing a satisfactory delivery lies in the proper antenatal preparation for the event.

The first interview. Contact should be made with the patient, and every possible step taken to put her completely at ease. As in every other kind of hypnotic work, this is of vital importance, for if you have failed to gain the patient's complete confidence by the end of the first session, it is most unlikely that you will ever be able to achieve really satisfying results. In the course of general conversation, directed towards the discovery of her ideas and attitudes concerning pregnancy and childbirth, you should try to assess her potentialities, both as a possible hypnotic subject, and with regard to motherhood. I usually introduce the possibilities of hypnosis, and explain its many advantages. At the same time, I am equally frank concerning its limitations.

I begin by telling the patient that since childbirth is a perfectly natural process, there is no reason why it should be either painful or unpleasant. That pain only occurs because the patient expects it, and is afraid of it, and because she is unable to prevent all her muscles from becoming rigid and tense. I point out that since hypnosis will teach her to be able to get rid of all this tension by relaxing her muscles during her confinement, there will be no reason why she should expect to have pain, and that she should consequently have a much easier time. I tell her that if she wishes hypnosis to be used it can help her greatly, but that she must not expect magical results. What can be achieved will depend firstly upon her own desire and ability to co-operate, and secondly upon the depth of hypnosis she can achieve with training.

I never make any over-enthusiastic promises, nor do I give any guarantee that I shall be able to be present at her confinement, even though such may be my intention if possible. I try to discover her own ideas, fears and reservations concerning hypnosis, and deal with these by explaining, as simply as possible what hypnosis is really like, and how it works. In this connection I emphasize the fact that there is not the slightest question of domination, and that it is purely a matter of team work. That the part she has to play is, in fact, every bit as important as mine.

I tell her that it will probably take two or three sessions to discover the greatest depth of hypnosis that she is capable of achieving. If she can go very deeply, then it should be possible to render her confinement almost painless. This, however, must not be relied upon since only about 20 per cent of women are capable of this depth. She can, however, be sure of one thing. Even as a result of the lighter stages, she will be able to relax, both mentally and physically, so much more successfully during her labour that she will certainly have a much easier time than she would otherwise have done.

Never, under any circumstances, do I make any attempt to induce hypnosis in the course of this first interview. I confine myself to the facts, to the removal of doubts and fears, and to the encouragement of the patient's motivation. I invite her to think over carefully, during the forthcoming week, all that she has been told, and to ask any questions that may occur to her next time.

The second interview. I begin by asking the patient whether she has been thinking about last week's discussion, and whether there are any questions she would like to ask. I deal with these first in order to dispel as far as possible any remaining doubts and uncertainties. I then explain, in the simplest possible terms, the method of inducing hypnosis, and tell the patient exactly what she has to do and what she may expect to happen. I follow by inducing hypnosis for the first time but make no attempt to gain real depth. I awaken the patient and discuss with her in some detail her own subjective sensations and reactions. I explain to her that learning hypnosis is just like learning to ride a bicycle for the first time. On the first occasion, somebody has to give support by holding the saddle all the time. On the next occasion, this support can be withdrawn for brief periods, during which the patient would be able to proceed on her course, wobbly and uncertain though this progress might be, to be supported only if there was any danger of falling off. On subsequent occasions the rider would do more and more on her own, until eventually riding would become just as natural an act as walking.

I tell the patient that, as soon as she has achieved the necessary depth, she will be taught how to use hypnosis herself, during her confinement. It is always important to obtain the husband's consent, before hypnosis is induced for the first time.

Subsequent interviews. I deepen the hypnosis until the patient has achieved the greatest depth of which she is capable. Should this prove insufficient for any marked degree of analgesia, I constantly instill into the patient's mind, under hypnosis, the following idea.

During your confinement . . . *you will feel so very relaxed . . . so very, very sleepy and drowsy . . . that you will feel much less discomfort than if you were wide awake.*

In all future discussions with the patient, it is wise to avoid the words ' pain ' or ' labour pains ', when referring to uterine contractions, which should be simply described as such, even in connection with the actual confinement. The word pressure is infinitely preferable.

When it is possible to induce localized analgesia to a painful stimulus such as a pin-prick, I test for somnambulism (by getting the patient to open her eyes without awakening from the trance) and for amnesia. If these are successful the labour can be rendered entirely painless throughout, provided that I am able to be present. This can still occur in my absence, but there is a risk of the patient's control breaking down at the worst moment just as the head is about to emerge. This will be the only point at which some form of supplementary anaesthesia may be needed.

If localized analgesia can be produced by suggestion, it is useful to demonstrate to the patient how it can be transferred to any region of the body. Deep subjects can be taught how to produce it for themselves, at will, under certain restricted circumstances which must also be clearly defined when the appropriate post-hypnotic suggestion is given. Such patients as these, however, will unfortunately always be in the minority. Nevertheless, the majority will still be able to attain a calmness of mind, and a satisfactory relaxation during light- or medium-depth hypnosis to serve them well at their confinement.

The fact that it may prove impossible to produce any marked degree of analgesia to pin-prick does not mean that the patient will be unable to exercise a considerable amount of control over physiological pain in her confinement. But it will naturally be necessary for the patient to attend more frequently for antenatal training (preferably at weekly intervals in the initial stages) than if complete somnambulism were achieved. In the latter case, not only need the prenatal training be less prolonged, but much greater use may be made of direct suggestion and post-hypnotic suggestion in the conduct of the labour itself. Moreover, it is possible for analgesia to be produced very rapidly indeed, either upon word of command or as the result of a predetermined signal. The question has been raised as to whether hypnotic analgesia is, in effect, nothing but amnesia. This seems to be disproved by the fact that analgesia can often be obtained in waking hypnosis, when no amnesia at all has been secured.

The Use of Auto-hypnosis in Labour

The teaching of auto-hypnosis can prove to be an invaluable asset in all cases in which sufficient depth has been obtained. In medium depth, the patient can usually be taught to produce a trance state herself at will, and to produce complete mental and physical relaxation by self-suggestion. Whilst the average depth of such auto-hypnosis is not great, it is quite sufficient to be of material assistance, particularly in the first stage of labour. The resulting analgesia is due to relaxation, and the relief of tension, fear and anxiety rather than to direct suggestion. The technique should be taught as early as possible and the patient encouraged to use it daily in her own home throughout her antenatal period. In this way she gradually gains confidence, not only in her own power of control, but also in her ability to secure complete relaxation and diminution of pain and discomfort during her confinement.

During her labour, the patient can make use of self-hypnosis in one of two ways:

1. She can induce it shortly after the onset of labour, and maintain the trance state undisturbed for considerable periods of time.

2. She can induce it each time she feels a contraction, and maintain it solely for the duration of each contraction.

She may elect to use either method or both alternately according to circumstances. I have found that the medium-depth patient usually appears to derive most benefit from the first procedure, and it is only the somnambule who is likely to achieve complete success and relief from the second.

The patient using auto-hypnosis will generally ' sleep ' or relax continuously throughout the earlier stages. She will often lie quite motionless and will require no attention other than routine care and observation. She will be able to converse, to urinate or defaecate, or to be fed at her own request. The midwife should be instructed not to talk to her or disturb her unnecessarily at this stage. An understanding and sympathetic midwife can greatly enhance the effectiveness of auto-hypnosis, indeed it may even be said that her attitude may well determine the difference between success and failure.

Somnambulistic patients, however, can be taught to induce a deep trance state, a complete analgesia and often, amnesia, within a matter of 5 to 10 seconds. This speed is essential if the patient is to retain full control during the height of delivery, when there is little intermission between the strong and frequent uterine contractions. In these cases I teach auto-hypnosis through post-hypnotic suggestion.

*In a few moments . . . when I count up to seven . . . you will open your
eyes and be wide awake, again.*
After I have wakened you up, I shall talk to you for a minute or two.
*You will then put yourself straight off to sleep again . . . into a sleep, just as
deep as this one.*
*You will lie back, comfortably . . . fix your eyes on a spot upon the ceiling . . .
and count slowly up to five.*
*As you count . . . your eyes will become more and more tired . . . you will feel
drowsier and drowsier . . . and, the moment you have reached five . . . your eyes
will close immediately . . . and you will fall immediately into a sleep, just as deep
as this one.*

I then waken the patient, chat to her briefly, and tell her to put herself
to sleep again. This she does without difficulty, and I tell her that,
whenever she needs to put herself to sleep, particularly during her
confinement, she will always be able to do so immediately by counting
up to five. I subsequently teach her how to produce complete mental
and physical relaxation through appropriate self-suggestions, and how to
induce localized analgesia whenever she needs to do so, by simply suggesting to herself that all pain will completely disappear the moment
she counts up to three. For obvious reasons, however, she must *not* be
left with the ability to do this with regard to each and every kind of
pain. Strictly limited conditions must be clearly defined, and she must
be told that she will be able to remove pain in this way only during her
confinement: no other type of pain will respond and on no other
occasion will this method achieve the slightest success.

I instruct the patient to practise this self-hypnosis regularly in her own
home to produce complete mental and physical relaxation, and I renew
the post-hypnotic suggestions that she will be able to exercise complete
control over pain *during her confinement* at each subsequent prenatal
training session.

The Management of Antenatal Hypnotic Training

Once satisfactory trance depth has been obtained and the technique
of auto-hypnosis mastered, whenever this is possible, the next most
important step is to give the patient as simple an explanation as possible
of the three stages of labour, and what she may expect to feel or to happen
in each of these stages. I usually explain it to the patient in the following
manner.

In every confinement, there are three separate and distinct stages. The first and longest of these is concerned with the necessary preparation for the birth of the child. This could not occur unless time were given for all the muscles to relax, and the passages to widen and dilate sufficiently to permit the passage of the baby.

Once these are wide open, the second and more active stage occurs. During this, the child descends through the passages, and eventually emerges and is born. When this has happened, there is still the final stage, which is not completed until the afterbirth has come away.

Now, probably the first sign that you will have that labour has started is a slight show of blood, almost as if a monthly period were beginning. With this you will feel some weak contractions of the womb, with long intervals between them. Sometimes, the show does not occur, and the only sign of commencing labour is the presence of these weak, infrequent, but regular uterine contractions. When you first feel these, look at the clock and time them. No matter how long elapses between them, if they are occurring at regular intervals, you have probably started in labour, so either send for the midwife, or go straight into hospital according to your previous arrangements.

You must not induce any hypnotic trance until this has been done.

During this first stage, you will find that the contractions will be weak, and will not occur very often. They will gradually cause the passages to open up, but this is a slow process and takes time. They will cause so little discomfort to begin with, that the only thing you will need to do is to sleep as much as possible, and to relax. You will be able to do this by putting yourself to sleep and relaxing as you have been taught to do. Because of this, you will feel the contractions merely as pressure in your stomach, and they will not distress you at all. If anything, or anyone disturbs you, you will immediately put yourself straight off to sleep again, as a result of which your labour will progress more steadily and easily. You will remain perfectly calm and unworried, and not in the least bit afraid.

Later, as the passages open up, the contractions will become stronger, heavier, and more frequent. You will not become frightened or try to resist this, because if it did not happen, your baby could never be born. This is a sign that your labour is progressing well. You will be able to stay in your trance and remain relaxed by taking a series of deep, rapid, rhythmic breaths. With each of these, you will relax more and more completely. All tension will disappear and you will feel only the discomfort of heavier pressure from each contraction. You will not lose control, and will remain perfectly passive, allowing the contractions to do their own work, without trying to assist in any way.

A short pause may occur, after which the contractions will recommence with increased strength. About this time, the membranes rupture and the waters escape. There is no need to become worried or alarmed about this. It merely means that that you have entered into the second stage of your labour, and the actual birth and expulsion of your child is about to begin. Although the contractions become much heavier and more frequent, they will not frighten you, because soon it will be necessary for you to co-operate and help in getting your baby born. As the contractions continue, you will begin to feel an almost irresistible desire to assist by bearing-down. No matter when this occurs, *you must not give way to it, until you are told to do so.*

If you do, you will delay the birth of your child, render it more difficult, and wear yourself out unnecessarily, without doing a scrap of good. As soon as you feel this urge, tell the midwife or nurse, but do not give way to it until she tells you to. When she does, take a deep breath, hold it as long as you can, and push down as hard as you can as long as each contraction lasts. If you have to breathe out before the contraction is over, take another deep breath as quickly as possible and continue to hold it and push down, since it is usually the last part of the contraction that produces most progress. You will find that this will greatly reduce the discomfort. Remember, as you bear down and push, how much you are helping to bring your baby into the world, because this could not be done without some hard work and physical exertion. It will be well worth while. In each interval, between the contractions, you will be able to relax completely, and sleep.

As the baby's head descends, and appears at the outlet, the final process of delivery is about to begin. At this point, you will be able to obey all instructions implicitly. Whenever you are told to stop pushing, you will stop pushing immediately, and indulge in rapid deep breathing instead. As a result of this you will relax more and more completely, and as the head presses down harder and harder on the outlet, the whole area will become quite numb and insensitive. You will experience an uncomfortable feeling of stretching, and the sensation of something passing through the outlet. Although you will probably need no extra help, suitable drugs or anaesthetics will be available if you feel the need of them. They will not be given to you unless you require them. You have only to ask. If, on the other hand, you wish to remain awake as your baby is born, you have only to say so. When you have seen the baby, and the afterbirth has come away, you will fall into a deep refreshing sleep. You will wake up from this feeling really fit and well, and remembering very little of what has occurred.

Throughout the whole of your labour, you will be able to talk, or answer questions if necessary, without waking up from your deep, relaxed, hypnotic sleep. You will be able to co-operate in every way, but you will feel far too sleepy and drowsy to become disturbed. You will carry out faithfully every instruction that you are given, just as effectively as if I had given them, myself.

The main object of subsequent antenatal hypnotic training sessions is to condition the patient to become completely relaxed, both mentally and physically, whenever she enters the trance state; to remove fear and apprehension, and to instil suggestions of confidence and general and physical well-being. This conditioning is more effective if the patient is taught auto-hypnosis and practises it regularly at home, thereby gaining much more confidence in her own power to control her reactions during the confinement.

When teaching auto-hypnosis and in the course of each ordinary hypnotic induction, it is always advisable to couple suggestions of increased relaxation with deep, rhythmic breathing. Once this technique has been mastered by the patient, it will prove invaluable in the alleviation of pain and distress during her actual labour.

The suggestions to be impressed upon the patient's mind at each training session can easily be constructed from the detailed description of labour under hypnosis which has already been given to her. These should be selected and phrased to suit each individual case, in accordance with certain general principles:

1. Suggestions that the patient will continue to keep fit and well throughout her pregnancy.

2. That she will look forward to her confinement with pleasure and happiness, and not with dread and apprehension.

3. That everything is perfectly normal (provided, of course, that this fact has been clinically established).

4. That, during her labour, she will fall into a deep hypnotic sleep whenever she is told to do so, or upon a pre-arranged signal she gives herself to induce auto-hypnosis, and all subsequent suggestions will be both accepted and acted upon.

5. That each contraction of the womb will be felt as a not altogether unpleasant sensation. Even during the second stage, the feelings experienced will be simply those of increasing pressure, comparable in every way to ordinary physical exertion.

Care must be taken not to abolish *all* her sensations, otherwise labour might well commence without the patient becoming aware of the fact.

6. That every time she puts herself into a deep hypnotic sleep, she will be able to relax her muscles and relieve tension so completely that she will

feel much less discomfort. The contractions will bother her very much less, and the delivery of the baby will become much easier.

7. That subsequently her breasts will produce plenty of milk, so that she will be able to breast-feed her child without difficulty.

This last suggestion is likely to be extremely successful since the commonest causes of deficient lactation are worry and fear. Hypnosis seems to abolish these by inducing an attitude of positive expectancy.

8. That once the confinement is over, and she has slept, she will wake up feeling perfectly fit and well, and may, if she so desires, remember little or nothing about it.

I precede these specialized suggestions by the usual ego-strengthening routine on every occasion. During the last six weeks of pregnancy, special emphasis is placed upon those suggestions relating to the patient's reactions and behaviour, and the instructions she is to follow during her confinement.

When the practitioner can not be present at the confinement, the patient can be placed post-hypnotically 'en rapport' with some other individual—doctor, nurse or midwife—with whose instructions she will comply as if they had been issued by the hypnotist. For this procedure to succeed, the deeper stages of hypnosis will have to be attained, and the individual to whom rapport is transferred fully informed as to the correct method of conducting a labour under hypnosis.

Hypnosis in Complicated or Obstructed Labour

Much has been written to advocate the use of hypnosis in obstetrics, but there are few authenticated reports of its possible dangers and disadvantages in any particular case. Attention should be drawn to certain practical difficulties that may arise in complicated cases if relations between hypnotist and obstetrician are not sufficiently close. The following case history should consequently prove of interest:

Case history. Mrs Blank, 25 years old, was referred to me on January 7th. She was expecting her first child in April and was anxious to gain any relief that hypnosis might offer her in the course of her confinement. Since there seemed to be some degree of pelvic contraction I sent her to a consultant obstetric and gynaecological surgeon, who arranged for her to be confined in the local maternity hospital. She subsequently visited me once a week for the first six weeks, and from then on once a fortnight until her confinement on April 15th.

I had no difficulty in inducing hypnosis, and by the end of several sessions she was trained to achieve reasonable depth and to enter the hypnotic state on a selected cue word. She never became completely somnambulistic, and she developed only a partial amnesia. At this depth her sensitivity to painful stimuli could be blunted but never completely abolished, so that absolute analgesia was never actually achieved.

Although I hoped to be present at her confinement, I thought it advisable to train her in auto-hypnosis. She learned the technique without difficulty and she was able, during antenatal training, to achieve complete relaxation and to gain some control over pain such as backache. But considering her repeated failure to produce satisfactory analgesia to painful stimuli artificially induced, I did not expect to be able to render her confinement completely painless, and I was doubtful as to how far she would be able to exercise her power of control over pain during labour.

At each antenatal session I continued, during hypnosis, to impress upon her the fact that she would be able during her confinement to put herself into a trance, to relax all her muscles and thus to remove her pains. She would *not*, however, be able to free herself entirely from sensations of discomfort, and she would always remain fully conscious of the pressure of her uterine contractions.

On one occasion she arrived with her arm in a sling. It appeared that she and her husband had been involved in a motor accident in which she had sustained injuries to her right arm and shoulder. When her husband extracted her from the car she was in great pain, and he went off to the nearest farm-house to seek assistance. On his return he found that she had put herself into a hypnotic trance and was completely free from pain.

The onset of labour occurred on April 14th. The patient was seen by her own doctor and admitted to hospital. When I visited her that evening she was fast asleep. I was told that she was quite comfortable, but that little progress had been made because her contractions were very poor. The following afternoon I was informed by telephone that a Caesarean section would almost certainly be necessary. The operation was performed successfully under ordinary anaesthesia and both mother and child subsequently did well.

In view of the difficulties in deciding upon surgical intervention in this case, the obstetrician involved has kindly supplied his own detailed account of the case:

Obstetrician's case history. I saw Mrs Blank on three occasions during the second half of pregnancy and she impressed me very much with her calm composure and happy anticipation of natural childbirth. She seemed entirely free from the physical and emotional strains that often complicate the antenatal period, and this may well have been partly due to her powers of inducing self-hypnosis. It became apparent from physical and X-ray examination that she was suffering from pelvic contraction which would undoubtedly lead to some degree of disproportion, but although she realized the implication of this it seemed to cause little, if any, anxiety.

Early labour. The onset of labour was marked by rupture of the membranes and regular uterine contractions which produced sensations of pressure, but no pain. It was thus difficult for her family doctor to advise that labour had started, and the same difficulty was encountered by the medical and nursing staff when she was admitted to the maternity hospital. It was unfortunate in view of the disproportion that she should suffer from primary uterine inertia with rather poor contractions, but it was confirmed by examination that labour had commenced although little progress was made during the first twenty-four hours.

Advanced labour. In order to ensure that a full trial of labour had been carried out, she was treated by an intravenous infusion of oxytocin, using 2 units in 500 ml. dextrose solution. This soon produced very strong uterine contractions which could be felt by observers, but there was still some doubt regarding their nature as Mrs Blank appeared to experience very little pain and repeatedly asked that they should be made more powerful to give her every chance of producing the baby naturally. It was only when a decision was reached some hours later that a Caesarean section would almost certainly be necessary that she lost her composure for the first time, indulging in a short fit of weeping and complaining of backache. There was still some doubt in the mind of at least one observer regarding the degree of uterine action that had in fact been achieved.

Delivery. When the uterus was explored and the baby delivered by lower segment Caesarean section, it was a surprise to find that the lower segment was very thin and that the retraction ring had risen almost to a dangerous height. It was clear that labour had advanced to a greater extent than had been apparent, due to the extreme composure of the patient and her failure to show any sign of systemic reaction to the strong contractions. There was in fact no danger to mother or child, but it is conceivable that in a multiparous patient labour might become dangerously advanced, possibly leading to some serious complications in similar circumstances.

Discussion. One difficulty of this case lay in arriving at an accurate decision as to when surgical intervention should be undertaken in the interests of both mother and child. This difficulty could have been minimized, and others eliminated, if conditions had permitted closer co-operation between us as hypnotist and obstetrician, and if it had been possible for the hospital staff to have been fully instructed regarding the changed conditions imposed by hypnosis on the course of labour.

The ideal situation would be for the obstetrician himself to undertake the induction of hypnosis and the prenatal training of the patient and to conduct the confinement. In practice one must often be content with the closest co-operation between the obstetrician and the medical hypnotist concerned. The fact that such a difficulty can arise as that in the case described above leads us to underline the positive dangers that may occur when expectant mothers are trained to produce auto-hypnosis and analgesia by unqualified hypnotists. We agree in drawing the following conclusions:

1. Where the medical hypnotist undertaking obstetric work is not himself conducting the confinement he should at all times be readily available for consultation during the labour, *and it is desirable that he should be present at the actual delivery.*

2. In complicated obstetrical cases hypnotic analgesia should only be employed after full investigations have been undertaken and when the closest co-operation between medical hypnotist and obstetrician can be ensured.

3. In multiparous or complicated obstetrical cases it is unwise and possibly dangerous to instruct the patient in the technique of auto-hypnosis unless the above safeguards can be guaranteed.

4. Whenever the technique of auto-hypnosis is taught, it is advisable that both the attending obstetrician and midwife should be warned that the signs and symptoms of maternal distress or impending catastrophe may be dangerously masked, or even absent.

5. Ideally, any physician wishing to utilize the benefits of hypnosis for patients in his special field of training should properly be the one to induce the hypnosis in the patient.

CHAPTER 22

The Hypnotic Treatment of Psychosomatic Symptoms and Psychological Illness

Both in general medical and hospital practice one regularly meets the patient who claims to be ill, suffering from a variety of pains and symptoms, although every possible investigation has failed to reveal any sign whatever of physical disease. Dealing with these people is difficult, for the doctor is usually so busy that he has little time or patience to sit and listen to an interminable list of apparently baseless complaints.

In such cases it is generally considered that the patient is either ' putting it on ' or is imagining his aches and pains. Consequently his friends and relatives, and sometimes even his doctor, tell him to pull himself together and snap out of it: to use a little will-power and he will soon be well again. Such advice is useless and it is likely to do more harm than good. The patient is seldom believed when he says that he has often tried without success, yet this is undoubtedly true. The fact that he has always failed despite every effort has only increased his feelings of hopelessness, and he no longer knows where to turn for help.

Let us examine this question more closely. Under normal circumstances, the self-starter of a motor-car is only used for a few seconds to start up the engine. If this can only be kept running by constant use of the self-starter, then there is something wrong. The battery will eventually become so run-down that the self-starter will no longer work. Similarly, when an individual can only keep going through the excessive use of will-power there is something wrong that requires investigation. Failing this, prolonged efforts to continue working are certain to lead to complete break-down. The fallacy of the assumption that the neurotic patient will not try to help herself was once expressed by a famous physician in the following terms: ' The patient says that she cannot— the nurse says that she will not—the truth is that she *cannot will.*'

T. A. Ross pointed out that there is no such thing as an imaginary pain, and that when a person complains of pain he is either suffering from real pain or he is lying about it. In the latter case, he is malingering.

But it is absurd to suggest that all patients with complaints for which there is no apparent physical basis fall into this category. The truth is that *pain, indistinguishable from that caused by physical ailments, can arise solely from psychological disturbances.* This can be shown convincingly by a simple hypnotic experiment:

A subject is hypnotized so deeply that he develops a complete amnesia for everything that occurs during the trance state. He is then given the post-hypnotic suggestion that, after he wakes up, he will be unable to move his left arm, which will be completely paralysed. He is also told that when anyone else tries to raise it for him he will experience severe pain in his shoulder. When he is awakened, he will not remember anything that has been said to him. He will consequently express the greatest surprise and concern when he finds that he cannot move his left arm. And should anyone try to lift his paralysed arm, his reactions and the expression on his face will leave no room for doubt as to the reality of the pain he is feeling.

Three important conclusions can be drawn from this experiment:

1. The paralysis and susceptibility to pain have been produced by the fact that an implicit belief has been implanted in the subject's mind that they are bound to happen.

2. In the waking state, the subject has no idea that any such belief does exist in his mind, and has no conscious knowledge of the incident that planted it in his unconscious mind.

3. The pain that he felt when he was wide awake again was just as real as if it had been caused by some physical disability.

Many other neurotic symptoms such as headaches, sickness, dyspnoea and itching, with which the general practitioner is painfully familiar, arise from unconscious beliefs and ideas in the patient's mind. One of the objects of modern psychological treatment is to discover the kind of unconscious beliefs and ideas that underlie the patient's symptoms and the manner in which they arose in any given case. When these hidden facts can be brought into the patient's consciousness, he will understand for the first time how and why his illness occurred, and this insight usually speeds up the removal of his symptoms.

An important question remains to be answered. How does the neurotic patient acquire these unconscious beliefs and ideas? In the experiment just described they were introduced by a hypnotist; it is unlikely that they normally result from auto-suggestion, since we are all capable at times of suggesting things to ourselves without developing neurotic symptoms.

Many pioneers in the psychological field tried to shed light upon this problem. Pierre Janet's conclusion that most neurotic symptoms had a hidden meaning was paralleled by Charcot's very apposite quotation from Shakespeare: 'Though this be madness, yet there's method in it.' But it was Breuer's work, about 1880, that provided the missing clue. He described how one of his patients, during a hypnotic trance, began spontaneously to talk about her symptoms in the minutest detail. The remarkable fact was that once she had unburdened herself of everything connected with a particular symptom, *while simultaneously giving vent to the feelings that were originally connected with the episode*, the symptom usually disappeared. Subsequently Freud questioned all his patients under hypnosis, about the origin of their symptoms, and since his results confirmed those obtained by Breuer, they jointly published papers on their work. In these they expressed the opinion that the recovery of such buried memories removed the emotion that was originally attached to them. Since they considered that the patient was being purged of the casual emotion, they called the process *abreaction*, or the working off of suppressed emotion.

Bernheim, in France, hypnotized a subject so deeply that he produced a complete amnesia for the events of the trance state, and gave him the post-hypnotic suggestion: 'When the clock strikes twelve, you will open the window.' He awakened the subject who opened the window promptly when the clock struck twelve. Bernheim asked why he had done this. Because of his amnesia the subject was unable to give the true reply and instead gave an explanation entirely satisfactory to himself: 'I thought it was getting too hot in here.' Bernheim insisted that this was not the correct reason, and told the subject that he would be able to remember the real one if only he tried hard enough. He continued to urge the subject to greater and greater efforts until he finally succeeded in eliciting the recollection of the original instruction. In this way, he had managed to connect an idea that was formerly unconscious with the main stream of consciousness, so that eventually the subject was able to admit that he knew he had been told to open the window.

Freud, who knew of Bernheim's experiment, realized that one could never accept the patient's own explanation of his illness because he was consciously unaware of the real cause of his symptoms, which was locked away deeply in his unconscious mind. But even more important, Freud had discovered how to rescue such ideas from oblivion. *One must persist and persist until the barrier is finally broken down.*

However, Freud's new method was not as successful as he had hoped, since too few patients could achieve the necessary depth of hypnosis. For this reason he discarded hypnosis altogether and allowed the patient to talk at random, telling everything that came into his mind whether it seemed to be significant or not. The patient was warned not to criticize, but to speak aloud each successive thought as it came into his mind. These free-associations gradually but invariably led to the origin of the symptom. He soon found that the very things of which the patient was most reluctant to speak were those of most importance in the causation of his illness, and that the so-called free-associations were not really free, but were determined by unconscious material that had to be analysed and interpreted.

The more Freud explored the mind by means of these free-associations —*psycho-analysis*—the more he wondered why patients ever lost track of their forgotten experiences. He eventually discovered that the memory of such experiences was painful, terrifying or humiliating to the patient. Indeed, many of our own lapses of memory may be explained by their connection with something that we do not care to remember, since recollection would be both painful and distressing.

This often occurs in certain mental conflicts. We refuse to solve them on the conscious plane because whatever solution we arrived at would be unpleasant. This form of forgetting is known as *repression*. It is a commonplace occurrence in every normal individual, but plays a tremendously important part in the causation of neurotic illness. Repression is the process whereby painful or unpleasant memories, together with their attached emotions and associations, are thrust out of consciousness and buried deeply in the unconscious mind where they become entirely forgotten and inaccessible.

We can find many examples of this mechanism operating in everyday life. We receive bills by the morning post and put them aside, fully intending to pay them the same night. Yet we forget them completely, and at the end of a week they are still unpaid. But the cheques we received by the same post are rarely overlooked, and are usually paid into the bank without delay. We also tend to forget to post other people's letters, but seldom forget to post our own no matter how busy we may be.

Even in such trivial cases of forgetting (through repression) a conflict arises between the conscious and the unconscious parts of the mind. The conscious mind tries to remember, while the unconscious mind successfully opposes all its efforts on the grounds that the matter is either unpleasant or troublesome, and consequently must not be remembered.

In neurotic illness with the development of psychosomatic symptoms, the mechanism is of the greatest significance and acts in the following way:

The patient is faced with some intolerably difficult situation in his everyday life which he just can't cope with. The tensions that this sets up in his mind cause so much anxiety that he has to find some way of escape, so he pushes it out of his conscious mind and escapes from it that way. This is what we call *repression*. Not only does he forget his present difficulties, but he simultaneously represses all strong emotions associated with them to which he was unable to react adequately at the time. This repressed emotion underlying his conflict provides the energy that is constantly trying to force it back into consciousness. On no account must this be allowed to happen since it could only cause mental pain and distress. So when repression can no longer hold it back, this energy becomes diverted into another channel and discharges itself in the form of physical symptoms.

In this way, psychosomatic symptoms arise as a defence against intolerable anxiety. It is hardly surprising that they are often so difficult to get rid of no matter how incapacitating they may be, since unconsciously they serve a useful purpose. It is important to realize that it is not the act of repression itself that causes the trouble, for *it is only when repression threatens to become ineffective that the physical symptoms arise*. In the more severe psychoneuroses it is usually some frightening and highly emotional experience that has become repressed, often dating back to the patient's early childhood.

When treatment succeeds in restoring the buried memories to consciousness and this is accompanied by a working-off of the emotions to which the patient was unable to give vent at the time, complete recovery usually follows. If abreactive techniques are used, this may occasionally be dramatic. The recovery of the buried memories alone, however, if unaccompanied by an adequate emotional response is not likely to bring the patient relief from his symptoms. Drug abreactions, hypnotic abreactions, hypno-analysis and even psycho-analysis are different psychiatric methods of tackling this fundamental problem.

There is hardly a physical symptom encountered in organic disease that could not originate at times from psychological disturbances. What, then, determines the appearance of one symptom rather than another in any particular case?

Many healthy individuals entertain a secret fear that some day they might contract a specific illness. The business man whose brother died unexpectedly from a coronary attack will be most likely to produce cardiac symptoms himself, should he subsequently develop a neurosis. At other times, the symptom may be connected with the patient's own emotional reaction to difficulties that he is reluctant to admit, even to himself. A husband is most unlikely to say that he feels ill because his wife's behaviour gives him a pain in the neck; instead he will complain of a functional torticollis. Similarly, a wife will never say that her husband is so exasperating at times that she could scratch his eyes out; she will suffer from a severe neurodermatitis with intolerable itching which she is able to scratch to her heart's content.

The protective function of symptoms is commonly seen. The business executive would rather develop a duodenal ulcer and blame it for his inefficiency than admit that his responsibilities are getting too much for him. A woman will develop a headache that prevents her from going to tea with an acquaintance for whom she does not care. But the headache and the ulcers are real enough; they have been unconsciously produced so as to avoid a situation that was unpleasant, while simultaneously concealing the real reason for distress.

Besides the knowledge of these mechanisms, one must also understand how a neurotic illness develops in the first place, and why its duration is so often prolonged. From the moment of birth, life demands continual re-adjustment to changes in our environment. A man's capacity for this adjustment depends on factors which may relate to his early infancy. A normal person, in this context is one capable of making this continual adjustment to himself and his environment without causing distress to himself or others. A neurotic person is one who is continually mal-adjusted to his environment, and it is this flaw in his capacity to respond adequately to changing circumstances that is the root cause of his illness.

Neurotic illness always represents an unconscious escape through illness from the difficulties, real or imaginary, that life has to offer. The important thing to realize is the fact that, to the neurotic, imaginary difficulties are just as real as if they actually existed.

A man capable of standing up to his difficulties directly, even if he fails to resolve them, will not become ill and will retain his self-respect. A man who continually evades them is certain to lose it in the end. The neurotic patient knows this as well as anyone, and adopts a different solution altogether. He becomes ill, so that at one stroke he not only avoids facing up to his problems, but also succeeds in retaining his self-respect, since nobody expects a sick man to be able to cope with difficulties. This is an entirely unconscious solution as the patient never realizes that his illness has enabled him to escape from anything, so it is wrong to regard him as a malingerer.

Onę should never condemn the neurotic for solving his problems in this way. Even the strongest of us has his 'breaking-point' when subjected to sufficient stress and strain. Most neurotics have a strong sense of inferiority and are certainly less adequately equipped to face life's difficulties than the average healthy individual. They tend to reach their breaking-point with surprising rapidity. There is no question of blaming them for this. In childhood they may have had the kind of up-bringing which has never given them the chance to learn to adjust.

The reason why neurosis is so difficult to cure is that the patient always gains some unconscious advantage from his illness: recovery would force him to face up to those very difficulties from which his illness provides a temporary refuge. *The neurotic feels that nobody understands him and is constantly seeking for someone who will listen to him sympathetically.* If you are prepared to fulfil this role, one of the greater obstacles to his recovery will disappear.

Encourage him to tell you his troubles in his own words, and you should not interrupt him until he has finished his story. Then question him closely about his domestic circumstances, business relationships and possible financial worries. He will rarely mention these himself since he is convinced that his illness is a physical one, so they will consequently seem to have no significance.

He must be assured that everything he says will be treated in strict confidence. His anxieties will sometimes revolve around such intimate matters that he will subsequently feel ashamed at having discussed them. For this reason, you should never criticize or express disapproval of his behaviour, however shocking it may have been. At this point, if he is to unburden himself freely, morals and ethics must not be allowed to come into the picture. You must, however, do all that you can to encourage his self-respect, but you must never let him feel that you consider yourself to be superior in any way. He is already painfully aware of his own feelings of inferiority, and much harm can be done by rubbing it in.

It is wrong and harmful to tell him to pull himself together, or that recovery depends upon himself. He will then become convinced that he is being completely misunderstood, and any power you may have had to influence him will vanish immediately. You must also remember that his pains and symptoms are real and not imaginary, and that he is suffering just as much as if they were caused by organic disease. The neurotic patient can only be helped if the reality of his sufferings is accepted. Only genuine sympathy, tolerance and a better understanding of his difficulties will really assist him on the long road to recovery.

The Use of Hypnosis in Psychosomatic and Neurotic Conditions

Unless he possesses a sound working knowledge of both normal and abnormal psychology, the general practitioner must obviously exercise the greatest care in selecting the cases he is going to treat by hypnosis. The mechanisms that have just been discussed should make it clear that indiscriminate symptom-removal is not without its dangers. Neurotic symptoms that seem to be purely physical in nature are neither chaotic or meaningless. They are often the surface expressions of deep, fundamental conflicts, and the removal of such symptoms alone resembles blowing away the smoke instead of seeking and putting out the fire. An imaginary example can be quoted to illustrate the importance of this:

Suppose a patient becomes afraid that he might one day commit suicide. Every time he sees a knife, he becomes terrified lest he should give way to this impulse. He subsequently has a slight fall or accident and bruises his right arm. Despite the trivial nature of this injury, his right arm and hand become completely paralysed. This, of course, is a hysterical paralysis. But note that as long as he cannot use his arm or hand, he will lose his fear of knives completely and will no longer feel in danger of taking his own life. He will consequently repress and forget all his old fears and will worry instead about the incapacity caused by his paralysis.

A hypnotist might easily succeed in removing the paralysis quickly and dramatically by the use of hypnotic suggestion alone. However the patient has been summarily stripped of his only defence against intolerable anxiety, and before long all his old fears and impulses will return. If he is not given further treatment, the so-called cure will probably result in yet another suicide since the patient will end up by cutting his throat.

In general practice it is usually unwise to try to tackle cases that fall into this category. The release of anxiety following the removal of the defensive symptoms calls for expert psychiatric knowledge and treatment. However, many of the milder psychosomatic and neurotic conditions fall well within the scope of the general practitioner. Deep psychotherapy is not necessarily required, and questioning in the hypnotic state will often suffice to reveal the superficial conflicts underlying the illness. Once the patient realizes these and is encouraged to face his real difficulties, his condition will rapidly improve.

One thing must be clearly understood. If you do decide to treat such cases by hypnosis, you are liable to become involved in any situation that may subsequently arise. Even in mild cases the symptom is a defence against something with which the patient cannot cope, and its mere removal may lead to a recurrence of anxiety. He will be in no better position to deal with this anxiety than before, so if you are not prepared to continue to help him—don't use hypnosis.

The treatment of many of the psychosomatic conditions that respond satisfactorily to hypnosis has already been described, but some of the less severe neurotic illnesses can also be treated with safety. Great discrimination, however, must always be exercised in making the choice.

Anxiety states. Hypnosis can be extremely useful in the milder cases, particularly those in which lack of self-confidence, excessive self-consciousness and a hesitancy to meet other people are prominent symptoms. Mild phobic and tension states also will often respond well to treatment. But the more severe anxiety states with profound phobias and obsessions should always be avoided as their treatment will present too many difficult problems and will be too time-consuming for the general practitioner. They should be left to the psychiatrist.

Hysteria and hysterical symptoms. Whenever deep hypnosis can be achieved, it is easy to get rid of hysterical symptoms such as paralyses or contractures, even long-standing ones; indeed recovery is often dramatic. The temptation to treat these cases should be resisted, however, for the deep underlying conflicts that may be uncovered will require expert psychiatric treatment.

The dental surgeon also would be wise to avoid using hypnosis in the hysterical type of patient, even though his sole purpose is the production of analgesia. He might not only find himself in grave difficulties, but could easily become subject to totally unfounded accusations.

Obsessional states. The treatment of these is always difficult and often unsatisfactory. In my experience, hypnosis is seldom more successful than other methods of treatment, and since an analytical approach is necessary, these cases are best considered unsuitable.

Depressions. It is not easy to assess the degree of suicidal risk involved in depressional states. Danger lies in the fact that it may be much less in the deeply depressed patient who has become lethargic and apathetic, than in milder, ambulant cases that have retained initiative. I consider that hypnosis should *never* be used in depressional states in which suicidal impulses are present unless the patient is an in-patient under hospital supervision, when it can safely be employed in conjunction with other measures. In the absence of suicidal impulses, it can be effectively used along with the anti-depressive drugs, provided that the patient can be kept under a reasonable degree of observation.

Hypnosis in Simple Psychotherapy

This will usually be the method of choice for the general practitioner who wishes to treat psychological conditions. Many different techniques are available, but I propose to deal only with those that are most applicable in general practice.

The first step in the treatment of the neurotic patient is to try to discover the probable cause of his disorder. Careful case-taking, followed by simple questioning under hypnosis, will usually shed a good deal of light upon causation. It is also important to try to form some opinion of the patient's individual assets and liabilities. Treatment is then aimed at helping the patient to regulate his life, and restoring his ability to cope with it. No attempt whatever is made to alter his personality —simply to modify his reactions to his difficulties. Several different methods of approach can help considerably in the accomplishment of this task.

Guidance. The neurotic patient is usually a rather helpless and inadequate individual with a strong feeling of inferiority. Because he lacks the capacity to adjust himself to circumstances, he finds that he cannot cope with life's difficulties on his own. He is consequently always looking for someone in authority to help him solve his problems.

He may need advice about his job. He may have difficulties arising from his relationships with business colleagues, friends, relatives or his wife and children. He will often display faulty attitudes towards sex and marriage that will need correction. Often he will tend to isolate himself and withdraw from other people. It will then be necessary to encourage him to take up some hobby, recreation or social activity that will take him amongst others, to counteract this tendency and widen his interests.

Many of these matters will naturally be discussed and suitable advice given in the waking state, and appropriate suggestions during hypnosis can be used to emphasize it and help the patient to act upon it more readily. The ego-strengthening routine will form a sound basis for treatment and should be extended to include any specific suggestions required in each case. It is most important to avoid a dictatorial attitude, for a persuasive approach is much more likely to succeed.

Reassurance. This is always necessary in every form of psychotherapy. The neurotic patient has worried about his symptoms until they have become grossly exaggerated and have caused numerous fears to arise. But he will usually accept reassurance from a doctor whom he believes to be sincere and to possess the necessary knowledge to understand his complaints. Such reassurance will naturally be accepted more rapidly in the hypnotic than in the waking state.

Most neurotic patients are afraid that their symptoms are caused by some serious organic disease. There are few who are not secretly afraid that, should their worries continue indefinitely, they will eventually become insane. Others dread the results of masturbation, or of sexual impulses and relationships. All these various fears will have to be dealt with by the strongest reassurance.

Persuasion. This involves the correction of the patient's mistaken ideas regarding his illness by appealing to his reason and intelligence. He is shown that he has been thinking along the wrong lines, and an attempt is made to convince him of the real nature of his illness and the way in which it arose. The true facts of the case are placed before him, and he is shown that there is no reason for him to continue to be ill. Once he begins to think in terms of getting well he will begin to improve: as long as he remains convinced that he will continue to suffer pain or other symptoms the more he will be bound to feel them. When ideas of health can be instilled into his mind ideas of disease will disappear.

Reconditioning. This technique is generally used when dealing with habits which the patient finds difficult to break, such as excessive smoking, over-indulgence in alcohol, over-eating, nail-biting and bed-wetting. The object is to replace the satisfaction derived from such habits with unpleasant emotions or experiences. This greatly assists the patient in his efforts to give them up. Even when this procedure is used, it is still necessary to try to supply or increase the patient's motivation to get rid of his habit.

Reconditioning will seldom succeed when the symptom has a strong defensive value against anxiety unless the patient has first gained some emotional insight into his difficulties.

CHAPTER 23

Hypno-analysis and Analytical Psychotherapy

We have seen how, in psychosomatic, neurotic and psychoneurotic illness, the patient's symptoms are maintained as a defence against unconscious mental conflicts, which may be either superficial or deep. The problem, particularly in the more severe cases, is to 'uncover' these conflicts and the associated emotional difficulties underlying the illness, and to help the patient to recognize and deal with them.

As I have already pointed out, many of the milder psychosomatic and neurotic illnesses, where the conflicts involved are relatively superficial and amenable to some of the simpler forms of investigation, can be treated successfully by the general practitioner. Others, however, arising from deeper conflicts and personality defects, will require a more penetrating form of analysis, conducted in accordance with orthodox psycho-analytical principles. The object is to purge the unconscious of repressed inner strivings and conflicts often arising from inimical experiences and conditionings in the past, so that the individual is no longer threatened by anxiety and his ego is strengthened to the point where it can cope realistically with both external and internal stresses. Psycho-analytic therapy thus involves a drastic re-organization of the patient's psychic apparatus so that, freed from the need to maintain repression, he is enabled to adapt himself to reality and to fulfil his basic psychological needs. Unfortunately, psycho-analysis has to be continued over long periods of time, even years, because of the patient's resistance to abandoning his defences or relinquishing the advantages he is deriving from his neurosis.

Obviously, the scope of psycho-analysis is strictly limited in private practice by the expense and duration of the treatment and in out-patient clinics by the time-factor. Moreover, although the root causes of the patient's illness are to be found in the past, many of the immediate difficulties for which he is anxiously seeking relief are situated in the present. Consequently, the ideal treatment would be relatively short, a matter of months rather than years, and would afford the patient speedy relief from his symptoms through the alleviation of his current problems.

It would also deal to a limited extent with some of the personality problems that have contributed to his illness.

Such a treatment has not yet been discovered, but there is little doubt that hypnotherapy and hypno-analysis constitute the nearest approach. Even Freud in his later years indicated that the eventual solution to the problem might well lie within the field of hypnosis.

Unfortunately, many psycho-analysts object to short-term psychotherapy on the grounds that it leaves the deepest personality problems untouched. Wolberg, however, has pointed out that psychotherapy is no mining operation that depends for its results entirely upon excavated psychic ore. He defines it as a human interaction embracing a variety of dimensions, psychological and social, verbal and non-verbal. Such complex elements as ' *faith* ', ' *hope* ', ' *trust* ', ' *acquisition of insight* ', ' *restoration of confidence and self-control* ', ' *self-realization* ', and the ' *development of the capacity to love* ' all enter into it. This probably explains the value of the regular use of an ' ego-strengthening' technique at the beginning of each hypnotherapeutic session.

Although in short-term psychotherapy we are mainly dealing with immediate and superficial problems, we may still succeed in influencing the total personality in depth, including the unconscious. Indeed, the human warmth and feeling experienced by a patient in a single session with a sympathetic therapist may often achieve more profound alterations than years of probing by a detached therapist intent upon wearing out resistance. Nor is the unconscious being entirely neglected, for even during short-term therapy, repressed psychic material may still be uncovered and dealt with.

Nevertheless, in short-term therapy we must be prepared to accept limited goals. It requires a great deal of time to alter deep-seated personality problems, and thus we may have to content ourselves with the immediate objective of symptom-relief and rehabilitation of the patient. Wolberg considers that we can reasonably expect short-term psychotherapy to succeed in achieving the following results in the average patient:

1. The relief of symptoms.
2. Restoration to the level of functioning that existed prior to the present illness.
3. An understanding of some of the forces that precipitated the illness.
4. Recognition of some of the personality defects that prevent the patient from adjusting to himself and to his environment.

5. A knowledge of how these arose from past experiences and child-hood conditionings.

6. Recognition of the relationship between such defects and the present illness.

If these tasks are successfully accomplished (and they may be considerably facilitated by the employment of hypno-analysis), we may often expect even greater developments as the patient applies himself to making the necessary adjustments he has learned during treatment.

Hypno-analysis, like psycho-analysis, can be divided into two stages. The first is analytic and relates to the uncovering of unconscious fears, impulses and memories and the way in which they prevent the patient from adjusting to himself and his surroundings. The second stage is synthetic in the sense that through insight and re-education the patient is helped to establish new habits of thought, new patterns of behaviour, and consequently to build up his self-confidence and control in order to face life anew. We must remember, however, that hypno-analysis differs from psycho-analysis in that *the therapist must on no account remain passive.* In any form of short-term therapy, one cannot permit the patient to become bogged down in resistance until somehow or other he muddles through. Resistances have to be dealt with by an active frontal attack before they paralyse progress, and it is in situations such as these that hypnosis can prove invaluable.

Regarding the selection of cases for hypnotherapy or short-term psychotherapy, Wolberg considers it best to assume that every patient is capable of benefiting from short-term treatment unless he proves refractory to it. If the therapist approaches each patient with the intention of doing as much as he can in up to 20 sessions, he will enable the patient to take advantage of short-term therapy up to the limit of his ability to profit therefrom. Should this fail to produce the necessary degree of improvement, prolonged therapy can always follow.

At this point, I should like to make it clear that in advocating the use of hypno-analysis in psychiatric work, I am not trying to peddle a new and original treatment. I am simply trying to show how the treatment of certain selected cases can be facilitated and shortened by the use of hypnosis. Indeed, the methods employed are largely those with which psychiatrists are already well-acquainted. They can, however, be rendered more rapid and effective through the simultaneous use of the hypnotic state and certain of its special techniques.

Whenever it is proposed to use hypno-analysis, it is always advisable to induce as deep a hypnotic state as possible. With gradual training, many patients can be taught to enter a sufficiently deep trance to permit the use of some, if not all, of the following techniques. The best results will naturally be obtained when the hypnosis is deep enough to enable the patient to recover forgotten memories of his earlier life or childhood. It will be much easier for him to do this if he is able to develop a post-hypnotic amnesia, which will temporarily protect him from the unpleasant necessity of having to face up to painful memories and experiences upon awakening. These can subsequently be restored to consciousness, as and when he feels strong enough to cope with them. In inducing such an amnesia, I rarely use direct suggestion. I find it more effective to employ a permissive method. During the trance, I tell the patient that after he awakens, *he will be able to remember just as much as he wishes, but that anything that he does not want to remember, he will be able to forget.*

Some hypno-analytical methods—free association, dream induction and automatic writing—often need only a light or medium trance. Other procedures such as hypnotic drawing, play therapy, dramatic recall, crystal- or mirror-gazing, age-regression and experimental conflicts will invariably require deep or somnambulistic trances. It is always imperative, however, that the patient should be able to talk and answer questions during hypnosis without awakening from the trance.

More detailed descriptions of the following techniques may be found in the many publications of Wolberg, Erickson and others.

Free Association

The induction of the hypnotic state itself will often remove many resistances to free association. The material tends to flow much more readily and a single session will often produce more information than several in the waking state. Medium-depth hypnosis will sometimes suffice, but the deeper the trance the more easily will resistance be overcome.

The patient is told to allow his mind to wander and to report each consecutive thought or idea that enters his mind, no matter how trivial or irrelevant it may seem. Some apparently insignificant things are often most important, so he must not withhold anything at all. Should he feel reluctant to talk, he is to mention it and describe any emotions such as fear or resentment that he may be feeling at the time.

The analyst should listen passively and avoid interrupting the patient's train of thought. But he should note carefully not only what the patient says but how he says it, for his mood, facial expression and tone of voice will often betray the presence of conflicts that he has not thought fit to mention. Should this occur, his attention should be drawn to his behaviour and he should be questioned about it in order to direct his further associations into the required channel.

Not every patient will display the same ability to express thoughts freely, without restraint. It may sometimes be very difficult, for such thoughts are often distressing recollections or things that the patient feels too ashamed to mention. Only training will enable him to learn how to associate freely. Occasionally encouragement and even urgent commands from the analyst will not succeed in overcoming the block in his associations. In such cases, one may try to circumvent the resistance by placing one's hand on the patient's forehead and telling him that at the count of five he will think of a word or get a mental picture of something connected with the material under discussion.

Dream Induction

The patient may be stimulated to dream on command during the hypnotic session, or it may be suggested to him post-hypnotically that he will dream at night during his normal sleep. The nature of the problems to be dreamed about can be suggested. Hypnotic dreams have all the characteristics of spontaneous dreams, and are dynamically just as significant. Wolberg emphasizes the fact that the dreams that follow the first attempts at hypnosis are tremendously significant and often contain the essence of the patient's problem.

Either a medium or deep trance will usually be necessary and the patient gradually trained to develop this ability to dream in response to hypnotic suggestion. At first it is probably best to suggest during hypnosis that he will have a dream the same night, during his sleep, and that he will report it at his next session. If successful these instructions are repeated, but in addition the patient will be instructed to dream about a specific subject. He is then told that he will have a dream immediately before awakening from his trance. Finally, he is instructed to dream during his trance and to relate it and discuss it without waking up.

Dreams that are revealed under hypnosis should not usually be interpreted in the waking state. The patient will often be able to interpret his own spontaneous or hypnotic dreams much more accurately while in a trance, since the dream symbolism is much more apparent during the hypnotic state.

Automatic Writing

The technique of automatic writing is taught by placing a pencil in the patient's hand during his trance and suggesting that his hand and arm feel as if they are completely detached and no longer belong to him. It is then suggested that his hand will begin to write and will move along quite automatically so that he will not be aware of what he is writing.

The product of such writing is usually quite different from the patient's normal writing. It is often quite undecipherable. Letters are badly formed, words run together and sentences are incomplete and fragmented. Whenever the patient is able to open his eyes without awakening from his trance, he can be instructed to write the full meaning of his communication underneath the automatic writing. If he is unable to open his eyes without awakening, he can be given the post-hypnotic suggestion that the meaning of his automatic writing will be quite clear to him after he awakens. It is always best to let the patient translate it for himself since he alone is able to supply the material that has been omitted or condensed beyond recognition.

Although the first attempts may end in failure, gradual training may often result in success. Some patients can acquire the technique in very light trances. A few may even be able to write automatically upon suggestion in the waking state. The disadvantage is that such patients may be quite unable to give the real meaning of their communications, which would only become apparent in the deep hypnotic state.

Hypnotic Drawing

The best results will only be obtained when the patient can achieve a somnambulistic trance in which he is able to open his eyes without awakening. He may either be instructed to draw whatever he likes, or subjects may be suggested to him by the therapist.

In his drawings, the patient may reveal unconscious attitudes towards members of his family, his wife and children or even the physician. Sometimes he can be requested to illustrate some specific dream or experience that he has had. Even more information can often be obtained if the patient is asked to make up a story about his drawing.

The technique of hypnotic drawing may also be advantageously combined with age-regression. Under these circumstances the patient will frequently be able to express in his drawings attitudes and feelings that are deeply repressed at the adult level.

Play Therapy

Again the patient must be able to open his eyes and handle the materials without awakening from his trance. Many of the resistances that adults display towards play therapy are eliminated in the hypnotic state. Indeed, as soon as the patient realizes that he is not expected to remain passive, and need not wait for directions from the therapist, he usually plays with the materials with great enthusiasm. Play therapy is particularly useful to the patient as a means of expressing unconscious aggression or jealousy towards parents or other children.

The usual equipment consists of a series of dolls representing an adult man and woman, an old man and woman, a boy and a girl about 10 years of age, a boy and a girl of 4, and a baby. Various animals, articles of furniture (including a bed large enough to accommodate the dolls), trains, cars, guns, soldiers, together with crayons, paper and pencils are useful additions. 'Plasticine' may often afford the patient useful outlet for displaying aggressive or destructive tendencies. The patient should be told to play or build as he likes and to talk about what he is doing. Sometimes the therapist himself will select what is to be used, and will suggest situations based upon material that has been obtained through free association. The patient projects his feelings on to the dolls because he is able, in this way, to dissociate himself from them.

When information is required about conflicts from which the patient suffered in childhood, play therapy can usefully be employed at regressed age levels. Whenever one has gained a general idea of the chief incidents in the patient's life, regression to the age at which these incidents occurred and setting the stage with appropriate materials, will greatly facilitate the therapeutic process.

Dramatic Techniques

In deep hypnosis the waking resistances to dramatization are readily removed. The patient is instructed to reproduce traumatic incidents and to act out emotional situations and experiences as if he were living through them once again. He usually does this so vividly that he feels as though he were actually participating in the experience. Indeed the emotional reaction may be so intense that considerable abreaction may be achieved.

The best example of dramatization used in this way is found in the treatment of war neuroses. When the patient is told to relive the traumatic scene, he responds with intense fear and rage in a most realistic manner. He will often scream with terror or pain, and will vigorously protect himself by shooting or bayoneting his enemies. Occasionally the same reaction may be produced in re-enacting traumatic incidents that have occurred in civilian life. When it is possible to regress the patient to the age or period at which he suffered the traumatic experience, this technique will become even more effective.

Sometimes the analyst remains passive after setting the scene and encouraging the patient to re-enact the incident, at other times he may have to take a more active role and represent one of the characters in the dramatic scene. Dramatics are particularly successful in affording the patient the opportunity to express repressed aggression.

Regression

During hypnosis, two distinct types of regression may be induced. In the first type, the patient acts in accordance with his current adult conception of himself at an earlier age period. He behaves as he believes he would have done as a child of the suggested age level. This is consequently a simulated reproduction of a past period of life.

The second type is entirely different both in character and in significance. This involves an actual return to an earlier age period, with a true revivification of the same patterns of behaviour that originally existed at that particular time. It does not depend upon current memories, recollections or reconstructions of a bygone age. It is as though the present and all life's experiences subsequent to the suggested age have been blotted out completely. This will include the hypnotist himself, who will consequently have to assume the role of someone known to the patient during this earlier period, such as a teacher, a relative or a neighbour, for it will obviously be difficult for the patient to converse with someone he will not meet until years later on. This is regression in a true sense, and in this state the patient is able to recapture memories and relive events and impulses that have long been forgotten and repressed.

Regression may often be usefully combined with other hypno-analytical techniques such as dream induction, play therapy, drawing, dramatics, automatic writing and crystal- or mirror-gazing. When these methods are employed at a regressed age level, material emerges that would otherwise be quite unobtainable at an adult age level.

A somnambulistic trance is usually essential and post-hypnotic amnesia can be a great asset. There are two main methods of producing regression:

1. The patient is slowly disorientated as to time and place, first as regards the day of the week, then the week itself, and finally the month and the year. When he is sufficiently confused, he is re-orientated to any desired period of his life. When it is necessary to investigate any particular symptom, he is told to remember and to live through the time when he first developed the symptom.

2. In very good subjects, the patient may be brought directly to the required age level without this preliminary disorientation. He is told that he is going back into the past and that he will feel as if he were once again living in the periods suggested to him. As he goes back, he will feel himself getting smaller and smaller. His arms and legs are getting smaller and smaller, and he is going back to the time when he was ten years old. As soon as he feels that he is exactly ten years old, he is to raise his hand.

Before awakening the patient, it is always best to tell him that he will forget everything that has occurred. The memories and material that have been recovered may be too distressing and painful for him to face right away in the waking state. He can be told that as soon as he feels able to tolerate this material, he will gradually bring it back into consciousness.

Crystal- and Mirror-gazing

This technique can only be employed when the patient enters a sufficiently deep hypnotic state to permit him to open his eyes without awakening. The patient is told that he will be able to open his eyes and see quite clearly, although he will still remain deeply asleep. He will look into the crystal or mirror (which is so placed as to reflect a blank ceiling), and will see things before him. He is then instructed to describe exactly what he sees.

In this connection, it is interesting to note that *imaginative aids are often more effective than material procedures*. Indeed, it has been found that on numerous occasions, when a patient has been instructed to imagine himself or visualize himself looking into a crystal ball or mirror, much better results were obtained.

This technique is often extremely successful in recovering buried memories. The patient will frequently be able to reconstruct scenes from his past life by hallucinating them exactly as they occurred. These arise more readily since the patient is dissociating himself from them and describing events as if he were watching actors on a stage. Nevertheless, intense emotional reactions are often associated with the recall of such material, and a considerable degree of abreaction can sometimes be produced.

Experimental Conflicts

Many patients have so rationalized their behaviour that they are unwilling to admit that anything can influence their conduct outside of awareness. They greatly resent the fact that they have impulses of which they are ashamed. Consequently, no matter how convincing the evidence may be, they firmly refuse to admit it. In these cases, the induction of an experimental conflict will often succeed in demonstrating to the patient the influence exerted by his own unconscious mind, and enable him to gain insight when every other method has failed.

The object is to show the patient how unconscious impulses and emotions can actually cause his symptoms to arise. For instance, situations may occur from time to time that cause the patient to feel hostility which his circumstances forbid him to express. He consequently turns this hostility back on himself and develops a psychosomatic symptom. During his treatment he may become aware of the fact that he feels hostile, and yet be quite incapable of realizing that this suppressed hostility is actually producing his symptom.

The technique involves the creation of an experimental conflict during the hypnotic state, which must be deep enough to ensure post-hypnotic amnesia. An entirely fictitious situation is suggested to him that will arouse hostility that he will be unable to express, possibly one in which he has been unfairly treated. He will feel this emotion acutely, but will be unable to give vent to it and will have to suppress it. The patient is then told that when he has awakened, this situation will come to mind. He will not consciously know what it is, but it will still be on his mind. It will worry him and influence his actions and his speech, but he will be quite unaware that it is doing so. When he wakens the unconscious conflict that is thus provoked will produce the same psychosomatic symptoms that arise whenever he spontaneously feels hostility. In this way, it becomes possible to demonstrate to the patient how certain emotions are responsible for his symptoms. Finally, an explanation may be given to the patient, in a further trance state, of the meaning of this experimental conflict. Directions to recall it in the waking state will often give him considerable insight into his problem.

Principles Underlying Special Hypno-analytical Techniques

Hypnosis is a state which easily lends itself to the production of 'dissociative' phenomena even in normal subjects, and these can be employed very effectively in exploratory, in confronting, and in therapeutic ways in hypnotherapy and hypno-analysis. Dr Erika Fromm gives a clear account of the principles involved. She points out that the major areas of dissociation commonly used for this purpose are:

1. Dissociating the 'observing' ego from the 'experiencing' ego.
2. De-egotizing parts of the body to express unconscious wishes, thoughts and feelings—as in automatic writing, hypnotic drawing and painting.
3. Dissociating various ego-states, processes and functions and helping the patient to re-integrate them in healthier ways.

In any kind of psychotherapy, particularly psycho-analysis, the patient has to learn to observe himself while he experiences affect. In hypnosis, this occurs spontaneously. The patient experiences strong affects, thoughts and hypermnesia and is aware that he does. He has thus dissociated the 'observing' part of the ego from the 'experiencing' or 'behaving' part. For instance, in hypno-analysis, the patient can be told to watch himself making a decision, or to hallucinate a person who looks exactly like him and who feels just as angry as he unconsciously does, come into the room and act exactly as he wants to, without feeling fear or guilt. In fact, in a deep somnambulistic trance, a patient who has to undergo surgery can even be told that another man who looks just like him, steps out of him and lies on the operating table whilst he, himself, sits over there in a chair in the corner of the theatre and watches that other man being operated upon. The patient's 'observing' ego in this case retains 'ego-cathexis' whilst the 'experiencing' ego is de-cathected. Because the 'observing' ego is separated from the 'experiencing' ego, and because the 'observing' ego alone retains the ego-cathexis—*that man, not I*—the patient does not feel any pain and can be operated upon without any anaesthetic. This technique is not infrequently used in obstetrical work in America to secure painless confinements.

Then again, in hypnosis we can often 'de-egotize' certain parts of the body to enable them to express unconscious wishes, thoughts and feelings. One of the easiest ways of producing automatic writing is to induce a 'glove-anaesthesia' in the patient's hand. He is then told that his hand is separating from his body, that it is beginning to experience a life of its own, and that it knows the patient's unconscious thoughts and wishes and can write them down. In this case, the ' conscious ' ego has become separated from the ' unconscious ' ego, and has afforded the latter a direct means of expression. If such a patient is asked a question, he may answer verbally with a ' yes ' or a ' no ', according to what he consciously feels. Simultaneously, his hand will write the real or unconscious answer, often a ' no ' when the answer verbally given is ' yes '. The hand can also write events, thoughts and feelings that have been repressed and are unavailable to the conscious memory. Drawing and painting can be similarly used in hypnotherapy, and you will notice that the same principle underlies the ' ideomotor finger-signalling technique ', described on page 356. Thus, it may reasonably be concluded that in the trance state the patient is in a state of regression in the service of the ego.

Hypno-analytical Methods and General Practice

Before discussing this question it is necessary to refer briefly to the transference situation, which plays such an important part in psycho-analysis, and to the resistances that are frequently encountered.

Freud noticed that when a patient had been freely associating for some time he began to display emotional attitudes towards the analyst. These emotions might be either love or hate, but although they were never expressed in so many words they became more or less obvious from the patient's behaviour. The patient who wished to express love would often forget something—possibly his gloves or umbrella—at the end of his consultation so that he had an excuse to return, or he would become increasingly solicitous in his attitude toward the analyst. On the other hand, if he began to feel hatred, he would show his hostility indirectly by praising some other psychiatrist, by forgetting to pay for his consultation, or by speaking disparagingly of the analyst.

Eventually Freud made the surprising discovery that his patients were behaving towards him as if he were someone they had loved or hated in the past, usually a parent. The patient was therefore ' transferring ' to Freud emotional attitudes toward the parents that had actually been repressed in childhood. Freud called this manifestation of emotion the *transference*, and the analyst can only deal with it by continually referring it back to its source. It must always be strictly controlled, and this calls for a great deal of psychiatric knowledge and experience. The analyst who allows the transference to get out of hand will deserve what he gets.

If the patient's love for the analyst remains unchecked, the analysis will get nowhere. If he hates the analyst too much, he may even become provoked to physical violence.

Transference is a most valuable instrument in psychoanalysis. Since the analyst is unconsciously identified by the patient with someone from the past towards whom he felt strong emotions that had to be repressed at the time, he becomes able to project these upon the analyst without feelings of guilt, thereby releasing much material that would otherwise have remained inaccessible. This has to be interpreted most carefully and handled with extreme delicacy until its true meaning can be accepted by the patient.

In hypno-analysis, as in psycho-analysis, two main kinds of resistance are commonly encountered. The first revolves around the patient's unwillingness to acknowledge unconscious drives and impulses and repressed traumatic memories and experiences; the second arises from the transference itself.

In the first type, the patient is either too afraid or too ashamed of his inner conflicts and memories to allow them to enter consciousness. Tension and panic cause him to erect barriers which succeed in blocking his train of thought whenever he approaches painful material. Sometimes he will even seek refuge in amnesia. Since hypnosis renders the unconscious mind of the individual much more accessible, it can help greatly in resolving such resistances.

Resistance arising from the transference situation is not so easily dealt with. The patient may become so frightened of his unconscious impulses that he seeks not only reassurance and support, but also affection from the analyst. In order to secure this he will adopt an attitude of helplessness to enlist sympathy, and will often refuse to work out his own problems until the analyst has first removed his symptoms. Alternatively, resistance may show itself in the form of hostility. If he finds it impossible to express his feelings of aggression, he may conceal them by becoming depressed and discouraged and will often wish to terminate his treatment. On the other hand, if he is able to display his hostile feelings openly, he may become critical or defiant, ridiculing the explanations and inter-pretations the analyst makes. Transference resistance may manifest itself in many other ways, details of which may be found in many authors' writings. They can only be dealt with by analysing them and interpreting them to the patient. showing him their purpose and how they are affecting his relationships with the analyst and with other

people. This is often a long and tedious task which can only be undertaken by those with the necessary psycho-analytical training and
experience.

In view of these difficulties and complications, the mishandling of
which may easily lead to grave repercussions, it is best to avoid the use
of most of the hypno-analytical techniques in general practice. Indeed,
they should normally only be undertaken when the doctor is sufficiently
well-versed in abnormal psychology to be able to deal effectively with
any situations that may arise. The patients who can achieve a sufficiently
deep trance state to secure the release of highly charged emotions will
certainly require a fully trained psychotherapist to interpret the material
produced, and to deal promptly with any acute anxieties or fears that
may follow in its train.

The therapeutic use of hypno-analysis *always* demands a specialized
training in psychiatric techniques in order to cope with transference
situations and resistances. But when hypno-analytical methods are
restricted to the recovery of buried memories and experiences, as in the
treatment of war or traumatic neuroses, this kind of training is less
essential. One or two of the simpler techniques can prove exceptionally
valuable in uncovering the superficial conflicts that underlie many
psychosomatic symptoms. These can then be resolved and treated by
the general psychotherapeutic measures already described. *The safest
course to adopt in general practice is to restrict the use of hypno-analytical
techniques to diagnostic purposes only, and to shun them altogether as therapeutic
instruments.* How long treatment is likely to take or how successful it will
be depends entirely on the nature of the emotional problems involved.
Generally speaking, psychosomatic conditions are much more easily
influenced than character disorders, and it is largely with the former that
we are concerned here as the latter come within the realm of the psychiatrist.

When questioning under hypnosis fails to shed light upon the superficial conflicts and emotional attitudes underlying the patient's illness,
one or two of the simpler hypno-analytical methods may help to resolve
the problem.

Some patients respond readily to the direct suggestion that they will
be able to recall forgotten events and experiences: ' When I place my
hand on your forehead you will be able to remember what was happening
when you first began to suffer from your symptom.' Even if nothing
is remembered in detail, a clue will often emerge that can be used as the
starting-point for free association under hypnosis. This will sometimes

yield further valuable information. But once the general pattern of the patient's difficulties becomes clear, it is best to discontinue this and to proceed with treatment on the non-analytical psychotherapeutic lines already described.

Should these direct methods fail to overcome the patient's resistance, an indirect technique may prove more successful:

> In a few moments, I am going to count up to five. When I have reached the count of five, a number will come into your mind. This number will be the number of letters in an important word that is closely connected with your trouble. Through this word you will be able to remember many things that you have completely forgotten.
> One . . . two . . . three . . . four . . . five!
> What number are you thinking of?
> Now I am going to count up to five several times, and each time I reach the count of five, a letter will come into your mind. Each letter will be one of the letters in that significant word. They will probably be jumbled up at first and you may not be able to understand them, but don't let that worry you.
> Now I am going to count up to five several times more, and this time at each count of five, the letters will come into your mind in their correct order in that important word.

Once this word is obtained, it should be followed immediately by free association without awakening the patient. He should be told to concentrate upon the word, and that as he does so many thoughts and recollections will come into his mind. He is not to withhold anything, and is to report each consecutive thought or memory, however trivial or irrelevant it may seem, the moment it enters his mind. In many instances, this technique will prove invaluable in providing the missing key to the problem, as one of the cases from my files illustrates extremely well.

The patient was an ex-service man, aged 34. He was unable to travel either by bus or motor-car without becoming panic-stricken. Since his discharge from the army, he had been quite incapable of resuming his peace-time occupation as a driver. He was unmarried, and living in lodgings. In the course of taking his history it emerged that on one occasion, during his service in Italy, he and his section were fired upon by a German Tiger tank which appeared unexpectedly from an adjoining wood. This was his last recollection until he awoke 24 hours later to find himself in bed in hospital, well behind the lines. He had no idea how he got there.

It seemed impossible to fill this vital gap in his memory since not only did all routine methods of investigation fail, but even age-regression was unable to penetrate the barrier. He readily entered a somnambulistic trance, during which he could easily be regressed to any age *except* 28, the age at which this incident occurred.

Eventually I adopted the technique just described. The number of letters in the word was 7. They first appeared as follows: EQSSRIU. When arranged in their correct order they spelt: SQUIRES, and subsequent association to this key word produced the following story.

Squires was the name of a young soldier in the same platoon as the patient. He was aged 19 and had a wife and a young baby that he had never seen. He was not of the stuff of which heroes are made and became terrified when under fire. On one occasion he ran away from the firing-line, and his company commander ordered my patient to fetch him back. This was extremely risky as it involved crossing a stretch of ground which was under heavy bombardment at the time. Since he fought and struggled when caught, my patient stunned him with the butt of his rifle and carried him back to his lines.

Being incensed at having had to risk his own life, my patient set himself out to make this lad's life a misery, taunting him, bullying him and even hitting him whenever he could get away with it. Then came the explosion of the shell from the Tiger tank. When my patient regained consciousness, he found that he was the only survivor of his section and that the mangled remains of the lad lay almost at his feet. He felt overcome with guilt and remorse but even now his ordeal was not ended, for on the journey back to hospital the ambulance in which he was travelling was blown off the road by a shell-burst. He once again became unconscious and woke up about 24 hours later without the slightest recollection of what had occurred.

Wolberg's ' Theatre-visualization ' Technique

Another useful indirect technique may prove equally effective in giving a lead, even in the more frequently encountered non-traumatic type of case. This consists of dream or fantasy induction in the hypnotic state. Wolberg gives many interesting examples of this method and the way in which it is employed, and it is one that I myself have found most valuable and informative.

The patient is told to imagine that he is sitting in the stalls at a theatre. As soon as he can picture himself quite clearly sitting there watching the closed curtains, waiting for the performance to begin, he is to raise his right hand. When this occurs, he is told that he can see a man (or woman) standing on the side of the stage, and peeping behind the closed curtains. He can see what is taking place on the stage behind the closed curtains—the patient cannot—and what this man sees is making him look very frightened or unhappy. As the patient watches, the curtains open and he can now see what is actually causing the man to look unhappy and frightened. As soon as the patient can see the little play that is occurring on the stage, he is to raise his hand. As soon as this happens, he is told to describe the action that is taking place on the stage.

Almost always, the situation that the patient describes will be one that is connected either with childhood memories, or with the difficulties of which he is consciously unaware. This technique is successful in enabling him to recover them because, in fantasy, he is dissociating himself from them and describing them as if they were applicable to other people and not to himself.

The patient is then told that he will see the curtains close, and that what the man at the side of the stage can see behind the curtain is now making him look extremely happy, as if his dearest wishes had been fulfilled. The patient will wonder what it is that is making this man feel so happy, and as the curtains open once more, he will be able to see the action on the stage that is causing this. As soon as he can see this, he is to raise his hand. He is then asked to describe exactly what he can see.

Redlich's ' Jig-saw Puzzle Visualization ' Technique

A more recent yet extremely effective investigatory technique is that devised by Dr Elizabeth Redlich, now widely known as the ' jig-saw puzzle visualization technique '. The effectiveness and simplicity of this method renders it of great value, not only to the psychiatrist but also to the general medical practitioner and dental surgeon. Moreover, deep trances are certainly not essential (though naturally desirable whenever possible) and in the average adult, a medium depth trance is usually all that is required.

Since the success of the technique depends upon the patient's capacity for visual imagery, it is always wise to test this, immediately after the induction and deepening of the trance. Say to him:

I am going to test your powers of imagination . . . so, whilst you are lying comfortably relaxed in the chair . . . I want you to try to imagine that you can see a pair of shoes.

Just visualize them . . . and try to picture them quite clearly in your mind's eye.
Tell me . . . what colour are those shoes?
What material are they made of?
What kind of heels have they?
Do they fasten up . . . and if so . . . how?

Most patients seem to have no difficulty at all in answering these questions. Therefore, you can feel quite confident that they possess a sufficient capacity for visual imagery to justify proceeding with the technique itself. If they fail in this test, however, it will be prudent to select some alternative method of investigation that does *not* depend upon visual imagery. On the other hand, when the test succeeds, you can proceed in the following manner:

I want you to sit upright in the chair . . . and picture a small table standing in front of you. On that table . . . there are several coloured boxes . . . red . . . green . . . yellow . . . and blue. Each of these contains the pieces of a separate jig-saw puzzle.
As soon as you can see yourself sitting at this table . . . with its different coloured boxes . . . your right hand will rise.
That's fine.
Now . . . I want you to choose one of those boxes . . . any colour that you prefer . . . and turn out the pieces of the jig-saw puzzle on the table.
You will notice that there is no picture on the lid of the box.
I don't know what picture will eventually emerge . . . neither do you . . . but it will be the picture of a scene or incident that is closely connected with your present illness.
Your unconscious mind knows . . . and will help you to fit those pieces of the jig-saw puzzle together . . . so that we shall be able to see what this picture is.
Now . . . start fitting the pieces together . . . you will be able to do so much more quickly than when you are wide-awake . . . and tell me what you can see . . . as the picture gradually builds up.

You will note that in the above description, I have specified the kind of picture that is to be produced, but this is not always necessary or even advisable. It may be better at first to leave the choice of the picture to the patient himself, until he has become familiar with the technique. If you wish, you can suggest that the picture he sees will be one that will cause him either distress or pleasure, as in Wolberg's ' theatre-visualization ' technique.

Prolonged observation has led me to believe that the colour of the box selected is not entirely without significance. Four boxes are generally specified—red, green, yellow, and blue. When the red box is chosen, it not infrequently happens that the picture, together with the patient's associations to it, reveals the presence of unconscious dangers, phobias, and even aggressive sexual conflicts. The green box is often connected with conflicts in which jealousy (particularly sibling jealousy) plays an important part, the yellow one with cowardice and feelings of inadequacy, and the blue box with conflicts centred around problems of frigidity and lack of feeling. I do not claim that this is invariably the case, and much more prolonged use and experience of the technique will be necessary before arriving at any definite conclusions.

Should the patient achieve a deep or somnambulistic trance, you will notice that he will enact the whole process of picking up the pieces of the puzzle and fitting them together. This, however, is certainly not essential. All that is really required is that the patient should be able to *imagine himself doing the appointed task*, and to describe whatever he sees. This is the more usual reaction.

If at any stage the patient says he can see nothing more, he can be told that the picture is not yet complete, and that as he continues to fit more of the pieces together he will be able to describe what else he sees.

Patients usually begin by describing scenes containing meadows, water, trees and houses (that is when the choice of picture has been left to them) and seem curiously hesitant at first to include people or animals. In this case, a discreet question such as ' Can you see any people or children there ? ' will generally stimulate them to open up with little difficulty. One then asks whether they can remember having seen this before, whether it reminds them of certain places, people, etc., whether they have any idea as to what is going on, and what the people are thinking or doing.

At this point, the patient often drifts off into free association, which can be followed up very advantageously. In special instances it may be wise to suggest to the patient that there is no need for him to acquaint you with the content of the picture as long as he takes a good look at it himself, and works out its significance.

When using this technique, you will notice that the patient sometimes produces a spontaneous abreaction to the content of the picture he is describing, without any stimulation whatever on the part of the therapist. This can prove both informative and helpful, and there is no danger of it getting out of hand since it can be terminated immediately by telling the patient to break up the picture and restore the pieces to the box.

On one occasion, this happened quite suddenly and unexpectedly when

I was demonstrating this technique upon a previously unknown volunteer subject before an audience of doctors and dental surgeons, the choice of picture being left entirely to the subject. When asked to describe what she could see, she surprised everybody by abreacting violently, shrieking out ' Cats . . . cats . . . I hate them '. She was told immediately to break up the picture and to put the pieces back in the box, whereupon she calmed down almost instantaneously. She was then told to select a different box which would contain a picture which would give her pleasure, and the demonstration proceeded successfully without further difficulty.

Whether an abreaction occurs or not, it is usually wise to tell the patient that after he awakens, he will be able to remember just as much as he wishes of what has transpired, but that anything that he does not wish to remember, he will be able to forget.

The ' Ideomotor Finger-signalling ' Technique

Milton H. Erickson was the first to describe the use of symbolic movements of the head for ' yes ' and ' no ' answers when patients found it difficult to talk whilst in a trance state. Le Cron found that he could employ a Chevreul pendulum for the same purpose, and subsequently added the use of unconsciously controlled finger movements to obtain ' yes ', ' no ' and ' I don't want to answer ' responses. This has since been used extensively and its many possibilities widely explored by Dr David Cheek. In numerous instances it can be used effectively to investigate the presence and nature of unconscious material, and the principle upon which it depends can best be described as follows:

When we prepare a patient's mind for the acceptance of hypnosis, we show him how to pay attention to some part of the body, and *not* to pay attention to another. We show him how to relax his muscles—and that muscles that are contracted constantly in fear will begin to hurt because of the restricted circulation of blood through those muscles. We can then go on to teach him how muscles can react ' unconsciously ', and thus establish a method of communication at an unconscious level by using the unconscious movements of the finger-muscles to indicate the answers ' yes ', ' no ', or ' I don't want to answer ' to the questions that are put to him. I have found the following approach to be most effective:

> I want you to put both hands on your lap . . . and I'll show you how you can learn to answer questions at an unconscious level.
> When you are talking to people . . . you have often seen them nod their heads when they agree with you . . . and shake their heads when they disagree with what you are saying.

And they don't even know they are doing so.

The movement is completely unconscious.

Now . . . I'm going to teach your unconscious mind how it can answer questions by causing one finger to rise for the answer ' Yes '—a different one for the answer ' No ', etc.

Just let your hands lie idly upon your lap.

I want you to think the thought . . . ' yes ' . . . ' yes ' . . . ' yes ' . . . over and over again.

And as you do so . . . you will soon feel one of your fingers beginning to lift up on its own . . . from your lap.

It's just like getting a swing going . . . you have to keep pushing it at intervals.

You do this by keeping on thinking . . . ' yes '.

And whilst you keep on thinking . . . ' yes ' . . . you are not thinking of ' no ' . . . or of any other answer.

Just keep on thinking . . . ' yes ' . . . ' yes ' . . . ' yes '.

There . . . you see.

The fore-finger of your *right* hand is slowly lifting up.

Put it down again.

Now . . . think the thought . . . ' no ' . . . ' no ' . . . ' no ' . . . over and over again.

And . . . as you do so . . . one of your other fingers will slowly rise.

It may be on the same hand . . . or it may be on the other hand.

There you are.

It's the fore-finger of your *left* hand.

So . . . if I ask your unconscious mind a question . . . and the answer is ' yes ' . . . after it has considered the question . . . it will cause your *right* fore-finger to rise.

If . . . on the other hand . . . the answer is ' no ' . . . your *left* fore-finger will rise.

A third finger may, of course, be conditioned to signify the response ' I *would prefer not to answer* ', should this be considered desirable.

Now . . . I'm going to ask your unconscious mind one or two questions.

Your conscious mind doesn't know the real cause of your illness.

Neither does mine.

But your own ' *unconscious* ' mind does.

And it can help us . . . in this way . . . to get to the real root of your trouble.

Is your unconscious mind ready to help?

The *right* fore-finger slowly rises . . . ' Yes '.

Does it object to being questioned in this way?

The *left* fore-finger slowly rises . . . ' No '.

As an example of the usefulness of this technique, let us suppose that we have reason to believe that our patient suffered some traumatic experience in childhood, which has been repressed and which consequently he is quite unable to remember. The precise age can often be pin-pointed in the following manner:

Did something unpleasant happen to you before you were 15 years old?

(Finger signals . . . ' Yes '.)

Did it happen before you were 10 years old?

(Finger signals . . . ' Yes '.)

Did it happen before you were 5 years old?

(Finger signals . . . ' No '.)

Did it happen when you were 9?

(Finger signals . . . ' No '.)

Did it happen when you were 8?

(Finger signals . . . ' No '.)

Did it happen when you were 7?

(Finger signals . . . ' Yes '.)

Provided that you ask the right questions, all of which must be capable of being answered by a simple ' Yes ' or ' No ', it is surprising how much valuable information you can obtain in this way.

It is not difficult to tell whether such answers are really unconsciously determined. Watch carefully the nature of the finger movement. An answer at a conscious level will result in an *immediate* movement, whereas an unconscious answer will be much more delayed and the consequent finger movement much slower and jerkier.

A convincing confirmation of the genuineness of such a reply was accidentally afforded by one of my patients. I had asked a particularly important and rather embarrassing question to which the ideomotor response signalled the answer ' Yes '. Upon awakening the patient, she expressed the greatest astonishment at what had occurred. She said ' When you asked me that question, I was quite sure that the answer was ' No ', yet despite this, my finger signalled the answer ' Yes '. I don't understand it at all .' Subsequent investigations proved beyond doubt the correctness of the ideomotor response.

Occasionally these techniques can be used successfully in general practice to uncover the nature of significant conflicts that lie just below the surface. Except in the case of war or traumatic neuroses, neither of them are likely to elicit a highly charged emotional release that might be too difficult to control. In the unlikely event of this occurring, the hypnosis should be terminated immediately and the patient referred to a psychiatrist for further treatment. Difficulties of this kind are much more likely to arise if the continued investigation of the material obtained, and its subsequent treatment, proceeds upon hypno-analytical rather than simple psychotherapeutic lines. Because of this, it is probably wisest for the general practitioner to confine himself to the simple techniques just described, and to avoid other hypno-analytical methods and even age-regression as means of further investigation.

CHAPTER 24

The Uses of Hypnosis in Dental Surgery

by

STANLEY TINKLER, L.D.S., R.C.S.(ENG.)

Whilst the use of hypnosis in dental surgery has been known and appreciated for many years, it has only recently assumed its rightful place. Many workers in this field, such as Radin, Becker, Frost and Wookey in this country, have written and lectured upon the subject, and in the United States, Moss, Secter, Heron and Weinstein are well known for the invaluable contributions they have made in furthering our knowledge in this respect.

Every dental surgeon is bound to encounter a limited number of patients who could successfully undergo all their dental operations, painful or otherwise, under hypnosis alone. Often, however, it is felt that many of the hypnotic procedures recommended for dentistry in the past are too time-consuming and laborious for the ordinary practitioner, working in his own surgery either privately or under the National Health Service. But in the light of what is known today about the number of patients who can be hypnotized into light, medium or even deep trances, it is gradually becoming realized to a greater and greater extent that the employment of these various trance states can afford the dentist considerable assistance in selected cases. Furthermore, in the Hospital Service, where the time factor is not so pressing and the condition of many patients is so serious that it requires more time to be spent upon them, hypnosis could well be used more widely than it is at the present time.

Deep Trance Hypnosis

Obviously with those patients who can achieve the deep trance state on the first or second attempt, dentistry will present no problems. Most of these will succeed in producing complete analgesia, and many will develop a total amnesia for such operations as are performed. In these circumstances there is no quicker or easier way of carrying out any dental operation. The patient can be seated in the chair and put into the trance state instantaneously by a conditioned signal, or within 10 seconds by a normal induction procedure. Anaesthesia of the intended area of operation can be obtained in a further 10 seconds, and the dentist can be proceeding about his business within 30 seconds of the patient entering the surgery. Unfortunately, this is only possible in a very small percentage of the total population and is consequently quite unattainable as a routine measure.

Medium Trance Hypnosis

A considerable number of patients can attain an intermediate stage of analgesia. Whilst they undoubtedly feel some pain, they feel much less under hypnosis than they would in the waking state. Although they are by no means completely analgesic, these patients can be considerably helped by hypnosis. My own feeling is that the prick of the needle when giving a hypodermic injection can be greatly mitigated by the direct suggestion under hypnosis that analgesia of the muco-periosteum in the area of the injection has been obtained.

Light Trance Hypnosis

By far the largest number of patients will achieve light or medium trances only unless the hypnotist is prepared to go to a great deal of time and trouble. Even under these circumstances, hypnosis can still prove to be a valuable supportive measure towards the completion of the treatment envisaged. We all know the type of patient who finds it difficult to pluck up his courage sufficiently to visit the dentist. We all know the type of patient who is overcome with anxiety and apprehension when he finally arrives in our consulting-rooms. We are also familiar with the patient who, whilst making strenuous efforts to control himself, is obviously finding it so difficult that he remains in a highly excitable and tensed-up state as long as we are operating upon him. In all these patients induction into the hypnotic state will alleviate their fears, reduce their anxiety and apprehension, and produce sensations of relaxation, comfort and well-being to a greater or lesser degree. Under hypnosis, the dentist can suggest directly to the patient that he will be able to relax, that there is no need for him to worry, that he will become less tense, less apprehensive, and that he will be able to try to assist the dentist in whatever procedure he is carrying out. Even this level of trance, at which suggestions can be quite potent and effective, constitutes one of the most valuable and widely applicable uses of hypnosis in dentistry.

As a dentist who regularly uses hypnotherapy on occasions, I feel I should warn the would-be dental hypnotist against the blandishments of patients who wish to undergo hypnosis unnecessarily, or request it for the relief of conditions that do not fit into the dental picture. It seems that the dental practitioner who is known to employ hypnosis tends to become the target for most of the cranks, medical and dental, in the area in which he practises. Thus it cannot be emphasized too strongly that the dentist who ventures outside the sphere of dentistry, in order to enhance his image or to oblige his patients, is doing so at considerable risk to himself. Regrettably, there do seem to be an appreciable number of such cranks in every area, and they seem to be attracted towards hypnosis as a bee is drawn to honey.

All attempts by such people or by the general public to ensnare the dental profession into using hypnosis for any other purpose than straight dental operations should be stoutly resisted. Most medical and dental practitioners who use hypnosis regularly consider that any attempt by a practitioner lacking psychiatric experience, to go outside his normal field of activity, is fraught with danger. The dentist should, therefore, confine his activities entirely to the dental field, and even at the risk of upsetting people he should decline to treat them for other conditions. For instance, dentists who practise hypnosis are constantly being asked to cure people of the habit of smoking. Whilst it is true that hypnotherapy can help to achieve this, it should still only be undertaken under competent medical guidance since there is always the danger that the addiction may become transferred from nicotine to something more dangerous.

The Main Uses of Hypnosis in Dentistry

1. Obtaining relaxation.
2. Ensuring co-operation from the otherwise unco-operative.
3. The reduction of anxiety and fear.
4. The preparation of the patient for local or general anaesthesia.
5. The production of analgesia.
6. The production of amnesia.
7. The control of fainting.
8. The control of bleeding.
9. The control of salivation.
10. The induction of muscular rigidity of the jaw and neck.
11. The extension of the period of analgesia.
12. The toleration of impression-taking without gagging or sickness.

13. Improvement of the effort necessary to learn the wearing of prosthetic or orthodontic appliances.

This list constitutes a fairly complete catalogue of most of the uses to which dentists put hypnosis in the course of their normal practice.

1. *Obtaining relaxation.* It is well known that the highly nervous patient invariably has a lower threshold of pain, and will consequently be under increasing tension as the operation proceeds. It is also recognized that if this state of tension in the patient can be reduced either by drugs or, in the case of dental hypnosis, by suggestion, the patient's pain threshold will be elevated to such an extent that simple operations not involving too much pain will become tolerable to that patient.

2. *Ensuring co-operation.* Even without the induction of hypnosis, it has been found that many patients who are reassured and talked to quietly in the waking state as their treatment progresses will become much more relaxed and co-operative, thus rendering the whole procedure very much easier. In the light and medium trance states, this effect can be tremendously enhanced.

3. *The reduction of anxiety and fear.* Most normal patients who visit their dentist are in some condition of fear. Those who have been coming for a long time probably do not fear us any more. But newer patients whose confidence we have not fully gained through lack of opportunity, and those who have experienced somewhat unsuccessful sessions in the past will exhibit a very active fear. If suitable steps can be taken to eliminate this, a state of mind will be produced in which treatment will become much more acceptable, and the pain threshold will once again be elevated. This can sometimes be achieved by a straightforward talk in the waking state, in the course of which the confidence of the patient is obtained. On other occasions, hypnosis can be used to great advantage since it can be directly suggested to the patient that his fears of a dental appointment will cease to exist ; that he will be able to allow the necessary treatment to be carried out ; and that he will experience no fear whatever during the whole of the time he spends with the dentist. In a similar manner, direct suggestion under hypnosis can be employed to reduce the fear of any particular operation that is contemplated. Fortunately, suggestions of this kind can prove very effective in the lightest stages of hypnosis, so that the vast majority of our patients can actually be helped in this way. Indeed, in so far as the reduction of anxiety and fear, and the attaining of relaxation

are concerned, I would say that at least nine out of ten patients can be assisted by the use of hypnosis.

4. *Preparation for local or general anaesthesia.* Most specialist anaesthetists are in the habit of using a relaxing technique in talking to their patients before inducing anaesthesia. In the dental surgery this method can usefully be adopted before giving nitrous-oxide and oxygen, and possibly some of the intravenous anaesthetic agents. Appropriate suggestions are made in a quiet, drowsy voice, and the monotony is maintained throughout the actual induction of anaesthesia. Hypnosis often supervenes well before anaesthetization is complete. Should local anaesthesia only be required, an extremely relaxed, sleepy state of mind can be induced by using a similar hypnotic technique, and it is interesting to note that under these circumstances the quantity of local anaesthetic necessary to obtain adequate anaesthesia for the operation contemplated can often be substantially reduced.

5. *The production of analgesia.* Some degree of analgesia, partial or complete, is obtainable in no more than 30 per cent of patients, but complete analgesia will only be obtainable in some 10 per cent, and even then will often require several visits to achieve. Thus complete analgesia, whilst being delightful to work with when it can be secured, must be regarded as the exception rather than the rule, whereas varying degrees of partial analgesia can often be attained.

6. *The production of amnesia.* A complete loss of memory for a dental procedure can often be induced in those deep-trance subjects who are capable of high degrees of analgesia. This can be utilized with great benefit to the patient whenever an operation has been protracted or particularly unpleasant. Under such circumstances, one can try to increase the patient's susceptibility to amnesia by various subterfuges such as the suggestion that the mind is going blank.

7. *The control of fainting.* This is readily susceptible to treatment by hypnotic methods. We are all only too familiar with the type of patient who, during a hypodermic injection or immediately following it, breaks out in beads of perspiration, blanches or goes grey, and in next to no time passes out in the chair. If, at the onset of the attack, he is told with confidence and authority to place his head between his knees, thereby compressing the abdominal viscera, his colour will return in a matter of seconds and the whole episode will be over within a minute or two. Any recurrence of this can be guarded against and avoided by

hypnotizing such patients and making strong, positive and authoritative suggestions that fainting will *not* occur on any future occasion. This is particularly effective if it is also explained to the patient that fainting is directly due to fear, and that next time he will no longer be afraid.

8. *The control of bleeding.* Bleeding from a post-extraction wound or immediately following an extraction can be controlled if a strong suggestion is given to the deeply hypnotized patient that the blood-flow in the particular area will be reduced for some hours. Under these circumstances, the bleeding will often cease completely. An extraction can frequently be performed without the loss of more than two or three drops of blood if the blood-flow is reduced by hypnotic suggestion before the extraction is made.

9. *The control of salivation.* In a similar manner, direct suggestions that the patient's saliva will dry up for a limited period will result in a definite lessening of the flow of saliva. This can be of great assistance in the type of patient who has a profuse or ropey saliva which constitutes an increasing hazard during the preparation of a cavity in a lower tooth.

10. *Induction of muscular rigidity of the jaw and neck.* This can be produced most efficiently in the hypnotic trance by simple, direct suggestion. This is usually done to a count of five, and it is suggested to the patient that the muscles of the jaw, head and neck will become completely stiff and rigid with the jaw locked widely open until the operation is completed. The rigidity is subsequently removed by a reverse count.

11. *Extension of the period of analgesia.* When it is anticipated that an operation will produce a certain amount of after-pain, it is quite reasonable to suggest to the patient that the area of operation will remain analgesic for the next twelve to twenty-four hours, thereby affording the patient a degree of post-operative comfort which would not exist nearly so long if an ordinary local anaesthetic had been used. Such instructions, however, must be strictly limited in application since severe pain following an operation may indicate the onset of a spreading infection, or that something else has gone wrong. In this case, it is essential that the patient should receive adequate warning of the necessity of revisiting the dentist.

12. *Impression tolerance and control of gagging.* The control of gagging and of sickness can undoubtedly be effected by hypnotic suggestion. The patient is told that the palate and upper portion of the pharynx

is becoming anaesthetized, and that he will consequently have no need to retch. This renders the taking of impressions which have to stay in the mouth for 3 minutes or more much easier in patients who are susceptible to this type of complaint.

13. *Tolerance of prosthetic and orthodontic appliances.* The co-operation of patients in the wearing of new dentures can be actively enlisted under hypnosis, and this is equally applicable to children in the wearing of fixed or removable orthodontic appliances. When suggestions to this effect are made, it is always wise to stress the reasons for the patient's co-operation and the benefits that are going to accrue from the wearing of the appliances. A further use of hypnosis in the field of orthodontics can be found in dealing with the normal thumb-sucking or tongue-thrusting type of child, whose dental abnormality is due to some extent to these two factors. A child can be instructed under hypnosis that if it must suck something, it will suck a finger rather than a thumb. This has the advantage of reducing considerably the size of the object that is sucked. The matter can be taken further and the patient can be told that any part of either hand which is placed in the mouth will taste so unpleasant that it will have to be removed. This has been known to occur after only one session of hypnosis.

All these applications of hypnosis in dentistry are directly beneficial both to the patient and to the operator. There is also an additional application which I have used with considerable success, which is of no direct benefit to the patient but is extremely helpful to the dentist. Under hypnosis, the patient is told quite firmly and authoritatively that he will not be late for future appointments and that he will leave his home or his place of business in ample time to arrive at the surgery some five minutes before his appointment is actually due. He will consequently not keep the practitioner waiting.

Techniques for the Induction of Hypnosis

The problems of hypnotic induction for dental purposes are rather different from those confronting the doctor or psychotherapist. In one sense, the dentist has a distinct advantage because the patient knows that hypnosis is only being used for a limited purpose, and consequently has the assurance that no exploration of his mind will be attempted. On the other hand, most dental patients suffer from the disadvantage that the fear and dread evoked by the prospect of dental treatment makes it more difficult for them to co-operate and relax. This can usually be overcome, however, provided that sufficient time and care are devoted to the preparation of the patient's mind before any attempt at induction is made. I cannot stress too strongly the importance of this step, which may well determine the difference between success and failure.

The Induction of Hypnosis in Adults

Any of the usual methods of induction are applicable to dental purposes. The choice should always be made with due regard to its suitability for the individual patient and the personality of the operator himself.

In the dental chair, I usually use the eye-fixation-distraction method (*see* p. 57) since I have found it to be both rapid and efficient.

> The patient is seated comfortably in the dental chair and his eyes are fixed either on a point on the ceiling or on the tip of a pen or pencil (the intra-oral lamp is a very suitable object upon which the patient can be asked to fix). The object is held above and slightly to the rear of the patient's eyes, so that a pronounced effort has to be made to keep it in view, and is sufficiently near for the eyes to focus convergently upon it (i.e. not more than a foot or eighteen inches away).
>
> The patient is asked to relax his muscles completely . . . to get really comfortable in the chair . . . and to fix his eyes upon the lamp.
>
> He is then told to count quietly to himself, backwards from 300.
>
> As he does this, suggestions are made of increasing heaviness of his eyes . . . of heaviness of the eyelids . . . and of a general feeling of lassitude.
>
> These suggestions are given in a monotonous tone of voice, and in a very short time, the eyes will appear to focus away in the distance and will become rather more moist than they normally are. Then the eyelids will begin to flicker a little, at which point the suggestions of heaviness are pressed with more emphasis and the patient told that his eyelids are wanting to close . . . that they are heavier and heavier . . . and are wanting to close, more and more. Eye-closure usually follows rapidly, and can be accelerated at the right moment by the instruction to go to sleep. The patient is then told that he will not want to open his eyes until instructed to do so.

Both the eye-fixation progressive relaxation method and Wolberg's hand-levitation method are equally suitable, but both require more time to be spent upon the actual induction.

The ' Dropped Coin ' Technique

Another simple and quick method of induction favoured by many dental surgeons is the ' *dropped coin technique* '. This is another ' eye-fixation' procedure, using the patient's thumb as a fixation point. Ideomotor activity in the actual opening of the fingers is also involved:

I want you to relax as much as possible . . . don't try to make anything happen . . . don't try to stop anything happening . . . just let everything happen . . . as it wants to happen.

All you have to do is to follow my instructions . . . and you will find it very easy to drift into a sleep-like state . . . but although your eyes will close . . . and will remain closed . . . you will not actually be asleep.

You will know everything that is going on . . . but you will not have the slightest desire to open your eyes . . . until I tell you to do so.

You could open them at any moment . . . if you wanted to . . . but you won't . . . simply because you will have no desire to do so.

Let us use this coin.

I am going to place this coin in your right hand . . . and I want you to close your fingers gently . . . so that when I turn your hand over . . . the coin does not fall.

Now . . . hold your right arm straight out . . . at shoulder-level . . . and stretch out your thumb.

Keep your eyes fixed on it . . . because I want you to follow these instructions carefully.

Fix your eyes upon your thumb-nail . . . and don't let them wander from it for a single moment.

Whilst your eyes are fixed upon your thumb-nail . . . I want you to pay close attention to your fingers . . . and to the coin . . . which is loosely held in the palm of your hand.

Notice the position of your fingers with regard to the coin . . . the position of your fingers with regard to each other . . . and to the palm of your hand. You can actually feel the coin . . . in the palm of your hand . . . and as you do so . . . you will become aware of a number of different sensations.

Now . . . I am going to start counting slowly upwards from *One.*

With each count . . . you will feel your fingers becoming more and more relaxed . . . more and more relaxed.

And as they do so . . . they will gradually straighten out to a point when the coin will drop out of your hand . . . and will fall on the floor.

When the coin drops . . . that will be a signal for three things to happen.

Your eyes will close . . . your whole body will sink back into the chair . . . and you will fall into a deep, deep sleep.

Your eyes may become so tired . . . through gazing at your thumb-nail . . . that they may even close before the coin drops.

If they do . . . that's fine.

Just keep them closed . . . and when the coin drops . . . let your whole body sink back comfortably into the chair . . . without bothering about your eyes which are already closed.

It may be . . . that as I count . . . your eyes will begin to blink.

If so . . . just let them blink as much as they want . . . and they will begin to feel so heavy . . . that it will be more comfortable to let them close on their own.

ONE . . . *Your fingers are beginning to relax . . . more . . . and more . . . and more. They are no longer touching the palm of your hand . . . and they are beginning to open . . . just a little bit.*

TWO . . . *Relaxing more . . . and more . . . and more.*

Your fingers are beginning to straighten out . . . they are opening more and more . . . so that the coin is now resting mainly on your fingers.

THREE . . . *You can notice quite a bit of movement now . . . in your fingers . . . and soon . . . that coin is going to drop to the floor . . . even sooner than you think.*

FOUR . . . *You're making excellent progress . . . just continue to relax . . . and let yourself go, completely.*

FIVE . . . *Your fingers are straightening out now . . . more . . . and more . . . and more. Soon . . . that coin will drop . . . and as it strikes the floor . . . let yourself slump limply down into the chair . . . let your eyes close . . . and enjoy that feeling of complete and utter relaxation.*

SIX . . . *You're doing splendidly . . . just let those fingers relax . . . more . . . and more . . . and more.*

SEVEN . . . *With each count . . . your fingers are relaxing . . . more and more . . . straightening out . . . more and more . . . so that your hand is slowly opening . . . and, very soon now . . . that coin will drop.*

(Suppose at this point, the coin drops.)

Deeply relaxed . . . deeply relaxed . . . go very, very deeply asleep.

The subject can then be told to take several very deep breaths . . . and that with each breath that he takes . . . he will become more and more deeply relaxed . . . deeper and deeper asleep. The hypnosis can be deepened by whatever method seems appropriate.

The Induction of Hypnosis in Children

Once a child's confidence has been gained, the induction of hypnosis becomes relatively easy since most children are readily susceptible unless they are exceptionally timid and nervous. The dentist's prestige will assist him in establishing satisfactory rapport, and in many cases, the deeper stages will be established without difficulty. The precise age of the child is not the most important factor. What does matter is whether the child's interest and attention can be held long enough for the suggestions to take effect. Consequently, the method may have to be varied from time to time in order to achieve this object. I find that provided that the child is able to count at all, a modified version of the eye-fixation-distraction method is usually most successful.

I tell the child to keep looking at the light, and to count slowly as far as it can. When it has reached this point, it is to start at the beginning again and repeat the count. In younger children it is often advisable to allow them to count out aloud, for this often seems to help considerably. During the count, the usual suggestions are made, suitably reworded and simplified, until the eyes close. This usually happens very quickly indeed.

If the very young child can be cajoled into keeping its eyes fixed upon the light, or dental mirror, the count can often be omitted for hypnosis will frequently supervene as a result of verbal suggestion alone.

The ' Picture Visualization ' Technique

Some dentists favour the picture-visualization technique described by Moss, an effective version of which is as follows:

Now it's time for us to play a game together . . . you'd like that, wouldn't you ?
I'll teach you what to do . . . and it's going to be a lot of fun . . . because all you have to do is to close your eyes . . . and pretend that you're asleep. You won't be really asleep, of course . . . but it will be most exciting . . . because during this ' pretend ' sleep, you can watch films . . . television . . . circuses . . . or anything else you enjoy.
So . . . make yourself as comfortable as possible . . . and start pretending, as soon as you're ready.
Close your eyes . . . and don't open them again until I ask you.
Now, I'd like you to pretend that you are back at home watching your favourite television programme.
I'm just going to lift up your hand . . . and as I lift it . . . the picture becomes sharper and clearer.
The better the picture . . . the higher your hand will rise . . . and the higher your hand rises . . . the better the picture will become.
And presently . . . you'll find that your elbow will begin to bend . . . and your hand will move towards your face.
And when your hand touches your face . . . that picture will be perfect. But don't let your hand touch your face . . . until you are satisfied with the picture. That's fine. Keep on watching the picture . . . and don't lose it . . . and you'll find that your hand will drop down to your lap . . . and as it does . . . you can pretend to be really asleep.
And notice how limp and slack your muscles have become.
Now, with television pictures . . . there is usually some music.
Just listen to that music . . . and as soon as you can hear it . . . start marking time to the music with your hand or finger.
Keep on watching the picture . . . and don't lose it.

As long as you have the picture . . . lift up the finger of your other hand . . .
and keep it up.
Then I'll know that this is the ' picture ' finger . . . and the other is the
' music ' finger.
What sort of picture are you looking at ?
Are there people or animals in it . . . or both ?
It really doesn't matter . . . because if you want to change the picture . . . you
can do so quite easily.
Don't lose the picture . . . or the music.
And I'd like you to know . . . that when you watch television like this . . .
you can feel things . . . but they won't bother you.
I can even pinch you . . . like this . . . and although you can feel the pinch
. . . it doesn't bother you at all. That's right . . . isn't it ?
Now I'm going to be working on your teeth . . . and although you can feel
something going on . . . as long as you go on watching the picture . . . and
listening to the music . . . it won't bother you . . . and really won't matter.
Is the picture still there ? Is the music still there ?
Just keep on watching . . . and listening.

Children have such vivid imaginations that one might almost say that
they spend a considerable part of their time in ' a world of pretence '.
Consequently, a technique of this kind is quite natural to them. You will
notice that whilst watching the picture and listening to the music, they
become completely relaxed and ' miles away ', so that it is quite easy to
work on them. They can still feel things, but it no longer matters or
bothers them.

To awaken the child, you can say that someone has turned the television
off, so it really isn't much use going on pretending. So tell it that it can
stop pretending now, open its eyes, and be wide-awake again.

Trance-deepening Procedures

I usually follow a similar trance-deepening routine to that which
has already been described. I begin by eliciting arm heaviness followed
by arm catalepsy (raising the arm and telling the patient it will remain
in the air without any conscious effort on his part, until he is told to lower
it). Deepening is then continued by the induction of automatic movement, either through the continuous rotation of the patient's hands,
one around the other, or through a to and fro movement of the forearm,
the patient being instructed to visualize a piece of cord pulling the hand
backwards and forwards. Should these tests prove successful, my final
deepening technique consists of dream induction. The patient is asked
to visualize in his mind some simple action such as combing the hair,

washing the face, or undoing a tie. He is then instructed to dream that he is performing this simple action, and as he does so, to act it out as he sits in the chair.

Tests for somnambulism can subsequently be applied. The patient can be told to open his eyes without awakening from the trance, and to rinse out his mouth, and that when he sits back in the chair again and his head touches the head-rest his eyes will close and he will remain in a very deep sleep. If he accomplishes this successfully, he has achieved the stage of somnambulism.

Several additional deepening techniques can be useful on occasions. The patient can be asked to picture himself descending in a lift, in some well-known shopping store. As he visualizes his descent and the lift passes the various floors, he is told that his sleep is becoming deeper and deeper. As an alternative, he can be asked to imagine that he is entering an underground station in London (provided that he has actually visited London) and that he is stepping on to the moving staircase. As he descends, his hypnosis will become deeper and deeper until he finds himself at the bottom of the escalator, when he will be in a very deep sleep.

The breathing technique is another useful deepening agent which seems to work extremely well with many patients. The patient is instructed to breathe in deeply . . . to hold his breath for two seconds . . . and as he breathes out, he will go into a deeper trance. This is repeated five times, and it is often quite dramatic to watch the patient deepening and relaxing, and his muscles becoming completely limp and flaccid as he breathes deeply in and out.

Dental Procedures at the Various Levels of Hypnosis

Even when the patient only succeeds in achieving light hypnosis, it should still be possible to enlist greater co-operation on his part and a considerable degree of relaxation. One can also expect to reduce his anxiety and fear, and to induce a certain amount of drowsiness and sleepiness in preparation for anaesthesia, either general or local. Moreover, the efforts made by the patient to tolerate the wearing of dentures or orthodontic appliances can often be improved.

In medium-depth hypnosis, all the above can be obtained even more easily and completely. Varying degrees of analgesia can also be produced, together with some control of fainting, bleeding and saliva flow. Gagging, during the taking of impressions, can be reduced, and muscular rigidity of the jaw and neck can be secured.

In deep hypnosis, in addition to the above, complete analgesia and possibly some amnesia can be obtained. In my experience, however, analgesia and amnesia are not necessarily both obtainable in every deep-trance subject. There may be complete analgesia without amnesia or the reverse. Unfortunately, the phenomena that can be elicited at different levels of hypnosis vary considerably from patient to patient, and it is fair to say that no general rules can be laid down as to what one can expect in any one individual.

The Time-factor in Dental Hypnosis

It is my practice to devote no more than three sessions to attempting to induce hypnosis. If satisfactory progress is not made within 3 to 5 minutes on each of these separate occasions, I do not consider the patient to be a suitable subject for hypnosis in a busy practice, since treatment will necessarily be both protracted and unremunerative.

It will be realized that nearly all dental patients could be assisted to some extent by hypnosis—at least 90 per cent—so that the use that any individual dentist makes of hypnosis in his own practice is bound to depend upon the amount of time he is prepared to devote to it, and whether the patient is strongly in favour of it and is willing to pay for his treatment on a time basis. When dentists take up hypnosis for the first time, they spend many unremunerative hours in attempting all the various phases of its application in dentistry, but most who have worked in this field for a number of years find it no longer necessary to employ hypnosis regularly, since many of the patients who were hypnotized in the first place have gained so much confidence that they do not require it any more.

Some patients are interested to have hypnotic treatment merely for the experience, and unless the dentist can see a real need for it, such requests should be firmly discouraged. On the other hand, there are a limited number of patients whom we should never be able to treat without the aid of hypnosis, used in one of the ways already mentioned. It is in such instances as these that I feel the greatest benefit is to be found, since these patients can be rendered quite amenable to treatment if a little time and care is taken in their preparation.

CHAPTER 25

General Observations on the Hypnotic State, its Induction, Deepening, and Utilization

As already stated in the introduction, my main object in writing this book has been to render the subject of hypnosis more intelligible to the uninitiated, to free it from the aura of mysticism which has so long impeded its progress and to stimulate interest and to encourage its use, particularly in the field of general practice. In so doing, I am aware that I have deliberately over-simplified the matter, so it would seem appropriate to conclude by drawing attention to a number of important principles and variables hitherto unmentioned in the text.

The Nature of the Hypnotic State

Although the 'suggestion' and 'dissociation' theories describe hypnosis in terms which make it more readily understandable even to the lay mind, and thus tend to overcome prejudice and misconception, I must strongly emphasize the fact that the '*hypersuggestibility*' that occurs is far from being the essence of the hypnotic state which depends primarily upon inter- and intrapersonal relationships. Hypnosis always involves a particular relationship between the hypnotist and his subject, and the trance, which is produced by the subject himself under the guidance and instruction of the hypnotist, affords a specialized means of communication between them. Jay Haley points out that in the old days, when hypnotists used to give authoritative 'sleep' commands to a completely passive subject, it was inevitable that the hypnotic situation should appear to be unique. Today, the hypnotic relationship can no longer be differentiated from other kinds of relationship by such obvious means. In fact, a trance can be induced during an apparently casual conversation. It can be induced in one member of an audience whilst the lecturer is talking to a group, or even in one person whilst the hypnotist is dealing with another. Surprisingly enough, a trance can sometimes be induced when the hypnotist does nothing. Thus, the hypnotic trance is intimately connected with the relationship existing between the hypnotist and his subject, to whom it is always a meaningful emotional experience. The hypnotist assumes responsibility for what happens during the trance. He initiates a series of messages, verbal and non-verbal, to which the subject, as long as he is willing, will respond. Even the prestige that he holds in the eyes of the subject only implies the readiness of the latter to accept the hypnotist as the person who will be responsible for initiating ideas and suggestions. Erickson has always stressed the importance of regarding hypnosis as a continuous process of communication, and has defined it in the following manner. *Hypnosis is the induction of special states of awareness, circumscribed in character, not easily intruded upon, and dependent upon the subject's own total experiential life, as selected by the subject and controlled and directed by the hypnotist.*

The Induction of Hypnosis

The induction of hypnotic states and phenomena is above all a matter of the communication of ideas and the eliciting of trains of thought and associations within the subject which ultimately lead to behavioural responses. Even when the hypnotist does something to the subject, or tells him what to do and how to do it, the trance that is produced is still the result of ideas, associations, mental processes and understandings that are already in existence in the subject's mind, and are consequently merely aroused within the subject himself. Far too many therapists in the hypnotic field regard their own activities, their intentions and desires, as the effective forces and uncritically believe that it is their own utterances to the subject that elicit or initiate specific responses. They fail to realize that what they say or do serves only as a means of stimulating or arousing within their subjects past learnings and understandings, some of which have been consciously and some unconsciously acquired.

Erickson considers that the best way to induce hypnosis is to casually present, in an apparently permissive fashion, a wealth of seemingly related ideas, in such a manner as to hold and fixate the subject's attention rather than his eyes, or by trying to induce special muscular states. Every effort should be made to direct the subject's attention to processes within himself, to his own body-sensations, his memories, emotions, thoughts, feelings, ideas, past learnings and past experiences. A good hypnotic technique organized in this way can be remarkably effective even under seemingly adverse circumstances. He also stresses the importance of taking advantage of, and making use of the subject's own behaviour patterns, rather than expecting him to conform to the hypnotist's own ideas. Rigidity in hypnotic techniques renders it impossible to secure controlled results, and an awareness of the variability of human behaviour and the need to meet it should form the basis of all such techniques. Too much emphasis is often placed upon external factors and the subject's responses to them, whereas it should rightly be placed upon the intra-psychic behaviour of the individual himself.

Before leaving this question of the induction of hypnosis, there are two points to which I would direct your attention, the importance of which are only too frequently underestimated. The first is ' *non-verbal communication* ' and the second ' *time-lag* '. In hypnosis, the first and most important task is to establish an immediate relationship with your subject to create the right atmosphere for securing his full co-operation. Then, during the subsequent process of induction, you should remember that your gestures and body-movements can be just as significant as what you are actually saying. As you suggest closure of the eyes, the strength of this suggestion can be reinforced considerably if you simultaneously allow your own eyes to slowly flutter and close. Also, if you take a deep breath yourself, and allow your own body to sag limply in the chair as you give suggestions of relaxation, you will find that the effect will become greatly enhanced.

The importance of ' *time-lag* ' is best illustrated by referring to the ' hand-levitation ' method of induction, in which the subject is gazing at his hands and is told that one of his fingers will jerk. It does not do so right away. There is a time-lag during which the subject mentally digests, understands and finally puts into action the idea that has been presented. Too many of us tend to work with a hypnotic subject and, having told him that ' so and so is going to happen ', expect him to comply without delay. He needs time. Indeed, this appreciation of time as a factor in itself is a vitally important consideration in trance induction. After all, if you were to administer a powerful drug, you would be prepared to wait a reasonable time for it to produce its effects. Time requirements may vary greatly from one type of behaviour to another. A subject who quickly develops visual hallucinations may require much more time to produce auditory ones. Time can also play an important part in trance-deepening, and in therapeutic suggestion. The interpolation of pauses and periods of silence of several minutes duration between successive steps will greatly facilitate the production of further depth and enhance the accept-ance of suggestion. Do not make the mistake, however, of believing that a subject who readily develops a deep trance is necessarily going to remain deeply hypnotized throughout the session. This is an unwarranted assumption which can seriously impair the validity of trance findings.

Most of us who are experienced in hypnosis have had ample proof of the extent to which trance-depth can fluctuate from time to time in the course of a single session.

The Deepening of Hypnosis

When you first begin to use hypnosis, you will find that the routine described on page , the induction of graded responses, will help to increase your confidence in yourself, since you can roughly estimate the progress you are making. But as you gain in proficiency and experience, you will find that this will no longer be necessary. You will no longer need to produce phenomena because of your uncertainty as to whether the patient has been hypnotized or not. I am in full agreement with Ainslie Meares when he expresses the view that the production of hypnotic phenomena tends to spoil the therapeutic milieu. Moreover, great depth is rarely necessary unless the production of extensive analgesias or the use of the more involved hypno-analytic techniques is required. Erickson's feeling is that the patient should go no deeper than he needs to go. He points out that some patients need to go very deeply into hypnosis, whilst others can accomplish all that they need to accomplish in a very light state of hypnosis. He says to the patient ' *Neither you nor I know what degree of hypnosis is necessary for you, but I think you are willing to develop that degree of hypnosis that is requisite for you to give your full attention to the therapeutic accomplishments that you need.*' The patient is thus left free to be in a light trance, a medium trance, or a deep trance, without making an issue out of it. He asks ' Why should a patient go any deeper than he needs to go ?' You can swim just as easily in five feet of water as you can in thirty feet, so why not let your patient have that same freedom. Fortunately, a great deal of useful therapeutic work can be successfully accomplished in the light and medium stages, and in my own practice I rarely find it necessary to test for depth.

The Utilization of Hypnosis

In the therapeutic application of hypnosis, I should like to correct any impression that hypnosis involves no more than the induction of a trance-state accompanied by ameliorative suggestions. There is, of course, much more to it than that. No matter whether the simpler psychotherapeutic measures or hypno-analytical techniques are employed, hypnosis is always an intense emotional experience meaningful to the patient. As Wolberg rightly says, it will often mobilize intense emotions and stir up latent conflicts, the manifestations of which yield clues to operative intrapsychic defences. Indeed, this is the very essence of the dynamic approach through hypno-analysis, which is considered by many hypnotherapists to be the most valuable contribution of hypnosis to psychiatry and one of the few really effective methods of employing short-term psychotherapy in place of the more expensive and protracted classical psycho-analysis. This technique, however, belongs properly to the realm of psychiatry rather than general practice.

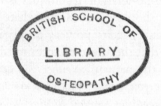

Bibliography

Allen, C. (1949). *Modern discoveries in medical psychology*, 2nd ed. London: Macmillan.

Ambrose, G. (1961). *Hypnotherapy with children*, 2nd ed. London: Staples Press.

—— (1953). 'Hypnosis in child psychiatry' in Schneck *Hypnosis in modern medicine*. Springfield, Illinois: Charles C. Thomas.

—— & Newbold, G. (1958). *A handbook of medical hypnosis*, 2nd ed. London: Baillière, Tindall & Cox.

Beck, L. F. (1938). 'Hypnotic identification of an amnesia victim', *Brit. J. med. Psychol.*, *16*, 1936.

Bernheim, H. (1957). *Suggestive therapeutics*. Westport, Conn.: Associated Booksellers.

Black, S., Humphrey, J. H. & Niven, J. S. F. (1963). 'Inhibition of Mantoux reaction by direct suggestion under hypnosis', *Brit. med. J.*, June 22nd.

Braid, J. (1960). *Braid on hypnotism*. New York: Julian Press Inc.

Bramwell, J. M. (1903). *Hypnotism, its history, practice and theory*. London: Grant Richards.

Brenman, M. & Gill, M. M. (1947). *Hypnotherapy*. London: The Pushkin Press.

Brill, A. A. (1944). *Freud's contribution to psychiatry*. New York: W. W. Norton Co.

Brown, W. (1938). *Psychological methods of healing*. University of London Press Ltd.

Cheek, D. P. & Le Cron, L. M. (1968). *Clinical hypnotherapy*. New York and London: Grune & Stratton.

Cooper, L. F. & Erickson, M. H. (1954). *Time-distortion in hypnosis*. Baltimore: The Williams & Wilkins Co.

Davis, L. W. & Husband, R. W. (1931). 'A study of hypnotic susceptibility in relation to personality traits', *J. abnorm. soc. Psychol.*

Dick-Read, G. (1944). *Child-birth without fear*. New York: Harper & Bros.

Erickson, M. H. (1952). 'Deep trance states and their induction' in Le Cron *Experimental hypnosis* (Ed.: Le Cron). New York: The Macmillan Co.

—— (1938). 'A study of clinical and experimental findings on hypnotic deafness', *J. gen. Psychol.*, *19*, 127.

—— (1939). 'An experimental investigation of the possible anti-social use of hypnosis', *Psychiatry*, *2*, 391.

—— (1939). 'The induction of colour-blindness by a technique of hypnotic suggestion', *J. gen. Psychol.*, *20*, 61.

—— (1944). 'The method employed to formulate a complex story for the induction of experimental neurosis in a hypnotic subject', *J. gen. Psychol.*, *31*, 67.

—— (1964). 'The confusion technique in hypnosis', *Amer. J. clin. Hypnosis*, 6, 183.

—— & Erickson, E. M. (1941). 'Concerning the nature and character of post-hypnotic behaviour', *J. gen. Psychol.*, 24, 95.

Erickson, M. & Kubie, L. S. (1941). 'The successful treatment of a case of acute hysterical depression by a return under hypnosis to a critical phase of childhood', *Psychoanal. Quart.*, 10, 583.

Estabrooks, G. H. (1957). *Hypnotism.* New York: E. P. Dutton & Co.

—— (1962). *Hypnosis: Current problems.* New York: Harper & Row.

Eysenck, H. J. (1943). 'Suggestibility and hypnosis. An experimental analysis', *Proc. roy. Soc. Med.*

Fisher, V. E. (1929). *An introduction to abnormal psychology.* New York: The Macmillan Co.

Forel, A. (1949). *Hypnotism.* New York: Allied Publications.

Freud, S. (1922). *Introductory lectures in psycho-analysis.* London: George Allen & Unwin.

—— (1938). *The basic writings of Sigmund Freud* (Ed.: A. A. Brill). New York: The Modern Library.

—— (1940). *Collected papers,* Vols I–V. London: Hogarth Press & Institute of Psycho-analysis.

—— & Breuer, J. (1940). *On the psychical mechanisms of hysterical phenomena* (Freud's collected papers). London: Hogarth Press & Institute of Psycho-analysis.

Fromm, E. (1968). 'Dissociative and integrative processes in hypnoanalysis', *Amer. J. clin. Hypnosis,* 10, 174.

Gindes, B. C. (1953). *New concepts of hypnosis.* London: George Allen & Unwin.

Goldie, L. (1957). 'The medical use of hypnotism', *Brit. med. J.,* 2.

Gordon, R. G. (1934). *The neurotic and his friends.* London: Methuen.

Haley, J. (1963). *Strategies of psychotherapy.* New York: Grune & Stratton.

—— (1968). *Advanced techniques of hypnosis and therapy: Selected papers of Milton Erickson.* New York & London: Grune & Stratton.

Hart, B. (1921). *The psychology of insanity.* Cambridge University Press.

Hartland, J. & Mills, W. (1964). 'The effects of hypnosis on a complicated obstetric case', *Amer. J. clin. Hypnosis,* 6, 348.

—— & Redlich, M. (1969), 'The "jig-saw puzzle" visualization technique', *Brit. J. clin. Hypnosis,* 1, 22.

Heron, W. T. (1957). *Clinical applications of suggestion and hypnosis.* Springfield, Illinois: Charles C. Thomas.

Heron, W. T. & Abramson, M. (1952). 'Hypnosis in obstetrics' in *Experimental hypnosis* (Ed.: Le Cron). New York: The Macmillan Co.

Hollander, B. (1935). *Methods and uses of hypnosis and self-hypnosis.* London: George Allen & Unwin.

Horsley, J. S. (1943). *Narco-analysis.* London: Oxford University Press.

Hull, C. L. (1935). *Hypnosis and suggestibility.* New York: Appleton Century Crofts.

Jackson, J. W. (1858). *Mesmerism.* London: H. Baillière.

Jacobson, E. (1938). *Progressive relaxation.* University of Chicago Press.

Janet, P. (1925). *Psychological healing,* Vols I and II. London: George Allen & Unwin.

Jones, E. (1913). *Papers on psycho-analysis.* London: Baillière, Tindall & Cox.

Kline, M. V. (1958). *Freud and hypnosis.* New York: Julian Press.

Kroger, W. S. (1962). *Psychosomatic obstetrics, gynaecology and endocrinology.* Springfield, Illinois: Charles C. Thomas.

—— (1965). *Clinical and experimental hypnosis.* Philadelphia: J. B. Lippincott.

Kubie, L. S. (1952). 'The use of hypnogogic reveries for the recovery of repressed data' in *Curative hypnosis* (Ed.: R. H. Rhodes). London: Elek.

Kuhn, L. & Russo, S. (1958). *Modern hypnosis*. Hollywood: Wiltshire Book Co.

Le Cron, L. M. (1952). *Experimental hypnosis*. New York: The Macmillan Co.

—— & Bordeaux, J. (1947). *Hypnotism today*. London: Heinemann Medical Books.

Lindner, R. M. (1944). *Rebel without cause*. New York: Grune & Stratton.

Maher-Loughnan, G. P., Macdonald, N., Mason, A. A. & Fry, L. (1962). 'Controlled trial of hypnosis in the symptomatic treatment of asthma', *Brit. med. J.*, August 11th.

Mangonet, A. P. (1952). *Hypnosis in medicine*. London: Heinemann Medical Books.

—— (1955). *Hypnosis in asthma*. London: Heinemann Medical Books.

—— (1959). *The healing voice*. London: Heinemann.

Mann, H. (1970). A.S.C.H. Lecture. *Hypnosis in the treatment of obesity*. University of Minnesota.

Marcuse, F. L. (1959). *Hypnosis: Fact and fiction*. London: Penguin Books.

Mason, A. A. (1960). *Hypnotism for medical and dental practitioners*. London: Secker & Warburg.

—— & Black, S. (1958). 'Allergic skin responses abolished under treatment of asthma and hay-fever by hypnosis', *Lancet*, ii, 877.

Meares, A. (1960). *A system of medical hypnosis*. Philadelphia: W. B. Saunders.

Mesmer, F. (1948). *Mesmerism*. London: Macdonald.

Moll, A. (1909). *Hypnotism*. London: Walter Scott Publishing Co.

Moodie, W. (1949). *Hypnosis in treatment*. London: Faber & Faber.

Moss, A. A. (1952). *Hypnodontics*. London: Henry Kimpton.

Muhl, A. (1952). 'Automatic writing and hypnosis' in *Experimental hypnosis* (Ed.: Le Cron). New York: The Macmillan Co.

Pattie, F. A. (1937). 'The genuineness of hypnotically produced anaesthesia of the skin', *J. gen. Psychol.*, *49*, 435.

—— (1941). 'The production of blisters by hypnotic suggestion. A review', *J. abnorm. soc. Psychol.*, *36*, 62.

Rhodes, R. H. (1952). *Curative hypnosis*. London: Elek.

Ross, T. A. (1923). *The common neuroses*. London: Edward Arnold.

—— (1932). *An introduction to analytical psychotherapy*. London: Edward Arnold.

Schilder, P. (1956). *The nature of hypnosis*. New York: International Universities Press.

Schneck, J. M. (1953). *Hypnosis in modern medicine*. Springfield, Illinois: Charles C. Thomas.

Schultz, J. H. & Luthe, W. (1959). *Autogenic training*. New York: Grune & Stratton.

Scott, M. (1960). *Hypnosis in skin and allergic diseases*. Springfield, Illinois: Charles C. Thomas.

Stein, C. (1969). *Practical psychotherapy in nonpsychiatric specialities*. Springfield, Illinois: Charles C. Thomas.

Teste, A. (1943). *Practical manual of animal magnetism*. London: H. Baillière.

Tuckey, C. L. (1921). *Treatment by hypnotism and suggestion*. London: Baillière, Tindall & Cox.

Van Pelt, S. J. (1950). *Hypnotism and the power within*. London: Skeffington & Son.

—— (1952). 'The control of the heart-rate by hypnotic suggestion' in *Experimental hypnosis* (Ed.: Le Cron). New York: The Macmillan Co.

Van Pelt, S. J., Ambrose, G. & Newbold, G. (1953). *Medical hypnosis.* London: Victor Gollancz.

Von Dedenroth, T. E. A. (1964). ' The use of hypnosis with " tobaccomaniacs " ', *Amer. J. clin. Hypnosis, 6,* 326.

Weitzenhoffer, A. M. (1953). *Hypnotism: An objective study in suggestibility.* London: Chapman & Hall.

—— (1957). *General techniques of hypnosis.* New York: Grune & Stratton.

Wells, W. R. (1940). ' The ability to resist artificially induced dissociation ', *J. abnorm. soc. Psychol., 35,* 261.

White, R. W. (1941). ' A preface to the theory of hypnotism ', *J. abnorm. soc. Psychol., 36,* 477.

—— (1941). ' An analysis of motivation in hypnosis ', *J. gen. Psychol., 21,* 145.

Whitlow, J. E. (1952). ' A rapid method for the induction of hypnosis ' in *Experimental hypnosis* (Ed.: Le Cron). New York: The Macmillan Co.

Wingfield, H. E. (1920). *Introduction to the study of hypnotism.* London: Baillière, Tindall & Cox.

Winn, R. B. (1958). *Scientific hypnotism.* London: Thorsons Publishers.

Wolberg, L. R. (1948). *Medical hypnosis* (2 vols). New York: Grune & Stratton.

—— (1946). *Hypno-analysis.* London: Heinemann Medical Books.

—— (1967). *The techniques of psychotherapy,* Vols I and II, 2nd ed. London: Heinemann Medical Books.

Wolfe, J. (1958). *Psychotherapy by reciprocal inhibition.* California: Stanford University Press.

Young, P. C. (1940). ' Hypnotic regression—fact or artefact? ', *J. abnorm. soc. Psychol., 35,* 273.

Index